WEIGHT LOSS, EXERCISE AND HEALTH RESEARCH

WEIGHT LOSS, EXERCISE AND HEALTH RESEARCH

CARRIE P. SAYLOR
EDITOR

Nova Science Publishers, Inc.
New York

NOTICE TO THE READER

The Publisher has taken reasonable care in the preparation of this book, but makes no expressed or implied warranty of any kind and assumes no responsibility for any errors or omissions. No liability is assumed for incidental or consequential damages in connection with or arising out of information contained in this book. The Publisher shall not be liable for any special, consequential, or exemplary damages resulting, in whole or in part, from the readers' use of, or reliance upon, this material.

This publication is designed to provide accurate and authoritative information with regard to the subject matter covered herein. It is sold with the clear understanding that the Publisher is not engaged in rendering legal or any other professional services. If legal or any other expert assistance is required, the services of a competent person should be sought. FROM A DECLARATION OF PARTICIPANTS JOINTLY ADOPTED BY A COMMITTEE OF THE AMERICAN BAR ASSOCIATION AND A COMMITTEE OF PUBLISHERS.

LIBRARY OF CONGRESS CATALOGING-IN-PUBLICATION DATA
Weight loss, exercise, and health research / Carrie P. Saylor (editor).
    p. ; cm.
Includes bibliographical references and index.
ISBN 1-60021-077-5
1. Weight loss. 2. Reducing diets. 3. Reducing exercises. 4. Exercise--Physiological aspects. 5. Health. I. Saylor, Carrie P.
[DNLM: 1. Obesity--prevention & control. 2. Weight Loss. 3. Diet. 4. Exercise. 5. Health. WD 210 W566 2006]
RM222.2.W2974   2006
613.2'5--dc22   2006007844

Published by Nova Science Publishers, Inc. ✤ New York

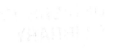

CONTENTS

PREFACE

Weight loss can be achieved in many ways including reduction of caloric intake, exercise and because of health reasons. This new book combines research from around the world in all three areas.

Short-term weight loss can be achieved by any means of reducing habitual calorie consumption to a level below calorie expenditure. Innumerable methods of weight loss are regularly employed; however, not all approaches are conducive to good health. There is persuasive scientific evidence characterizing the dietary pattern, or narrow range of dietary patterns- variations on a very clear theme- contributing to long-term health. Despite wide-spread claims to the contrary, this same basic dietary pattern is more consistently associated with long-term weight control than any other. Given that compelling evidence is available to guide dietary recommendations for health, studying alternatives is unlikely to be as helpful as studying methods of helping the public permanently adopt this approach. It is noteworthy that this is how we approach physical activity; our efforts are devoted to facilitating uptake of exercise, not to a systematic study of alternatives to it. Chapter one reviews four popular dietary approaches to weight loss with regard to both healthfulness and utility in weight loss and control. This review is unique in that it draws from various disciplines, providing insight from such diverse sources as anthropological accounts of "native" diets, trial data reporting links between dietary patterns and health outcomes in diverse cultures and populations, and an ongoing review of the public health/medical literature pertaining to diet and weight.

Obesity is an increasing health problem. As a consequence, many people attempt to lose weight by dieting or participation in weight loss programs. Weight loss is associated with an increased risk of gallstone formation: the incidence is 10-40%, of which 30-40% becomes symptomatic. This leads to substantial morbidity (cholecystitis, choledocholithiasis, biliary pancreatitis) and expensive treatments (hospital admission, endoscopic retrograde cholangiopancreatography, cholecystectomy). Weight reduction and fasting lead to bile lithogenicity through four mechanisms: biliary cholesterol oversaturation due to mobilisation of peripheral fat, increased production of mucine by the gallbladder, 40% increase of bile calcium concentration, and reduction of gallbladder motility. Risk factors for gallstone formation during weight reduction are: rate of weight loss > 1.5 kg/week, total weight loss > 25% of pre-existing weight, very low calorie (< 600 kcal/day) and low fat (< 2 g/day) diets and weight loss following bariatric surgery. Preventive measures include limiting the rate of weight loss to less than 1.5 kg per week, and providing a fat intake of at least 7 g/day. Randomized controlled trials have shown that ursodeoxycholic acid (600 mg daily) is effective for prevention of gallstones (risk reduction 25%). Aspirin is less effective than ursodeoxycholic acid; non-steroidal anti-inflammatory drugs (NSAIDs) have not proven effective. Prophylaxis with ursodeoxycholic acid should be considered in obese patients (BMI > 30 kg/m2) in whom the expected weight loss is rapid or difficult to control, for example after bariatric surgery. This is all discussed in chapter three.

Low body mass and weight loss are strong independent risk-factors for low bone mineral density (BMD) (osteoporosis) and bone loss among postmenopausal women. Although this relationship has fairly convincingly been demonstrated in recent studies the underlying contribution of fat tissue related estrogen production, bone effects of leptin, role of nutritional and mechanical factors remain to be resolved. The present study in chapter four reviews the recent findings on effects of body mass and weight loss on skeletal health in early postmenopause. Furthermore, it accompanies these findings with new unpublished research results on independent and interactive effects of body mass and weight change on bone loss in a prospective population based Osteoporosis Risk Factor and Prevention (OSTPRE) -study.

For the present study, the study population, 954 early postmenopausal women, was selected from a random sample (n=2025) of the OSTPRE study cohort (n=13 100) in Kuopio, Finland. Dual X-ray absorptiometry (DXA) bone mineral density (BMD; g/cm^2) at the lumbar spine (LS) and femoral neck (FN), and body mass (kg), were measured at baseline in 1989–91 and repeated at five-year follow-up in 1994–97. Women were divided into tertiles based on their baseline body mass: under 63 kg, 63-72 kg and over 72 kg.

The results indicate weight loss and low BMI were associated with higher bone loss, low BMD and increased risk of osteoporosis. Weight loss during the follow-up significantly predicted greater bone loss rate in FN in all baseline tertiles (p<0.02 in regression model). In LS, the women in the lowest tertile had significant negative relationship between bone loss and weight loss (p=0.031) but not in other tertiles (p=NS). This effect was independent of adjustments for age, use of HRT, calcium intake and other potential confounders. There were no differences between absolute body mass change values (kg) and percent change of body mass. The interaction analysis (regression model) showed significant interaction for bone loss between weight loss and baseline weight in LS (p=0.022) but not in FN (p=NS). This effect was also not affected by any adjustments.

In conclusion, body mass and weight change are the most important life-style determinants of postmenopausal bone density and rate of bone loss. According to present prospective study, weight change affects bone loss independently of start point body mass in FN but not in LS. This most likely represents differences in the structure of bone tissue in these areas and may suggest independent pathogenesis for weight change induced bone density changes.

Although numerous work-site obesity prevention programs have been widely promoted thus far, a majority of them have been unsuccessful. Problems of the previous programs are as follows. (1) Programs have a high rate of attrition. (2) Participants find it very difficult to maintain the decreased weight. (3) Many participants feel that the programs are not fit for them. These problems imply that it is necessary to develop effective work-site programs that match the type of intervention to the participants and offer the necessary support. In chapter five, the author will introduce a new approach to grouping participants for tailored work-site weight loss programs. Specifically, based upon the signal detection analysis, higher-order interaction of the causal factors of obesity are analyzed.

The subjects were male, white-collar workers (20 to 64 years of age), in Osaka, Japan. Since conventional methods, such as regression analysis or analysis of variance, cannot deal with the interaction of many variables, signal detection analysis by Kraemer was used to identify the higher-order interaction of multiple predictors of obesity.

Out of 15 independent variables, a higher-order interaction consisting of 8 significant variables was identified. Consequently, the subjects were categorized into nine subgroups. It was revealed that the obesity of two groups of workers, 40 or more years old with a high degree of obesity, had different causes: one was related to working conditions, and one was related to smoking cessation. For the other terminal groups, further factors related to obesity were revealed.

Although the applicability of the findings is limited, the methodology using signal detection analysis might be applicable to other weight loss programs as a way of facilitating the matching of the type of intervention and the target group. To verify the efficacy of this approach to grouping participants for tailored work-site weight loss programs, an intervention study for weight loss will be necessary.

Physical inactivity has been identified as a health care burden (Katzmarzyk, Gledhill, and Shephard, 2000). It is a primary risk factor for both psychological and physical ill health, including many disease states that often originate during childhood years yet only become apparent in adulthood (Malina, 1996). Community-based initiatives promoting physical activity to prevent chronic disease have been found to be highly cost effective relative to traditional care (Baxter , Milner, Wilson, et al., 1997; Segal, Dalton, and Richardson, 1998; Tuomilehto, Lindstrom, Eriksson, et al., 2001). Despite the irrefutable evidence linking physical activity with physiological and psycho-social health benefits throughout the lifecourse (Bouchard, 2001; The Surgeon General's Call to Action, 2001), North Americans find little time in their daily life to be physically active. Approximately 54-57% of all North Americans are not active enough to reap such health benefits (Centers for Disease Control and Prevention,1999a). While traditional interventions have encouraged people to add physical activity to their daily activities or to change their daily routines, little attention has been paid to the contexts within which these changes must be made (Giles-Corti, and Donovan, 2002). These established approaches have much to recommend them, but the success rate of individualized exercise prescription interventions can be very low (Dishman, 1994). People can slip back into their normal, less-healthy behavior patterns in environments that do not support an active lifestyle. Research on the barriers to physical activity reveals that, in addition to overcoming personal, social, and psychological hurdles, policy and environmental factors also impede individuals' efforts to be active (Canadian Fitness and Lifestyle Research Institute, 2004; Centers for Disease Control and Prevention, 2001; King, Hawe, and Corne, 1999; Mitchell, and Olds, 1999; Salmon, Owen, Crawford, and Bauman, and Sallis, 2003; Wen, Thomas, Jones et al., 2002). Although the research literature is replete with studies of the individual determinants of physical activity, there is a collective gap in our understanding of the connections between individual determinants and those in the social, physical, economic and cultural environments. Advances in personal treatment approaches are important, but they seem to have limited impact on populations that continue to live in physical environments that have been called, with justification, "obesogenic" (Swinburn, Egger, and Raza, 1999). Chapter six presents a socio-ecological framework for considering the multiple levels of influence on physical activity behavior, and provides some evidence that such comprehensive approaches are effective in promoting an active lifestyle

In chapter seven, this was a cross-cultural comparative study that examined college students' physical activity behavior in both the Republic of China (ROC) and United States of America (USA) on the basis of the full Transtheoretical Model (TTM) of behavior change. Although current investigations do support TTM as a powerful model of physical activity behavior change, there remains a need for examining other variables and constructs relative to those proposed in TTM. From a health promotion planning or intervention perspective, the integration of some of the PRECEDE/PROCEED (PRE) constructs might provide unique insight into physical activity behavior. A total of 1,132 participants were recruited into this study, with 531 coming from the ROC and 601 coming from the USA. In spite of similar recruitment techniques, the participants from the ROC were older and had lower BMIs than those in the USA. They also spent more time sitting in comparison to their American counterparts. The scales and subscales used in this study were completed in the participants' native language (i.e., Chinese or English). Prior to their use in this study, all of the questionnaires were translated into Chinese using a multiple-step methodology, including back translation, and they were found to have reasonable internal consistency. Results showed that the best predictive model for the stages of physical activity behavior change was based on concomitants coming from both TTM and PRE together. Specifically, the variables that contributed the most to the participants' stage of change for physical activity classification in a stepwise analysis, in order of entry, were the behavioral processes of change, nationality, predisposing, cognitive processes of change, and gender. The overall classification accuracy was 49%. Other than the maintenance stage (66%-68% classification accuracy), this study found that the preparation stage (65.5%-70.4% classification accuracy) was especially reliably predicted, which suggests that the preparation stage might be less transitory than previous thought. Furthermore, the concurrent validity of the stage of change measure used in this study was significantly related to the International Physical Activity Questionnaire (IPAQ). This is the first application of IPAQ in the ROC (Taiwan) and the results of the present study support its continued use as a physical activity measure within a new country. As nationality was a key concomitant of stage of change classification, the present study suggests there may be a need for more non-Eurocentric research with TTM before concluding that behavior change strategies and techniques hypothesized in the model (e.g., behavioral and cognitive processes of change, decisional balance, and self-efficacy) are fully generalizable in physical activity behavior change interventions using mixed culture samples. Likewise, there may be some unique contributions to such interventions by incorporating constructs from a broader health promotion planning or intervention model.

There is good evidence that regular physical activity has a protective effect against several chronic diseases, including coronary heart disease, hypertension, obesity, diabetes, osteoporosis, colon cancer, depression and anxiety. Physical activity levels, including occupational and commuting physical activity, have decreased in recent years in China as discussed in chapter eight. Physical activity among Chinese urban people is very different in comparison to the Western populations. Walking or cycling to and from work and school constituted a large component of daily activities among the majority of Chinese urban population. Low level of leisure time physical activity was common in Chinese urban population. People with more daily walking or cycling to and from work and leisure time physical activity had lower levels of cardiovascular risk factors, including low levels of body mass index, blood pressure, total and low-density lipoprotein cholesterol, and triglyceride, high level of high-density lipoprotein cholesterol, and low prevalence of overweight, hypertension, and smoking. Regular leisure time physical activity reduced the risk of total, cancer, respiratory and cardiovascular deaths and daily walking or cycling to and from work also decreased the risk of colon cancer.

Changes in the neutrophil degranulation process induced by physical exercise have not been studied sufficiently. It is not clear how degranulation affects other neutrophil functions. The purpose of this study in chapter nine was to examine the effects of intensive physical activity on human athletes and rat blood neutrophil degranulation by determining activities of myeloperoxidase (MPO) and lysozyme, to investigate an oxidative burst activity in parallel with the dynamics of blood neutrophil degranulation in trained human subjects, and to evaluate the possible associations between degranulation intensity and the athlete's individual work capacity. Treadmill running and rowing were exercises used in human study. Animal model of exercise used was swimming with weight added to the body mass. The rat myeloperoxidase (MPO), human lysozyme and corticosterone concentrations were determined by radioimmunoassais. Enzymatic lysozyme activity was measured by a turbidimetric assay with Micrococcus lysodeicticus.

The results indicate acute exercise stimulated neutrophil degranulation. Significant increases of myeloperoxidase (MPO) (+67%) and lysozyme (+51%) contents were found in rat blood plasma after swimming. Blood plasma lysozyme concentration increased by 41% during treadmill exercise in athletes. Blood concentrations of neutrophil proteins normalized both in humans and animals during first hours of rest. An increase in neutrophil protein concentrations in plasma was accompanied by a decrease of their level in neutrophils. This association was observed as well when enzyme lysozyme activity was determined in both blood plasma and leukocytes. A degree of neutrophil secretory reaction in athletes depended on the mode of physical load: it was higher when rowers performed rowing exercise as compared to treadmill running. Data suggest an influence of glucocorticoid in the observed activation of neutrophil secretion. The neutrophil capacity for an oxidative burst was not changed by exercise, but decreased for the first 3-6 h of the post-exercise period. This suggests a lack of association between the oxidative burst activity and the degranulation process.

In conclusion, intense exercise in human athletes and animals leads to activation of blood neutrophil secretory degranulation. There is no association between degranulation process and the neutrophil oxidative burst activity. As a result of degranulation there is neutrophil protein concentration increase in plasma and its decrease in neutrophils. The neutrophil proteins appeared in blood during degranulation can be involved in enhancement of bactericidal potency of blood, activation of granulopoeisis, neutrophil efflux from bone marrow, and conditioning of blood endothelium for leukocyte extravasation.

The aim of chapter ten is to examine the evidence in the literature with regard to the safety of exercise in pregnancy. A literature search revealed fourteen randomised controlled trials which were systematically reviewed. The outcome measures looked at were both short and long term consequences of training in healthy pregnant women.

The methodology of all included studies was qualitatively evaluated, though few were graded as good. The majority were small and had variable compliance from the volunteers. There was a lack of standardisation of the training schedules: the frequency ranged from 3 - 5 times per week, training intensities varied from age related maximal heart rates of 50 - 75% and exercise periods ranged from 20 – 60 minutes in length. Overall however, the exercise could be classified as moderate.

The literature revealed neither the fetus nor the mother derived harm from moderate exercise in pregnancy. Pregnant women who exercised in the above manner delivered normal healthy infants. With increasing intensity of exercise it appears the children are born with a lower percentage of body fat and thereby a lower birth weight, though still within normal range. This form of training does not appear to increase the incidence of preterm birth or caesarean section. The low number of studies and small patient numbers make it difficult to draw any conclusions with regard to teratogenic effects of hyperthermia. The exclusion of women who developed obstetric complications means it is not possible to draw any conclusions as regards exercise and the risk of placental abruption or bleeding.

In conclusion, moderate exercise seems to have positive effects on pregnancy by way of improved physical well being. Moderate exercise also appears to increase psychological well being – the women feel better. Children born to mothers who exercised regularly showed no significant difference to those born to sedentary mothers in either a positive or a negative way. There was no apparent positive or negative effect on the infant at birth. From currently available data it appears that regular exercise of moderate intensity is both safe and commendable in pregnancy.

Further research in this area is required to assess whether physical activity can increase the risks of obstetric complications or cause significant effects from hyperthermia, particularly where exercise intensity is greater than as described here.

Recent research, primarily in rodent models, has demonstrated that estrogen can diminish post-exercise skeletal muscle leukocyte infiltration, as well reduce a number of indices of muscle damage. Data on estrogen influence in humans, primarily based on male versus female comparisons, has produced more conflicting results. There are several mechanisms by which estrogen can potentially influence muscle damage and inflammatory responses following exercise-induced disruption. However, more research is necessary to determine the role of these mechanisms in estrogenic effects on skeletal muscle. Although some preliminary data is available, the physiological significance of the potential influence of estrogen on muscle damage and inflammatory responses has also yet to be characterized. In particular, the potential effects of estrogen on muscle repair mechanisms are just beginning to be explored. In addition, several human and animal studies have suggested that estrogen may also influence skeletal muscle strength, fatigue and function and that there may be interactive effects of estrogen and progesterone in these effects. This review in chapter eleven will provide an overview and summary of these estrogen and skeletal muscle related controversies. It will also discuss the potential implications of estrogenic influence on skeletal muscle damage, repair and function in humans. These issues are particularly relevant to post-menopausal females and relate to the health controversies associated with post-menopausal hormone replacement therapy.

In: Weight Loss, Exercise and Health Research
Editor: Carrie P. Saylor, pp. 1-27

ISBN 1-60021-077-5
© 2006 Nova Science Publishers, Inc.

Chapter 1

WEIGHT LOSS, WEIGHT MAINTENANCE, AND HEALTH: CAN WE FIND AND CLAIM THE COMMON GROUND?

David L. Katz and Meghan O'Connell

Yale Prevention Research Center Department of Epidemiology
and Public Health, Yale University School of Medicine, New Haven, CT

ABSTRACT

Short-term weight loss can be achieved by any means of reducing habitual calorie consumption to a level below calorie expenditure. Innumerable methods of weight loss are regularly employed; however, not all approaches are conducive to good health. There is persuasive scientific evidence characterizing the dietary pattern, or narrow range of dietary patterns- variations on a very clear theme- contributing to long-term health. Despite wide-spread claims to the contrary, this same basic dietary pattern is more consistently associated with long-term weight control than any other. Given that compelling evidence is available to guide dietary recommendations for health, studying alternatives is unlikely to be as helpful as studying methods of helping the public permanently adopt this approach. It is noteworthy that this is how we approach physical activity; our efforts are devoted to facilitating uptake of exercise, not to a systematic study of alternatives to it. This chapter reviews four popular dietary approaches to weight loss with regard to both healthfulness and utility in weight loss and control. This review is unique in that it draws from various disciplines, providing insight from such diverse sources as anthropological accounts of "native" diets, trial data reporting links between dietary patterns and health outcomes in diverse cultures and populations, and an ongoing review of the public health/medical literature pertaining to diet and weight.

INTRODUCTION

In the United States, obesity is not only epidemic, but arguably the gravest and most poorly controlled public health threat of our time.[1-3] Some 65-80% of adults in the US are overweight or obese.[4] While the mortality toll of obesity has been the subject of recent controversy (*http://health.yahoo.com/news/54598*), some 300,000 to 400,000 premature deaths each year are thought to result from direct and indirect effects of the obesity epidemic.[5] A linear relationship exists between BMI and all-cause mortality.[6] Obesity contributes substantially to cardiovascular risk, [7-9] and excess body weight is a potent risk factor for most cancers.[10]

The prevalence of dieting and the self-reported reasons for dieting (health improvement, weight loss) vary by socioeconomic status; a cross sectional study with over 10,000 participating US adults found that between 8-21% of the population were dieting.[11] Other research demonstrates that women with higher BMIs often started dieting at a younger age and diet more frequently compared to women with lower BMIs.[12] Dieting is also very common among young adults. A study of dieting behaviors among 324 college students showed that 38% and 13% of females and males respectively, were dieting to lose weight.[13]

There is persuasive scientific evidence characterizing the dietary pattern supporting good health throughout the lifespan. It is important to examine weight loss strategies with regard to not only weight, but also overall health over the short and long term. This chapter will summarize the existing literature defining an array of diets and the evidence assessing their health promoting qualities and utility for weight control. The review encompasses four principal areas within the expansive literature addressing diet and weight regulation, including the Mediterranean diet, Paleolithic diet, low-fat (conventional) diets and low-carbohydrate diets.

MEDITERRANEAN DIETS

The Mediterranean diet differs from the typical American diet in the quantity and quality of fat, and the quantity of unrefined grains, vegetables, fruit, and lean protein sources.[14] The Mediterranean diet is low in saturated fat and high in monounsaturated fatty acids, high in antioxidants especially vitamin C and E, and high in fiber and folic acid.[15] Olive oil is the dominant fat source, and consumption of fruit and vegetables, grains, fish and legumes are moderate to high. Wine is commonly served with meals.[15] Although there is variation in the Mediterranean diet depending on country and region due to cultural, ethnic, religious, economic and agricultural production differences[14, 16] and possibly even due to other elements that vary across culture, and are difficult to control for, such as stress, social bonds, familial support, and even spirituality,[17, 18] the dietary characteristics common to the region (described above) have been consistently associated with good health and longevity.

THE MEDITERRANEAN DIET AND HEALTH PROMOTION

Populations within Europe that consume the Mediterranean diet have lower incidences of major illnesses such as cancer and cardiovascular disease than their non-European Western counterparts. The health benefits of the Mediterranean diet are transferable to non-Mediterranean regions. Studies have demonstrated beneficial effects on the coronary risk profile among populations outside of the region adopting the Mediterranean diet.[15] Studies suggest that the health-conferring benefits of the Mediterranean diet are due mainly to a high consumption of fiber, fish, fruits and vegetables and possibly olive oil.[19] It should, however, be noted that many of the Mediterranean populations enjoying good health have traditionally high rates of physical activity compared to Western societies; this factor likely explains some of the health benefits enjoyed by Mediterranean peoples.

In a recent systematic review, Trichopoulou and Critselis reviewed data from five cohort studies exploring the association of Mediterranean diet with overall mortality. Findings suggest that although it is not yet clear which components in the Mediterranean diet are responsible for apparent health effects, the diet is likely to aid in the prevention of both coronary heart disease and cancer.[20] A longitudinal study of elderly subjects conducted in 11 European countries between 1988 and 2000 (the HALE Project) confirmed that adhering to a Mediterranean diet, along with moderate alcohol use, physical activity, and nonsmoking were associated (each independently) with a lower risk of all-cause mortality. The findings demonstrated that among individuals aged 70 to 90 years, adherence to a Mediterranean diet and healthful lifestyle was associated with a more than 50% lower rate of all-cause and cause-specific mortality.[21] Similarly, in reviewing data from four cohorts of elderly people in Greece, Spain, Denmark and Australia, Trichopoulou (2004) found that close adherence to the Mediterranean diet is positively associated with longevity.[20]

Computation of an index (the Mediterranean Adequacy Index) has recently allowed researchers to begin to determine how close or far the food intakes of population groups are from a reference Mediterranean dietary pattern.[22] The measure has been used in surveys of male participants in the Seven Countries Study; findings show that scores were inversely correlated with the 25-year death rates from coronary heart disease in the 16 cohorts (R = -0.72; p = 0.001).[23]

Intervention studies in East Finland and Southern Italy have convincingly shown that the coronary risk profile (lower LDL cholesterol and blood pressure levels) is improved by a Mediterranean diet.[15] A systematic review of the influence of the Mediterranean diet on the development and progression of coronary heart disease found that in all studies included in the review, benefits from the Mediterranean diet were significant, with the reduction in risk ranging from 8% to 45%. The authors concluded that the cardio-protective effect of the Mediterranean diet warrants promotion of the dietary pattern to meet public health objectives.[24]

Some of the most compelling evidence comes from the Lyon Diet Heart Study. In this study, the American Heart Association's Step I Diet used in clinical practice to lower cardiac risk factors was modified and made comparable to the Mediterranean pattern of dietary intake, but with higher α-linolenic acid. This RCT investigated the effect of the diet on coronary recurrence rates after a first myocardial infarction. Subjects following the Mediterranean diet had a 50-70% lower risk of recurrent heart disease compared to controls.

The study also demonstrated participants' ability to modify dietary fat and cholesterol consistent with the National Cholesterol Education program/AHA Step I diet, while consuming a Mediterranean style diet. This study raises questions about the possible independent benefits of increasing α-linolenic acid in the diet.[16, 25] Several additional studies dating back to the 1960s support the association between typical Mediterranean eating habits and protection against coronary heart disease.

In a recent review, Biesalski, et al (2004) reported that based on the Nurses Health and Physicians Health studies, a diet which is similar to the Mediterranean diet, combined with regular physical activity and weight regulation, is protective against the development of type 2 diabetes, despite a tendency for the diet to contain nutrients with a high glycemic index (the author states that this is likely due to high fiber content of the Mediterranean diet).[26] The Mediterranean diet has been found to improve glucose metabolism in healthy young men and women.[27] Among diabetic patients, the diet may provide protection against peripheral arterial disease; evidence from an Italian study of type 2 diabetics showed high dietary scores (higher quality of Mediterranean diet) were protective, while the use of butter increased risk.[28] Additional benefits among diabetics have been reported. Toobert, et al. (2003) tested the effectiveness of the Mediterranean Lifestyle Program, a comprehensive lifestyle self-management program including the Mediterranean diet, on cardiovascular risk factors in postmenopausal women with type 2 diabetes. Significant improvements in HbA(1c), BMI, plasma fatty acids, and quality of life were reported at the 6-month follow-up. Favorable patterns were seen in lipids, blood pressure, and flexibility but did not reach statistical significance.[29]

The incidence of certain cancers in the Mediterranean area is lower than in other areas of the world. The Mediterranean diet, rich in antioxidants, might be preventive; however, sound epidemiologic evidence about its ability to prevent the most frequent cancers is scarce. The role of particular antioxidants in the Mediterranean diet is unclear, but convincing data exist to support the contention that a diet low in saturated fat and alcohol and rich in plant food and whole grain, such as the traditional Mediterranean diet, is associated with lower risk of cancer.[30] La Vecchia (2004) analyzed the role of various aspects of the Mediterranean diet in several common epithelial cancers in over 12,000 cancer cases and 10,000 controls. For most epithelial cancers the risk decreased with increasing vegetable and fruit consumption, with relative risk (RR) between 0.3 and 0.7 for the highest versus the lowest tertile. A number of antioxidants and other micronutrients showed an inverse relationship with cancer risk and intake of whole-grain foods was related to a reduced risk of several types of cancer, particularly of the upper digestive tract.[31] In the same study, refined grain intake was associated with an increased risk of different types of cancer, including those of the upper digestive tract, colorectum, breast and endometrium. In other studies, the Mediterranean diet or elements of the diet have been shown to favorably affect the risk of cancers of the lung,[32] pancreas,[33] oral cavity and pharynx,[34] ovaries,[35] breast,[36] prostate,[37] and squamous cell esophageal cancer.[38] Randomized trials of the Mediterranean diet using a whole-diet approach, rather than focusing exclusively on antioxidants or micronutrients are needed.[39]

The Mediterranean Diet and Weight Control

The Med diet is relatively high in total fat. However, because of the overall pattern of foods in this diet, it is not based largely on energy-dense foods as most higher-fat diets tend to be. The evidence is convincing that energy dense foods generally contribute to weight gain.

However, it is also clear that when energy restriction can be achieved on a diet relatively high in fat content, weight loss is achieved.[40] A Mediterranean diet which is high in monounsaturated fatty acids but overall not predominantly comprised of energy-dense foods may be more effective at long-term weight loss than a low total fat diet, as it may be more palatable and therefore better sustained than a low fat diet.

McManus, et al (2001) evaluated a calorie controlled moderate fat Mediterranean diet compared to a standard low-fat diet (also calorie controlled). The Mediterranean diet resulted in superior long-term participation and adherence, leading to improvements in weight loss. The moderate-fat group lost a mean of 4.1 kg, body mass index of 1.6 kg/m(2), and waist circumference of 6.9 cm, compared to increases in the low-fat group of 2.9 kg, 1.4 kg/m(2) and 2.6 cm, respectively at 18 months; P < or = 0.001 between the groups.[41] A study by Flynn, et al (2004) demonstrated weight loss (and a strong reduction in cholesterol levels and increased feelings of well-being) among 115 postmenopausal women after 15 months of adopting the diet.[42] The intervention involved a weekly cooking class for 1 year, with professional chefs providing training in the correct use of natural ingredients of the traditional Mediterranean diet.

There is some evidence that in addition to facilitating weight loss, a moderately hypocaloric Mediterranean diet may also improve body composition among obese subjects. Using a diet based on the Italian Recommended Dietary Allowances and elaborated using available nutritional indices, De Lorenzo, et al demonstrated that a Mediterranean style diet with energy content (mean 6.5 MJ/day) matching the resting metabolic rate and with macronutrient breakdown of 55% carbohydrate, 25% fat, 20% protein and 30g fiber prevented loss of fat-free mass and improved metabolic parameters in 19 obese women. Following the diet, total and segmental fat mass decreased, while no significant loss of total and segmental lean body mass was observed. The study also resulted in significant improvements in metabolic profile.[43]

It is worth noting that although many studies have demonstrated successful weight control and health improvements with adoption of the Mediterranean diet, only one weight loss study with greater than 6 months follow-up has been undertaken in the United States.[41] This study demonstrated positive weight related results and superior adherence to a Mediterranean diet compared to a low fat diet. More research is needed to determine whether the diet can be implemented and sustained among free living populations in the U.S. given the current state of ubiquitous access to and American affinity for energy-dense snack and fast foods.

Paleolithic Diets

Quite distinct from biomedical research, a fairly extensive body of work characterizes what is known about the native nutritional habitat of our species. Knowledge of our ancestral dietary pattern is useful in explaining human dietary preferences and tendencies. The origins of human dietary behavior have been traced back at least four million years, while modern homo sapiens, our ancestors, date back approximately 30,000 years.[44] While there is debate about many details, there is general consensus that humanity adapted over eons to an environment in which calories were relatively scarce, and physical activity demands high.[45] Saturated and trans fat intake were low and negligible, respectively; micronutrient intake was high; intake of omega-3 and omega-6 fatty acids were high (omega-3 fatty acids were found in all foods consumed), and the ratio of the two was about equal; and protein intake was from lean sources.[46, 47] The traditional human diet was low in both starch and sugar, but rich in complex carbohydrate from a variety of plant foods.[46]

Many, but not all, anthropologists suggest we were more gatherers than hunters, and that meat likely contributed less to our subsistence than plant foods.[48, 49] Studies of fossil records and modern-day hunter-gatherers suggest the 30-40% of total calories were obtained from hunting (animal foods), while the remaining were obtained through gathering (plant foods). This partial reliance on meat did not expose our ancestors to the kinds of dietary fat linked to modern day chronic diseases. The fat content (by weight) of free living animals is estimated to have been approximately 4%, compared to modern beef cattle with 25-30% fat.[44]

The process of natural selection remains a pertinent consideration in our dietary behavior, as the human genome has remained unchanged for thousands of years, and our genes are very similar to the genes of our ancestors during the Paleolithic period 40,000 years ago.[46, 49-52] While changes in diet have occurred over the last 10,000 years (with the beginning of the Agricultural Revolution), with very dramatic changes experienced over the past 100 years, the diet of our distant ancestors still dictates our food preferences and aversions. Dependence on hunting meant the food supply was unreliable, with cyclical periods of feast and famine. This pattern of eating in excess during times of plenty conferred a survival advantage during periods of relative famine, but has predisposed modern day humans to excess weight gain. The current nutritional environment of sustained abundance is one that humans have not had adequate time to adjust to. In essence, modern day humans are programmed to "feast" while food is available, with no physiological mechanism for self-discipline in environments with unprecedented access to foods of all varieties. Genetic evolution and cultural history have cultivated human dietary preferences that are well suited for a world in which food is difficult to acquire. Thus, it is not surprising that our lack of defense against dietary excess makes us vulnerable to the most prevalent modern day chronic diseases.

THE PALEOLITHIC DIET AND EVIDENCE OF HEALTH PROMOTION

That the dietary pattern of early humans should be relevant to human health requires nothing more than acknowledging that human beings are creatures. For all other species under our care, epitomized by zoological parks, the diet we provide is an adaptation of the diet consumed in the wild. The "native" human diet appears to have provided roughly 25% of calories from fat, 20-25% of calories from protein, and the remainder from complex carbohydrates;[46] this pattern is remarkably confluent with that demonstrating compelling health benefit in clinical trials.[53, 54]

The Greek variant of the Mediterranean Diet has been identified as one of the most traditional and is associated with low rates of coronary and all-cause mortality.[15] The diet of Crete closely resembles the Paleolithic diet in regards to fiber, antioxidants, saturated fat, monounsaturated fat and the ratio of n-6 to n-3 fatty acids.[14] This type of diet also characterized the diet used in the Lyon Diet Heart Study, which demonstrated remarkable reduction in coronary events and related deaths in a cohort of patients who had previously suffered MI.[55] In general, the Paleolithic diet tends to be somewhat lower in fat than Mediterranean diets. This is of note in light of the fact that very low fat diets, too, have been shown to prevent and reverse cardiovascular disease.[56] The Paleolithic diet is situated between low-fat diets and the higher-fat intake of some Mediterranean diets, while falling within the recommended dietary intake ranges of the IOM.

However, the history of human diet through early evolution fails to identify the optimal diet for health. Early humans lived abbreviated lives by current standards. Although little is known about nutrition related health problems of the time, paleo-anthropologists concur that traditional man was free of degenerative illness; lifespans were short due to infections, childbirth, inter- and intra-clan conflict and predation.[57] Thus, while an appreciation for the 'native' nutritional habitat of Homo sapiens should inform consideration of the optimal dietary pattern, it should by no means supplant modern science.

The Paleolithic Diet and Weight Control

To our knowledge, the Paleolithic diet has not been tested for weight control. Many factors are thought to favor sustainable weight loss; an emphasis on energy-dilute, nutrient-dense foods; a balanced, and varied diet; a reliance on relatively unprocessed foods; a relatively high intake of fiber, plant foods, and lean protein; etc. The Paleolithic diet epitomizes many if not all of these characteristics. While there have been no formal trials of the Paleolithic diet per se, its characteristics are reflected in the diets of those successful at long-term maintenance of weight loss.[58]

FAT RESTRICTED DIETS

The Low-Fat Diet and Evidence of Health Promotion

A rich and varied literature argues that restriction of dietary fat is both conducive to weight loss, and health-promoting.[59, 60] Many cultures recognized for good health and longevity have native diets very low in fat.[61] The worst that can be said of fat restriction for weight loss is that if extreme, it may not be optimal for health.[62] Even critics of dietary fat restriction appear to agree that low-fat diets offer health benefits relative to the typical American diet, which is high in saturated and trans fat.

On the basis of evidence linking dietary pattern to health outcomes, national dietary guidelines have long emphasized consumption of specific low-fat foods, namely whole grains, vegetables, and fruits. *The United States Preventive Services Task Force* advises clinicians to endorse to all patients over the age of 2 a diet restricted in fat, particularly saturated fat, and abundant in fruits, vegetables, and grains.[63] These recommendations are highly concordant with those of the National Heart Lung and Blood Institute at the National Institutes of Health. The *United States Department of Agriculture* recommendations,[64] depicted in the USDA food guide pyramid,[65] also emphasize abundant intake of grains, vegetables, and fruits, with restricted intake of both simple sugars and total fat. The *National Cancer Institute* sponsors the "5-a-day" program encouraging fruit and vegetable intake, and endorses dietary guidelines that include 20-35 grams of fiber per day, with 30% or less of calories from fat.[66] The *American Heart Association* offers dietary guidelines that call for 55% or more of calories from carbohydrate, 30% or less from fat (7-10% saturated/trans fat, 10% polyunsaturated and 15% monounsaturated fats), and 15-20% from protein.[67] The *American Dietetic Association* supports the USDA Dietary Guidelines and recommends a variety of grains, at least 5 servings of fruits and vegetables daily, restriction of saturated fat and cholesterol, and limited sugar and sweet consumption.[68] The *American Diabetes Association* advocates 55% of calories from carbohydrate, up to 30% from fat (10% saturated/trans fat, 10% polyunsaturated fat), and 15-20% from protein.[69] In 2002, The National Academies of Science' Institute of Medicine (IOM) released dietary guidelines calling for 45-65% of calories from carbohydrate, 20-35% from fat, and 10-35% from protein, in conjunction with 60 minutes each day of moderately intense physical activity.[70] The Institute of Medicine guidelines further emphasize the restriction of saturated and trans fat and their replacement with monounsaturated and polyunsaturated fat.

Reviews of diet for optimal health do not necessarily demonstrate complete accord on all points, but are nonetheless substantially confluent with regard to fundamentals. Diets rich in naturally low-fat fruits, vegetables and whole grains; restricted in animal fats and trans fat from processed foods; limited in refined starches and sugar; providing protein principally from lean sources; and offering fat principally in the form of monounsaturated and polyunsaturated oils are linked to good health.[44, 71-77] With regard to diet and optimal health, debate is substantially limited to variations on this basic theme, rather than any fundamental departures from it.

Several studies have demonstrated improvements in, and in some cases prevention of chronic disease with reliance on a low-fat diet, and suggest that diets higher in saturated fat may pose a higher diabetes risk than those higher in unsaturated fat.[78] In the Diabetes Prevention Program, a calorie-controlled, relatively low-fat diet coupled with moderately intense physical activity for at least 150 minutes per week reduced the incidence of Type 2 diabetes by 58%.[53] The Finnish Diabetes Prevention Study also included the reduction of total and saturated fat as two main lifestyle change goals that contributed to reduced risk of diabetes. A recent systematic review reported that four studies found that low fat diets may prevent type 2 diabetes and reduce antihypertensive medication for up to 3 years.).[79] In contrast to these controlled trials, a 14 year epidemiological study of woman conducted at Harvard found that trans fat intake increased the risk of type 2 diabetes, while total, saturated and monounsaturated fat intake was not significantly associated with risk of type 2 diabetes.[80]

Reducing the amount of saturated fat and cholesterol in your diet helps lower your blood cholesterol level, thereby reducing cardiac risk.[81] Studies by Ornish, et al (1998) have demonstrated significant reduction in cardiac events without medication among participants enrolled in a lifestyle program incorporating a low fat diet with exercise, stress management and smoking cessation, compared to a control group.[56] Total dietary fat intake has been linked to hyperlipidemia and coronary disease for over 40 years while recent evidence suggests that saturated and transfat intake only need be restricted.[82] Hypertension is also a risk factor for cardiac disease. The DASH Collaborative Research Group has shown that hypertension can be prevented and treated by reducing intake of *saturated and total fat*, and adopting a diet rich in fruits, vegetables, grains and low-fat dairy.[54] A recent systematic review of weight loss trials lasting 1 year or more indicated that low fat diets not only produced significant weight losses up to 36 months, but resulted in improvements in blood pressure and lipids, as well as fasting plasma glucose after 12 months.

According to scientific review of available evidence at the National Cancer Institute, fat consumption is associated with increased risk of endometrial, breast, prostate, and stomach cancers.[83] Current evidence suggests that it might be the type of fat in the diet, rather than the total amount of fat, that is most pertinent to cancer risk.[84] The Mediterranean diet has been identified as one providing some degree of protection against several types of cancer (see *The Mediterranean Diet and Health Promotion*), while being relatively high in total fat due to moderate/high consumption of monounsaturated fats, but low in saturated and transfat. According to the American Cancer Society, controlling weight is also vital to reducing cancer risk, as overweight and obesity increase the risk of cancers of the breast (among women 50+), colon, endometrium, esophagus, and kidney.[84] Fat restriction may contribute to lowering cancer risk by facilitating weight control (see *Low-Fat Diets and Weight Control)*

Low-Fat Diets and Weight Control

There are numerous reviews on the subject of diet for weight loss.[79, 85-96] In the aggregate, this literature lends strongest support to diets abundant in fruits, vegetables and whole grains, and restricted in total fat.

High dietary fat intake is a powerful predictor of weight gain.[97] Transcultural comparisons dating back at least to the work of Ancel Keys consistently indicate that higher intake of dietary fat is associated with higher rates of obesity, and chronic disease.[98-100] Most authorities concur that high intake of dietary fat contributes to obesity at the individual and population levels. The theoretical basis for weight loss through dietary fat restriction is strong, given the widely acknowledged primacy of calories in weight governance, and the energy density of fat.[101] Dietary fat is the most energy dense and least satiating of the macronutrient classes.[102-104] When fat restriction is in accord with prevailing views on nutrition, i.e., achieved by shifting from foods high in fat to naturally low-fat foods, the results are consistently favorable with regard to energy balance and body weight.[105] The weight loss benefit of advice to follow fat-restricted diets is however, no more enduring than that of advice to restrict calories by any other means.[106]

Although the literature on *long-term* weight loss success is thin, the best available data are from observational studies,[107] trans-cultural comparison, and the National Weight Control Registry.[108] The Registry was established to characterize the behavioral patterns of individuals successful at long-term maintenance of considerable weight loss (an average loss of 30 lb maintained for over 5 years). Registry data indicate that a relatively low-fat, and therefore energy-dilute, diet is a mainstay of successful weight maintenance (as is regular physical activity).[58, 109, 110] The overall pattern of the diet reported in this registry shares much in common with the fundamentals of the Paleolithic diet.

Despite the extensive literature supporting dietary fat-restriction for weight loss and control, there are dissenting voices.[111] For the most part, dissent is predicated on the failure of dietary fat restriction to achieve population-level weight control in the United States. Recent trends in the US suggest that fat intake over recent decades was held constant, not reduced, and that intake of total calories has risen to dilute down the percent of food energy derived from fat; increased consumption of highly processed, fat-reduced foods is the principal basis for these trends.[112] Thus, the failure of dietary fat restriction to facilitate weight control is more a problem of adherence than effectiveness.[113]

In response to the public's interest in fat restriction, the food industry generated a vast array of low-fat, but not necessarily low-calorie, foods over the past two decades, prototypical of which is Snackwell® cookies. The increase in calories was driven by increased consumption of calorie-dense, nutrient-dilute, fat-restricted foods, contemporaneous with a trend toward increasing portion sizes in general.[114-118] Lowering the fat content of processed foods while increasing consumption of simple sugars and starch is not consistent with the long-standing recommendations of nutrition authorities to moderate intake of dietary fat. Yet it is this distorted approach to dietary fat "restriction" that best characterizes secular trends in dietary intake at the population level, and that subtends the contention that dietary fat is unrelated to obesity.

CARBOHYDRATE RESTRICTED DIETS

Although the popularity of carbohydrate-restricted diets for weight loss appears to be waning, they have been trendy for several years, so much so that they have reshaped the American food supply. Therefore, an assessment of diet, health and weight loss thus requires particular consideration of entries in this category. Review of low-carbohydrate diets to date suggests that short-term weight loss is consistently achieved, but that neither weight loss sustainability, nor long-term effects on overall health, has yet been determined. A recent systematic review published in Lancet, found that weight loss achieved while on low-carbohydrate diets is associated with the duration of the diet and restriction of energy intake, but not with restriction of carbohydrates. Evidence supporting and refuting this claim and preliminary evidence related to the health impact of low-carbohydrate diets will be discussed in this section.

THE LOW-CARBOHYDRATE DIET AND EVIDENCE
OF HEALTH PROMOTION

Research regarding the safety of low carbohydrate diets is limited; to date studies have been of short duration and have relied on small sample sizes and often experienced high attrition. Regardless of the state of new research in this area, many scientists believe that ample evidence exists to warrant cautioning the public against use of low carbohydrate diets. In 2002, on the basis of consensus opinion, the *American College of Preventive Medicine* formally adopted a position in support of dietary recommendations within the IOM ranges (described in *Low-Fat Diet and Evidence of Health Promotion*), and in opposition to carbohydrate restriction for purposes of weight control.[119]

In contrast to fat restriction, carbohydrate restriction is potentially linked to an array of adverse health effects.[120] There is evidence that weight loss attributable to carbohydrate restriction is in part body water loss. Gluconeogenesis consumes water along with glycogen, and ketone bodies cause increased renal excretion of sodium and water.[121] Studies indicate dizziness, fatigue and headache are common side effects[122]of ketosis.

Ketosis is potentially harmful, with possible long-term sequelae including hyperlipidemia, impaired neutrophil function, optic neuropathy, osteoporosis, and protein deficiency as well as alterations in cognitive function.[121] Children on ketogenic diets as part of an anti-seizure regimen have developed dehydration, constipation and kidney stones. In response to ketosis, renal calcium excretion increases. To make up for the loss of calcium in urine, it is mobilized from bone to circulation.[121] One study of adolescents on a ketogenic diet showed decreased bone mineral density after just 3 months, despite vitamin D and calcium supplementation.[122] Sustained ketosis causes bone resorption, suggesting a risk for osteoporosis.[123]

Comparison of eight high-protein, low-carbohydrate diets indicates that the Atkins diet had the highest level of total fat, saturated fat, and cholesterol.[122] Consuming a diet high in saturated fat may raise total and low-density lipoprotein cholesterol levels, both of which contribute to cardiovascular disease. A significant increase in LDL has been reported among subjects on the Atkins diet,[121] although this finding is inconsistent. An increase in C-reactive protein (CRP) on the Atkins diet has been observed as well,[122] suggesting an inflammatory response. A high intake of saturated fat increases the risk of insulin resistance,[122] contradicting the contention of low-carbohydrate diet proponents that carbohydrates are to blame for insulin resistance.[124] High fat diets may also predispose to cancer.[125]

High-protein intake may negatively affect renal function in healthy individuals, and certainly accelerates renal disease in diabetes. In patients with renal dysfunction on a high-protein diet, there is glomerular damage causing spillage of plasma proteins and resultant tubular injury and fibrosis.[122] As noted, urinary calcium excretion is also increased and hypercalciuria may ensue, predisposing to calcium stone formation.[121] High-protein intake imposes a metabolic burden on both the liver and kidneys, requiring additional excretion of urea and ammonia.[126]

Extreme carbohydrate restriction is potentially associated with increased risk of dysthymia, if not depression, through a serotonergic mechanism.[127] The production of serotonin in the brain requires delivery and uptake of tryptophan, which is influenced by both the availability of tryptophan and the actions of insulin. With very low carbohydrate intake and blunted insulin release, tryptophan delivery to the brain is impaired, serotonin production is limited, and mood instability has been reported to ensue;[128] the public health significance of this mechanism remains uncertain.

Finally, high-protein, low-carbohydrate diets simply don't allow for adequate intake of fruits and vegetables, restricting nutrient and fiber-rich foods shown to be protective against cancer, cardiovascular disease, diabetes and diverticular disease.[129-132] Fiber lowers cholesterol, reducing the risk for cardiovascular disease, and lowers insulin secretion after meals by slowing nutrient absorption.[122 , 133]

In comparison to the litany of potential hazards associated with a low carbohydrate diet, some studies have demonstrated benefits accompanying weight loss on low carbohydrate diets in the short-term. There is some evidence to suggest that dietary protein may preserve resting energy expenditure following weight loss.[134] This, together with protein's high satiety index, suggest a benefit of protein intake at the high end of the range advisable for overall health as an aid to weight loss and control efforts.[135, 136]

Some studies have reported greater reductions in triglycerides among subjects following low carbohydrate diets in comparison to low fat diets.[137-141] Others have demonstrated greater reductions in LDL and total cholesterol with increases in HDL; however, findings are inconsistent across studies. Favorable effects on markers of inflammation have been reported.[142-144]

It is unclear whether weight loss, which is powerfully beneficial for health, rather than carbohydrate restriction may be responsible for health improvements reported in short-term studies. Low carbohydrate studies have consistently resulted in weight loss; however, current data do not adequately illustrate the safety and efficacy of the diet in relation to lifetime chronic disease risk.

LOW-CARBOHYDRATE DIETS AND WEIGHT CONTROL

There is insufficient data to assess long-term efficacy of low carbohydrate diets in terms of weight control. The 8 studies of longest duration are described below.

In a widely publicized recent study comparing the effectiveness and adherence rates of four popular weight loss diets among overweight subjects with hypertension, dyslipidemia or fasting hyperglycemia, Dansinger, et al (2005) found no significant difference in mean weight loss between groups at one-year.[144] Predictably, the study reported no significant differences in mean total calorie reduction between groups, lending support to the widely accepted notion that total calorie consumption, regardless of macronutrient content, is of prime importance in weight loss efforts. Further studies discussed in this section also support this contention. All diet groups (Atkins, Weight Watchers, Ornish and Zone) had poor adherence rates, with no significant difference between groups. In all diet groups, greater adherence to the diet resulted in improved weight outcomes; participants in the top tertile of adherence had a mean loss of 7% body weight. No significant differences in cardiac risk factors were noted between groups; in each group the amount of weight loss predicted improvements in several risk factors.

Two studies of low-carbohydrate diets that received widespread attention are those by Samaha et al.[145] and Foster et al.,[146] published in the same issue of the New England Journal of Medicine in 2003. Samaha and colleagues compared a very low carbohydrate diet (<30gm carbohydrate per day) to a fat and calorie restricted diet in 132 adults with a BMI of 35 or above over a 6-month period. The carbohydrate restricted diet resulted in greater weight loss at 6 months than the low-fat diet, but was also associated with a far greater reduction in daily calorie intake (a mean reduction of 271kcal per day for the low fat diet, and 460kcal for the low carbohydrate diet). Results at 12 month follow-up indicate no significant difference in weight loss between groups; however, the low-carbohydrate group resulted in some more favorable changes in fasting glucose concentrations and insulin sensitivity.[138] Foster et al.

compared the Atkins' diet as described in *Dr. Atkins' New Diet Revolution*[147] to a fat and calorie restricted diet in 63 obese adults followed for 12 months. The low carbohydrate diet produced significantly greater weight loss at 6 months, but not 12 months. Calorie intake was not reported. In both studies, attrition and recidivism were high; Samaha and colleagues noted that their trial was unblinded, whereas Foster et al. made no mention of blinding.

Brehm and colleagues[148] examined weight loss, cardiac risk factors, and body composition in 53 obese women randomly assigned to a very low carbohydrate diet, or a calorie-restricted, balanced diet with 30% of calories from fat. At 6 months follow-up, subjects assigned to the very low carbohydrate diet group lost more weight (8.5 +/- 1.0 vs. 3.9 +/- 1.0 kg; P < 0.001) and more body fat (4.8 +/- 0.67 vs. 2.0 +/- 0.75 kg; P < 0.01) than those assigned to the low fat diet group; cardiac risk measures improved comparably in both groups. Adherence to the diet was low in the very low carbohydrate group.

In 1999, Skov et al. reported an interesting variation on the low-carbohydrate diet theme by comparing two fat-restricted (30% of calories) diets, one high in carbohydrate (58% of calories), the other high in protein (25% of calories).[136] Subjects were 65 overweight adults followed for 6 months, and were provided diets strictly controlled with regard to nutritional composition, but unrestricted in calories. More weight was lost with high protein (8.9 kg) intake than with high carbohydrate (5.1 kg) intake; no weight loss occurred in a control group.

In a 6 month non-controlled trial, Westman, et al (2002) assessed the effects of a very low carbohydrate diet among 51 overweight or obese adults. Carbohydrate intake of less than 25 grams per day was recommended to start and was increased to 50 grams upon achievement of 40% of target weight loss. Mean daily calorie consumption at follow-up was 1447 ± 350, but was not measured at baseline. Calories restrictions were not prearranged; however, subjects were instructed to eat only until hunger was relieved. All subjects available for follow-up (41) developed ketonuria; levels were used to verify self-reported carbohydrate intake. Subjects lost a mean of 10.3% ± 5.9% body weight. Significant decreases in total cholesterol, LDL and trigylceride levels as well as increases in HDL were reported.[140]

Yancy, et al (2004) compared a low-carbohydrate diet plus nutritional supplementation to low fat diet with calorie deficit of 500-1000 calories/day among 120 overweight, hyperlipidemic subjects. Both groups received exercise recommendation and attended group meetings. The low fat diet group lost significantly less weight than the low-carbohydrate diet group at 6 months (mean change, -12.9% vs. -6.7%; P < 0.001). Reductions in fat mass were similar between groups. The low carbohydrate group had lower attrition, yet the low fat group appeared to have better adherence to the diet.[139]

Brinkworth, et al (2004) compared the effectiveness at 68 weeks of two calorie and fat controlled 12 week diets: a standard protein group (15% protein, 55% carbohydrate) and high-protein group (30% protein, 40% carbohydrate). Results indicated no significant difference in weight loss between groups; however neither group had high compliance to the diet. Both diets significantly increased HDL cholesterol concentrations (P<0.001) and decreased fasting insulin, insulin resistance, sICAM-1 and CRP levels (P<0.05).[149]

Several other studies comparing low carbohydrate to low-fat or conventional diets with durations ranging from 6-12 weeks were reviewed. Studies using comparable energy intake among subjects across groups consistently reported no significant difference in weight loss regardless of the target population,[150-154] but measured various other outcomes with some positive results attributed to low carbohydrate intake.

LOW GLYCEMIC INDEX AND GLYCEMIC LOAD DIETS

Advocates of low carbohydrate diets often share a common rationale pertaining to glycemic index (GI) or glycemic load (GL). The glycemic index of a food is a measure of how quickly its ingestion results in a rise in blood glucose levels, and the height of that response,[155] Carbohydrate containing foods can be ranked according to their postprandial glycemic response.[156] It is only possible to apply GI analysis to foods containing at least 50 grams of available carbohydrates, while foods are commonly consumed in varying amounts and may not meet this threshold. Using GI alone, high GI foods that are consumed in small amounts (carrots, for example) can be labeled hazardous.

This deficit led to the development of the glycemic load. Taking both GI and reasonable serving sizes into account, the GL is the weighted average GI of a food multiplied by the percent of energy from carbohydrate[157] and is believed to better predict the glycemic impact of foods.[156]

The role of glycemic index and glycemic load in weight control is not clear and is a new area of research. Few studies have been conducted and all have been short-term. These are described below.

A recent trial by Ebbeling et al.[158] reveals some of the potential distortions introduced when means of improving dietary intake pattern are considered as mutually exclusive of one another. This group of investigators compared a diet reduced in glycemic load, with 30-35% of calories from fat, to a diet termed "conventional" in which fat was restricted to 25-30% of calories, but the quality of the carbohydrate choices was unaddressed. The reduced glycemic load diet resulted in slightly greater weight loss, and control of insulin resistance, than the control diet in the 16 obese adolescents followed. What seems most noteworthy, however, is that the range of fat intake for the low-fat and low-glycemic load diets are actually contiguous. Thus, this study actually compared two diets that differed little with regard to fat content, one in which glycemic load was controlled, the other in which it was not. This is very much like comparing complex to simple carbohydrate, and finding that complex carbohydrate has preferable health effects. Regrettably, in the rush to defend competing dietary claims, this simple message is obscured.

In a 10-week trial, Sloth, et al (2004)[159] investigated the role of glycemic index in on energy intake, weight and risk factors for chronic disease in 45 healthy women by comparing a low fat high carbohydrate/GI diet to a low fat high carbohydrate/low GI diet. No significant differences were observed between groups in energy intake, body weight or fat mass. The study found some beneficial effects of low GI diet on risk factors for ischemic heart disease.

In 2000, Spieth and colleagues[160] reported the results of a retrospective cohort study comparing a low glycemic-index to a low fat diet for weight loss in 107 obese children.[160] Greater reduction in the BMI was observed at approximately 4 months in the low-GI group (-1.53 kg/m(2) [95% CI, -1.94 to -1.12]) as compared to the low-fat diet group (-0.06 kg/m(2) [-0.56 to + 0. 44], P<.001).

In a study by Heilbronn, et al (2002) 45 overweight subjects with type II diabetes were randomly assigned to either a high or low GI diet following four weeks of high saturated fat diet. All diets were energy restricted. Weight loss did not differ between groups; however, a significantly greater reduction in LDL was observed in subjects on the low GI diet, with low glucose tolerance.[161]

OTHER

Several behavioral strategies for controlling calorie intake have been devised. Some of the most exciting new research in the area focuses on how the properties of foods, namely energy density and portion size are important determinants of energy intake and can be manipulated to adjust intake.

Studies by Rolls and colleagues have demonstrated that increasing the volume of low energy foods consumed prior to a meal leads to decreased consumption overall. In a study comparing energy intake among subjects provided with low calorie salads in various sizes to those with no first course, inclusion of low calorie salads resulted in reduced meal energy intake (by 7% for the small portion and 12% for the large).[162]

Other studies have shown that increasing the energy density of foods while keeping the volume constant does not influence energy intake, suggesting that the volume of food that is consumed has a greater influence on perceptions of a food's pleasantness and increases in volume may accelerate termination of eating.[163] Increasing food volume while reducing or keeping calories constant can be accomplished by incorporating water[164] or air[165] into foods; however drinking water with or before meals may not result in similar reduced energy consumption.[164] Incorporating fruits and vegetables into the diet may also decrease energy intake, given their low energy density and high concentration of water and fiber.[87]

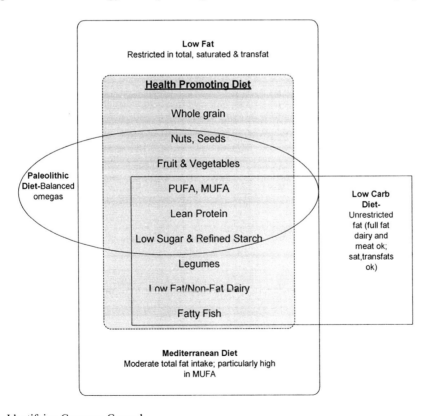

Figure 1. Identifying Common Ground

Evidence is clear that individuals under-estimate the calorie content of foods[166] and do not describe portion size accurately.[167] Increases in the size of meals and snacks reliably results in increased consumption.

In a study by Diliberti, et al (2004), restaurant customers who purchased oversized meals increased their calorie intake by 43%.[168] Rolls, et al (2004) investigated the effects of various portion size of sandwiches on calorie intake, showing that when served the 12-inch sandwich, compared with the 8-inch sandwich, females consumed 12% more energy (74 kcal) and males consumed 23% more energy (186 kcal). Importantly, increased consumption did not translate into differences in hunger and fullness ratings in this study[169] and others.[170] Adults also overeat when snacks sizes are large. A study by Rolls, et al (2004) showed that intake of potato chips was greater among study subjects receiving larger snack bags compared to subjects receiving smaller bags. Results showed that snack intake increased significantly as the package size increased for both males and females.[171] Rolls and colleagues have also recently demonstrated that children as young as 4 also overeat when served large portions, compared to smaller ones, as opposed to younger children who appear to rely on hunger as a cue for eating.

The commonalities of prevailing weight loss approaches include the acceptance of or emphasis on lean protein, low or non-fat dairy, fruits and vegetables, unsaturated fats and limits on sugar and refined starches (see Figure 1). These and other areas of overlap among various weight loss diets are concordant with scientifically sound dietary recommendations to promote health and are therefore, the most appropriate choice of diet to achieve both good health and weight control.

The 2005 Dietary Guidelines for Americans

The main tenets of the newly released Dietary Guidelines for Americans issued by the Departments of Health and Human Services (HHS) and Agriculture (USDA) are to choose a variety of nutrient-dense foods and beverages that limit the intake of saturated and trans fats, cholesterol, added sugars, salt, and alcohol. Specific advice on appropriate consumption by food grouping for an average 2,000-calorie daily diet include the following: two cups of fruit and 2½ cups of vegetables per day (including a wide variety of each weekly); three or more 1 ounce servings of whole-grain products per day (at least half of all grains should come from whole grains); three cups per day of fat-free or low-fat milk or equivalent dairy products; restriction of saturated and trans fatty acids to fewer than 10% of calories, with total fat intake less than 35% of calories (preferred fat sources are fish, nuts, and vegetable oils containing polyunsaturated and monounsaturated fatty acids) and lean, low-fat, or fat-free meats, poultry, dry beans are preferable protein sources. Additional recommendations to minimize added sugar, limit added salt in food preparation and consume less than 2,300 mg (approximately one teaspoon of salt) of sodium per day and limit alcohol to one and two drinks per day for women and men respectively, were provided. There is considerable overlap between these recommendations for a health promoting diet and the principal components of the diets reviewed in this chapter. Following these guidelines while monitoring and balancing calories consumed with calories expended in physical activity, represent the most prudent means of weight control.

CONCLUSION

Given that health improvements are the most important goal in weight loss efforts and that weight loss is achieved with any number of methods, it is common sense to take the approach that is most consistent with good health. We have substantial and compelling evidence regarding the basic dietary pattern conducive to human health. There is, as well, considerable evidence from multiple sources to suggest an association between a health-promoting diet and lifestyle, and sustainable weight control. A significant portion of the fundamental components of various diets that support weight loss are also concordant with what we know about diet and health; common elements in weight loss diets are described above (fruit, vegetables, limited fat, sugar and refined starches, etc.) This basic dietary pattern appropriate for both health and weight control is relatively clear (see Table 1); the current challenge lies in helping the public achieve and maintain a balanced, healthful diet sufficiently controlled in calories to be conducive to weight control.

Table 1. Recommended Way of Dietary Pattern for Optimal Health and Weight Control. Adapted from: _The Way to Eat_ [172]

Nutrient Class/Nutrient	Recommended Intake
Carbohydrate, predominately complex	Approximately 55-60% of total calories
Fiber, both soluble and insoluble	At least 25 grams per day, with additional potential benefit from up to 50 grams per day
Protein, predominantly plant-based sources	Up to 20% of total calories
Total Fat _Types of Fat_	Not more than 30%, and preferably 20-25% of total calories
Monounsaturated Fat	10% of total calories
Polyunsaturated Fat	10% of total calories
Omega-3 and Omega-6 fat	1:1 to 1:4 ratio
Saturated Fat and Trans fat (partially hydrogenated fat)	Ideally, less than 5% of total calories
Sugar	Less than 10% of total calories
Sodium	Up to 2400 mg per day
Cholesterol	Less than 300 mg a day
Water	8 glasses a day/64oz/2liters
Alcohol, moderate intake if desired	Up to one drink a day for women Up to two drinks a day for men
Calorie level	Adequate to achieve and maintain a healthy weight.
Physical Activity / Exercise	Daily moderate activity for 30 minutes Strength training twice weekly

The current focus on finding alternatives to the dietary pattern known to promote health, not only neglects the robust base of evidence validating the need for its widespread adoption, but it is a potential public health threat. For as long as we remain distracted by competing dietary claims, we fail to take the requisite steps or mobilize the requisite political will to make healthful eating more accessible to all. In other words, the more of our resources we devote to questioning where we ought to go, the longer it will take to get there.

Consider the state of both knowledge, and public health practice, with regard to physical activity. It is widely accepted that a lifetime of regular physical activity promotes health. On this basis, current effort is directed toward identifying practical means of raising daily activity levels. In other words, the 'what' is established, so we are grappling with the 'how'-from encouraging use of stairs, to making sure neighborhoods have sidewalks, to re-establishing physical education in our schools. We do this in spite of the fact that we do not know for certain that there is no alternative to regular physical activity. We have not systematically examined every conceivable means of being sedentary-different postures, different positions, different couches upon which to perch to prove that none has the same effects as being regularly active. This would be absurd. Yet it seems, if we were to apply the standard we are using for diet, that is exactly what we would do. Rather than work to promote the activity pattern abundant but not-truly-definitive evidence indicates promotes health, we would devote our resources to studying every conceivable alternative to that pattern.

We have, in the aggregate, as much evidence regarding the association between diet and health as we do regarding physical activity and health. Diet may be a more complex variable, but the parallel is still strong. The evidence we have in support of a particular dietary pattern for health suggests that our resources should be devoted to learning how best to achieve and maintain this dietary pattern, not looking for alternatives. The sooner we accept that we know where we should be going, the sooner we may actually hope to advance toward that destination.

REFERENCES

[1]   Tillotson JE. Pandemic Obesity: What Is the Solution? *Nutr Today*. 2004;39(1):6-9.
[2]   Mascie-Taylor CG, Karim E. The burden of chronic disease. *Science*. 2003;302:1921-2.
[3]   Jeffery RW, Utter J. The changing environment and population obesity in the United States. *Obes Res*. 2003;11:12S-22S.
[4]   Mokdad AH, Ford ES, Bowman BA, et al. Prevalence of obesity, diabetes, and obesity-related health risk factors, 2001. *JAMA*. 2003;289:76-9.
[5]   Mokdad AH, Marks JS, Stroup DF, Gerberding JL. Actual causes of death in the United States, 2000. *JAMA*. 2004;291(10):1238-45.
[6]   Calle EE, Thun MJ, Petrelli JM, Rodriguez C, Heath CW, Jr. Body-mass index and mortality in a prospective cohort of U.S. adults. *N Engl J Med*. 1999;341(15):1097-105.
[7]   Sowers JR, Frohlich ED. Insulin and insulin resistance: impact on blood pressure and cardiovascular disease. *Med Clin North Am*. 2004;88:63-82.
[8]   Lindsay RS, Howard BV. Cardiovascular risk associated with the metabolic syndrome. *Curr Diab Rep*. 2004;4:63-8.

[9]   Reaven G, Abbasi F, McLaughlin T. Obesity, insulin resistance, and cardiovascular disease. *Recent Prog Horm Res*. 2004;59:207-23.

[10]   Calle EE, Rodriguez C, Walker-Thurmond K, Thun MJ. Overweight, obesity, and mortality from cancer in a prospectively studied cohort of U.S. adults. *N Engl J Med*. 2003;348(17):1625-38.

[11]   Paeratakul S, York-Crowe EE, Williamson DA, Ryan DH, Bray GA. Americans on diet: results from the 1994-1996 Continuing Survey of Food Intakes by Individuals. *J Am Diet Assoc*. 2002;102:1247-51.

[12]   Ikeda JP, Lyons P, Schwartzman F, Mitchell RA. Self-reported dieting experiences of women with body mass indexes of 30 or more. *J Am Diet Assoc*. 2004;104(6):972-4.

[13]   Liebman M, Cameron BA, Carson DK, Brown DM, Meyer SS. Dietary fat reduction behaviors in college students: relationship to dieting status, gender and key psychosocial variables. *Appetite*. 2001;36(1):51-6.

[14]   Simopoulos AP. The Mediterranean diets: What is so special about the diet of Greece? The scientific evidence. *J Nutr*. 2001;131:3065S-73S.

[15]   Kok FJ, Kromhout D. Atherosclerosis--epidemiological studies on the health effects of a Mediterranean diet. *Eur J Nutr*. 2004;43(Suppl 1):2-5.

[16]   Kris-Etherton P, Eckel RH, Howard BV, S. St. Jeor, Bazzarre TL. Nutrition Committee Population Science Committee and Clinical Science Committee of the American Heart Association. AHA Science Advisory: Lyon Diet Heart Study. Benefits of a Mediterranean-style, National Cholesterol Education Program/ American Heart Association Step I Dietary Pattern on Cardiovascular Disease. *Circulation*. 2001;103(13):1823-5.

[17]   Cukur CS, de Guzman MR, Carlo G. Religiosity, values, and horizontal and vertical individualism-collectivism: a study of Turkey, the United States, and the Philippines. *J Soc Psychol*. 2004;144(6):613-34.

[18]   DeJong MJ, Chung ML, Roser LP, et al. A five-country comparison of anxiety early after acute myocardial infarction. *Eur J Cardiovasc Nurs*. 2004;3(2):129-34.

[19]   Owen RW, Haubner R, Wurtele G, Hull E, Spiegelhalder B, Bartsch H. Olives and olive oil in cancer prevention. *Eur J Cancer Prev*. 2004;13(4):319-26.

[20]   Trichopoulou A, Critselis E. Mediterranean diet and longevity. *Eur J Cancer Prev*. 2004;13(5):453-6.

[21]   Knoops KT, deGroot LC, Kromhout D, et al. Mediterranean diet, lifestyle factors, and 10-year mortality in elderly European men and women: the HALE project. *JAMA*. 2004;292(12):1433-9.

[22]   Alberti-Fidanza A, Fidanza F. Mediterranean Adequacy Index of Italian diets. *Public Health Nutr*. 2004;7(7):937-41.

[23]   Fidanza F, Alberti A, Lanti M, Menotti A. Mediterranean Adequacy Index: correlation with 25-year mortality from coronary heart disease in the Seven Countries Study. *Nutr Metab Cardiovasc Dis*. 2004;14(5):254-8.

[24]   Panagiotakos DB, Pitsavos C, Polychronopoulos E, Chrysohoou C, Zampelas A, Trichopoulou A. Can a Mediterranean diet moderate the development and clinical progression of coronary heart disease? A systematic review. *Med Sci Monit*. 2004;10(8):193-8.

[25] de Lorgeril M, Salen P, Martin JL, Boucher F, Paillard F, de Leiris J. Wine drinking and risks of cardiovascular complications after recent acute myocardial infarction. *Circulation.* 2002;106(12):1465-9.

[26] Biesalski HK. Diabetes preventive components in the Mediterranean diet. *Eur J Nutr.* 2004;43(Suppl 1):26-30.

[27] Perez-Jimenez F, Lopez-Miranda J, Pinillos MD, et al. A Mediterranean and a high-carbohydrate diet improve glucose metabolism in healthy young persons. *Diabetologia.* 2001;44(11):2038-43.

[28] Ciccarone E, Castelnuovo AD, Salcuni M, et al. A high-score Mediterranean dietary pattern is associated with a reduced risk of peripheral arterial disease in Italian patients with Type 2 diabetes. *J Thromb Haemost.* 2003;1(8):1744-52.

[29] Toobert DJ, Glasgow RE, Strycker LA, et al. Biologic and quality-of-life outcomes from the Mediterranean Lifestyle Program: a randomized clinical trial. *Diabetes Care.* 2003;26(8):2288-93.

[30] Visioli F, Grande S, Bogani P, Galli C. The role of antioxidants in the mediterranean diets: focus on cancer. *Eur J Cancer Prev.* 2004;13(4):337-43.

[31] La Vecchia C. Mediterranean diet and cancer. *Public Health Nutr.* 2004;7(7):965-8.

[32] Fortes C, Forastiere F, Farchi S, et al. The protective effect of the Mediterranean diet on lung cancer. *Nutr Cancer.* 2003;46(1):30-7.

[33] La Vecchia C, Negri E. Fats in seasoning and the relationship to pancreatic cancer. *Eur J Cancer Prev.* 1997;6(4):370-3.

[34] Franceschi S, Favero A, Conti E, et al. Food groups, oils and butter, and cancer of the oral cavity and pharynx. *Br J Cancer.* 1999;80(3-4):614-20.

[35] Bosetti C, Negri E, Franceschi S, et al. Olive oil, seed oils and other added fats in relation to ovarian cancer (Italy). *Cancer Causes Control.* 2002;13(5):465-70.

[36] Trichopoulou A, Katsouyanni K, Stuver S, et al. Consumption of olive oil and specific food groups in relation to breast cancer risk in Greece. *Natl Cancer Inst.* 1995;87(2):110-6.

[37] Trichopoulou A, Lagiou P, Kuper H, Trichopulos D. Cancer and Mediteranean dietary traditions. *Cancer Epidemiology Biomarkers Prev.* 2000;9(9):869-873.

[38] Bosetti C, La Vecchia C, Talamini R, et al. Food groups and risk of squamous cell esophageal cancer in northern Italy. *Int J Cancer.* 2000;87(2):289-94.

[39] Martinez-Gonzalez MA, Estruch R. Mediterranean diet, antioxidants and cancer: the need for randomized trials. *Eur J Cancer Prev.* 2004;13(4):327-35.

[40] Shah M, Garg A. High-fat and high-carbohydrate diets and energy balance. *Diabetes Care.* 1996;19:1142-52.

[41] McManus K, Antinoro L, Sacks F. A randomized controlled trial of a moderate-fat, low-energy diet compared with a low fat, low-energy diet for weight loss in overweight adults. *Int J Obes Relat Metab Disord.* 2001;25(10):1503-11.

[42] Flynn G, Colquhoun D. Successful long-term weight loss with a Mediterranean style diet in a primary care medical centre. *Asia Pac J Clin Nutr.* 2004;13:S139.

[43] De Lorenzo A, Petroni ML, deLuca PP, et al. Use of quality control indices in moderately hypocaloric Mediterranean diet for treatment of obesity. *Diabetes Nutr Metab.* 2001;14(4):181-8.

[44] Katz DL. *Nutrition in Clinical Practice* Philadelphia, PA: Lippincott Williams and Wilkins; 2001.

[45] Eaton SB, Strassman BI, Nesse RM, et al. Evolutionary health promotion. *Prev Med.* 2002;34:109-18.

[46] Eaton S, Eaton SB III, Konner M. Paleolithic nutrition revisited: A twelve-year retrospective on its nature and implications. *Eur J Clinical Nutrition.* 1997;51:207-216.

[47] Baschetti R. Paleolithic nutrition. *Eur J Clin Nutr.* 1997;51:715-6.

[48] Katz DL. Evoluationary Biology, Culture, and Determinants of Dietary Behavior. *Nutrition in Clinical Practice.* Philaelphia, PA: Lippincott Williams and Wilkins; 2001:279-90.

[49] Eaton S, Eaton SB III, Konner M, Shostak M. An Evolutionary Perspective Enhances Understanding of Human Nutritional Requirements. *J. Nutr.* 1996;126:1732-1740.

[50] Simopoulos AP. Evolutionary aspects of diet, essential fatty acids and cardiovascular disease. *European Heart Journal.* 2001;3(suppl D):D8-D21.

[51] Tannahill R. *Food in History* London, England: Penguin Books, Ltd; 1988.

[52] Neel J. *Physician to the gene pool.* New York, NY: John Wiley.; 1994.

[53] Knowler WC, Barrett-Connor E, Fowler SE, et al. Reduction in the incidence of type 2 diabetes with lifestyle intervention or metformin. *N Engl J Med.* 2002;346(6):393-403.

[54] Sacks FM, Svetkey LP, Vollmer WM, et al. Effects on blood pressure of reduced dietary sodium and the Dietary Approaches to Stop Hypertension (DASH) diet. DASH-Sodium Collaborative Research Group. *N Engl J Med.* 2001;344:3-10.

[55] de Lorgeril M, Renaud S, Mamelle N, et al. Mediterranean alpha-linolenic acid-rich diet in the secondary prevention of coronary heart disease. *Lancet.* 1994;343:1454-59.

[56] Ornish D, Scherwitz LW, Billings JH, et al. Intensive lifestyle changes for reversal of coronary heart disease. *JAMA.* 1998;280(23):2001-7.

[57] Solomons N. Nutritional dilemmas for long-term health. *Asia Pac J Clin Nutr.* 2004;13:S21-2.

[58] Klem ML, Wing RR, McGuire MT, Seagle HM, Hill JO. A descriptive study of individuals successful at long-term maintenance of substantial weight loss. *Am J Clin Nutr.* 1997;66(2):239-46.

[59] Astrup A. The role of dietary fat in the prevention and treatment of obesity. Efficacy and safety of low-fat diets. *Int J Obes Relat Metab Disord.* 2001;25(Suppl 1):S46-50.

[60] Connor W, Connor S. Should a low-fat, high-carbohydrate diet be recommended for everyone? The case for a low-fat, high-carbohydrate diet. *N Engl J Med.* 1997;337:562-563.

[61] Drewnowski A, Popkin BM. The nutrition transition: new trends in the global diet. *Nutrition Reviews.* 1997;55(2):31-43.

[62] Katan M, Grundy S, Willett W. Should a low-fat, high-carbohydrate diet be recommended for everyone? Beyond low-fat diets. *N Engl J Med.* 1997;337:563-6.

[63] US Preventive Services Task Force. Guide to Clinical Preventive Services. 2nd ed. Baltimore, MD: Williams and Wilkins; 1996.

[64] United States Department of Agriculture. Dietary guidelines for Americans 2000.: *http://www.health.gov/dietaryguidelines/dga2000/document/contents.htm*; 2000.

[65] U. S. Department of Agriculture. The Food Guide Pyramid. Washington, D.C.: *http://www.nal.usda.gov:8001/py/pmap.ht*m; 1992.

[66] National Cancer Institute. National Cancer Institute Dietary Guidelines.: *http://www.pueblo.gsa.gov/cic_text/food/guideeat/guidelns.htm*l.

[67] American Heart Association. Step I and step II diets.: *http://www.americanheart. org/presenter.jhtml?identifier=4764.*

[68] American Dietetic Association. Weight Management -- Position of ADA. *J Am Diet Assoc*. 2002;102:1145-1155.

[69] Franz MJ, Bantle JP, Beebe CA, et al. Evidence-based nutrition. Principles and recommendations for the treatment and prevention of diabetes and related complications. *Diabetes Care*. 2002;25:148-98.

[70] Institute of Medicine Food and Nutrition Board, National Academies of Science. *Dietary Reference Intakes for Energy, Carbohydrate, Fiber, Fat, Fatty Acids, Cholesterol, Protein, and Amino Acids (Macronutrients).* Washington, D.C.: National Academy Press; 2002.

[71] Hu FB, Willett WC. Optimal diets for prevention of coronary heart disease. *JAMA*. 2002;288:2569-78.

[72] Hu FB, Manson JE, Willett WC. Types of dietary fat and risk of coronary heart disease: a critical review. *J Am Coll Nutr*. 2001;20:5-19.

[73] Hu FB. Plant-based foods and prevention of cardiovascular disease: an overview. *Am J Clin Nutr*. 2003;78:544S-551S.

[74] Willet WC. *Eat, Drink, and Be Healthy* NY, NY: Simon and Schuster Source; 2001.

[75] Reddy KS, Katan MB. Diet, nutrition and the prevention of hypertension and cardiovascular diseases. *Public Health Nutr*. 2004;7(1A):167-86.

[76] Mathers JC. Nutrition and cancer prevention: diet-gene interactions. *Proc Nutr Soc*. 2003;62(3):605-10.

[77] Key TJ, Schatzkin A, Willett WC, Allen NE, Spencer EA, Travis RC. Diet, nutrition and the prevention of cancer. *Public Health Nutr*. 2004;7:187-200.

[78] Howard BV. Dietary fat as a risk factor for type 2 diabetes. *Ann N Y Acad Sci*. 2002;967:324-8.

[79] Moloney M. Dietary treatments of obesity. *Proc Nutr Soc*. 2000;59:601-8.

[80] Salmeron J, Hu FB, Manson JE, et al. Dietary fat intake and risk of type 2 diabetes in women. *Am J Clin Nutr*. 2001;73(6):1019-26.

[81] American Heart Association.: *www.eamericanheart.org.*; 2005.

[82] Katz D. Chapter 6: Diet, Atherosclerosis, and Ischemic Heart Disease. *Nutrition in Clinical Practice*. Philadelphia, PA: Lippincott, Williams and Wilkins; 2000:63-76.

[83] National Cancer Institute. Epidemiology: Diet and Cancer. Surveillance, Epidemiology and End Results (SEER).: *http://seer.cancer.gov/*; 2005.

[84] Byers T, Doyle C. Diet, Physical Activity and Cancer…What's the Connection? www.cancer.org ed: American Cancer Society.

[85] Astrup A. Dietary approaches to reducing body weight. *Baillieres Best Pract Res Clin Endocrinol Metab*. 1999;13:109-20.

[86] Astrup A, Ryan L, Grunwald GK, et al. The role of dietary fat in body fatness: evidence from a preliminary meta-analysis of ad libitum low-fat dietary intervention studies. *Br J Nutr*. 2000;83:S25-32.

[87] Rolls BJ, Ello-Martin JA, Tohill BC. What can intervention studies tell us about the relationship between fruit and vegetable consumption and weight management? *Nutr Rev*. 2004;62:1-17.

[88] Wadden TA, Butryn ML. Behavioral treatment of obesity. *Endocrinol Metab Clin North Am*. 2003;32:981-1003.

[89] Plodkowski RA, St.Jeor S. Medical nutrition therapy for the treatment of obesity. *Endocrinol Metab Clin North Am.* 2003;32:935-65.

[90] Bedno SA. Weight loss in diabetes management. *Nutr Clin Care.* 2003;6:62-72.

[91] Wing RR, Gorin AA. Behavioral techniques for treating the obese patient. *Prim Care.* 2003;30:375-91.

[92] Vermunt SH, Pasman WJ, Schaafsma G, Kardinaal AF. Effects of sugar intake on body weight: a review. *Obes Rev.* 2003;4:91-9.

[93] Pirozzo S, Summerbell C, Cameron C, Glasziou P. Should we recommend low-fat diets for obesity? *Obes Rev.* 2003;4:83-90.

[94] Drewnowski A. The role of energy density. *Lipids.* 2003;38:109-15.

[95] Cheuvront SN. The Zone Diet phenomenon: a closer look at the science behind the claims. *J Am Coll Nutr.* 2003;22(1):9-17.

[96] Jequier E, Bray GA. Low-fat diets are preferred. *Am J Med.* 2002;113(Suppl 9B):41S-46S.

[97] Schrauwen P, Westerterp KR. The role of high-fat diets and physical activity in the regulation of body weight. *Br J Nutr.* 2000;84:417-27.

[98] Keys A, Menotti A, Aravanis C, et al. The seven countries study: 2,289 deaths in 15 years. *Prev Med.* 1984;13:141-54.

[99] Keys A, Aravanis C, Blackburn H, et al. Coronary heart disease: overweight and obesity as risk factors. *Ann Intern Med.* 1972;77:15-27.

[100] Keys A. Relative obesity and its health significance. *Diabetes.* 1955;4:447-55.

[101] Katz DL. Clinically Relevant Fat Metabolism. *Nutrition in Clinical Practice.* Philadelphia, PA: Lippincott, Williams and Wilkins; 2001:9-15.

[102] Peters JC. Dietary fat and body weight control. *Lipids.* 2003;38:123-7.

[103] Hill JO, Melanson EL, Wyatt HT. Dietary fat intake and regulation of energy balance: implications for obesity. *J Nutr.* 2000;130:284S-288S.

[104] Schutz Y. Macronutrients and energy balance in obesity. *Metabolism.* 1995;44:7-11.

[105] Bray G, Popkin B. Dietary fat intake does affect obesity! *Am J Clin Nutr.* 1998;68:1157-1173.

[106] Pirozzo S, Summerbell C, Cameron C, Glasziou P. Advice on low-fat diets for obesity. *Cochrane Database Syst Rev.* 2002(2):CD003640.

[107] Mattes RD. Feeding behaviors and weight loss outcomes over 64 months. *Eat Behav.* 2002;3:191-204.

[108] Wing RR, Hill JO. Successful weight loss maintenance. *Annu Rev Nutr.* 2001;21:323-41.

[109] McGuire MT, Wing RR, Klem ML, Seagle HM, Hill JO. Long-term maintenance of weight loss: do people who lose weight through various weight loss methods use different behaviors to maintain their weight? *Int J Obes Relat Metab Disord.* 1998;22(6):572-7.

[110] Shick SM, Wing RR, Klem ML, McGuire MT, Hill JO, Seagle H. Persons successful at long-term weight loss and maintenance continue to consume a low-energy, low-fat diet. *J Am Diet Assoc.* 1998;98:408-13.

[111] Willett WC, Leibel RL. Dietary fat is not a major determinant of body fat. *Am J Med.* 2002;113(Suppl 9B):47S-59S.

[112] Wright JD, Kennedy-Stephenson J, Wang CY, et al. Trends in intake of energy and macronutrients --- United States, 1971-2000. *MMWR.* 2004;53:80-82.

[113] Jequier E. Pathways to obesity. *Int J Obes Relat Metab Disord.* 2002;26:S12-7.

[114] Astrup A. The American paradox: the role of energy-dense fat-reduced food in the increasing prevalence of obesity. *Curr Opin Clin Nutr Metab Care.* 1998;1(6):573-7.

[115] Rolls BJ, Miller DL. Is the low-fat message giving people a license to eat more? *J Am Coll Nutr.* 1997;16:535-43.

[116] Harnack LJ, Jeffery RW, Boutelle KN. Temporal trends in energy intake in the United States: an ecologic perspective. *Am J Clin Nutr.* 2000;71:1478-84.

[117] McCrory MA, Fuss PJ, Saltzman E, Roberts SB. Dietary determinants of energy intake and weight regulation in healthy adults. *J Nutr.* 2000;130:276S-279S.

[118] Nestle M. Increasing portion sizes in American diets: more calories, more obesity. *J Am Diet Assoc.* 2003;103(1):39-40.

[119] American College of Preventive Medicine Position Statement. Diet in the Prevention and Control of Obesity, Insulin Resistance, and Type II Diabetes.: *http://www.acpm. org/2002-057(F).htm.*

[120] Katz DL. Pandemic obesity and the contagion of nutritional nonsense. *Public Health Rev.* 2003;31:33-44.

[121] Denke M. Metabolic effects of high-protein, low-carbohydrate diets. *The American Journal of Cardiology.* 2001;88:59-61.

[122] Tapper-Gardzina Y, Cotugna N, Vickery C. Should you recommend a low-carb, high-protein diet? *The Nurse Practitioner.* 2002;27(4):52-57.

[123] Eisenstein J, Roberts SB, Dallal G, Saltzman E. High-protein weight-loss diets: are they safe and do they work? A review of the experimental and epidemiologic data. *Nutr Rev.* 2002;60:189-200.

[124] Atkins R. *Dr. Atkins' New Diet Revolution* New York, NY: HarperCollins Publishers, Inc.; 2002.

[125] Katz DL. Diet and Cancer. *Nutrition in Clinical Practice.* Philadelphia, PA: Lippincott Williams and Wilkins; 2000:114-126.

[126] St. Jeor S, Howard B, Prewitt E, Bovee V, Bazzarre T, Eckel R. Dietary Protein and Weight Reduction: A Statement for Healthcare Professionals From the Nutrition Committee of the Council on Nutrition, Physical Activity, and Metabolism of the American Heart Association. *Circulation.* 2001;104:1869-74.

[127] Katz DL. Diet, sleep-wake cycles, and mood. *Nutrition in Clinical Practice.* Philadelphia, PA: Lippincott Williams and Wilkins; 2001:243-7.

[128] Benton D. Carbohydrate ingestion, blood glucose and mood. *Neurosci Biobehav Rev.* 2002;26:293-308.

[129] Terry P, Terry JB, Wolk A. Fruit and vegetable consumption in the prevention of cancer: an update. *J Intern Med.* 2001;250:280-90.

[130] Van Duyn MA, Pivonka E. Overview of the health benefits of fruit and vegetable consumption for the dietetics professional: selected literature. *J Am Diet Assoc.* 2000;100(12):1511-21.

[131] Weisburger JH. Eat to live, not live to eat. *Nutrition.* 2000;16(9):767-73.

[132] Ornish D. Was Dr. Atkins Right? *Am J Diet Assoc.* 2004;104:537-42.

[133] Chandalia M, Garg A, Lutjohann D, von Bergmann K, Grundy SM, Brinkley LJ. Beneficial effects of high dietary fiber intake in patients with type 2 diabetes mellitus. *N Engl J Med.* 2000;342(19):1392-8.

[134] Westerterp-Plantenga MS, Lejeune MP, Nijs I, Ooijen Mv, Kovacs EM. High protein intake sustains weight maintenance after body weight loss in humans. *Int J Obes Relat Metab Disord.* 2004;28(1):57-64.

[135] Katz D. Diet, Obesity, and Weight Regulation. *Nutrition in Clinical Practice.* Philadelphia, PA: Lippincott Williams and Wilkins; 2000:37-62.

[136] Skov A, Toubro S, Ronn B, Holm L, Astrup A. Randomized trial on protein vs. carbohydrate in ad libitum fat reduced diet for the treatment of obesity. *Int J Obes Relat Metab Disord.* 1999;23:528-536.

[137] Volek JS, Sharman MJ, Gomez AL, Scheett TP, Kraemer WJ. An isoenergetic very low carbohydrate diet improves serum HDL cholesterol and triacylglycerol concentrations, the total cholesterol to HDL cholesterol ratio and postprandial pipemic responses compared with a low fat diet in normal weight, normolipidemic women. *J Nutr.* 2003;133(9):2756-61.

[138] Stern L, Iqbal N, Seshadri P, et al. The effects of low-carbohydrate versus conventional weight loss diets in severely obese adults: one-year follow-up of a randomized trial. *Ann Intern Med.* 2004;140(10):778-85.

[139] Yancy WS, Olsen MK, Guyton JR, Bakst RP, Westman EC. A low-carbohydrate, ketogenic diet versus a low-fat diet to treat obesity and hyperlipidemia: a randomized, controlled trial. *Ann Intern Med.* 2004;140(10):769-77.

[140] Westman EC, Yancy WS, Edman JS, Tomlin KF, Perkins CE. Effect of 6-month adherence to a very low carbohydrate diet program. *Am J Med.* 2002;113(1):30-6.

[141] Noakes M, Foster P, Keogh J, Clifton P. Very low carbohydrate diets for weight loss and cardiovascular risk. *Asia Pac J Clin Nutr.* 2004;13(Suppl):S64.

[142] Seshadri P, Iqbal N, Stern L, et al. A randomized study comparing the effects of a low-carbohydrate diet and a conventional diet on lipoprotein subfractions and C-reactive protein levels in patients with severe obesity. *Am J Med.* 2004;117(6):398-405.

[143] Sharman MJ, Volek JS. Weight loss leads to reductions in inflammatory biomarkers after a very-low-carbohydrate diet and a low-fat diet in overweight men. *Clin Sci (Lond).* 2004;107(4):365-9.

[144] Dansinger ML, Gleason JA, Griffith JL, Selker HP, Schaefer EJ. Comparison of the Atkins, Ornish, Weight Watchers, and Zone diets for weight loss and heart disease risk reduction: a randomized trial. *JAMA.* 2005;293(1):43-53.

[145] Samaha FF, Iqbal N, Seshadri P, et al. A low-carbohydrate as compared with a low-fat diet in severe obesity. *N Engl J Med.* 2003;348:2074-81.

[146] Foster GD, Wyatt HR, Hill JO, et al. A randomized trial of a low-carbohydrate diet for obesity. *N Engl J Med.* 2003;348(21):2082-90.

[147] Atkins R. *Atkins' New Diet Revolution* New York, NY.: M. Evans and Company, Inc.; 1999.

[148] Brehm BJ, Seeley RJ, Daniels SR, D'Alessio DA. A randomized trial comparing a very low carbohydrate diet and a calorie-restricted low fat diet on body weight and cardiovascular risk factors in healthy women. *J Clin Endocrinol Metab.* 2003;88:1617-23.

[149] Brinkworth GD, Noakes M, Keogh JB, Luscombe ND, Wittert GA, Clifton PM. Long-term effects of a high-protein, low-carbohydrate diet on weight control and cardiovascular risk markers in obese hyperinsulinemic subjects. *Int J Obes Relat Metab Disord.* 2004;28(5):661-70.

[150] Segal-Isaacson CJ, Johnson S, Tomuta V, Cowell B, Stein DT. A randomized trial comparing low-fat and low-carbohydrate diets matched for energy and protein. *Obes Res.* 2004;12(Suppl 2):130S-140S.

[151] Golay A, Allaz A, Morel Y, Tonnac Nd, Tankova S, Reaven G. Similar weight loss with low- and high-carbohydrate diets. *Am J Clin Nutr.* 1996;63:174-178.

[152] Golay A, Eigenheer C, Morel Y, Kujawski P, Lehmann T, Tonnac Nd. Weight-loss with low or high carbohydrate diet? *Int J Obes Relat Metab Disord.* 1996;20:1067-1072.

[153] Meckling KA, O'Sullivan C, Saari D. Comparison of a low-fat diet to a low-carbohydrate diet on weight loss, body composition, and risk factors for diabetes and cardiovascular disease in free-living, overweight men and women. *J Clin Endocrinol Metab.* 2004;89(6):2717-23.

[154] Miyashita Y, Koide N, Ohtsuka M, et al. Beneficial effect of low carbohydrate in low calorie diets on visceral fat reduction in type 2 diabetic patients with obesity. *Diabetes Res Clin Pract.* 2004;65(3):235-41.

[155] Ludwig DS. The glycemic index: Physiological mechanisms relating obesity, diabetes, and cardiovascular disease. *JAMA.* 2002;287:2414-2423.

[156] Colombani PC. Glycemic index and load-dynamic dietary guidelines in the context of disease. *Physiology and Behavior.* 2004;83:603-610.

[157] Moyad MA. Fad Diets and Obesity-Part II: An introduction to the theory behind low-carbohydrate diets. *Urologic Nursing.* 2004;24(3):442-445.

[158] Ebbeling CB, Leidig MM, Sinclair KB, Hangen JP, Ludwig DS. A reduced-glycemic load diet in the treatment of adolescent obesity. *Arch Pediatr Adolesc Med.* 2003;157:773-9.

[159] Sloth B, Krog-Mikkelsen I, Flint A, et al. No difference in body weight decrease between a low-glycemic-index and a high-glycemic-index diet but reduced LDL cholesterol after 10-wk ad libitum intake of the low-glycemic-index diet. *Am J Clin Nutr.* 2004;80(2):337-47.

[160] Spieth LE, Harnish JD, Lenders CM, et al. A low-glycemic index diet in the treatment of pediatric obesity. *Arch Pediatr Adolesc Med.* 2000;154(9):947-51.

[161] Heilbronn LK, Noakes M, Clifton PM. The effect of high- and low-glycemic index energy restricted diets on plasma lipid and glucose profiles in type 2 diabetic subjects with varying glycemic control. *J Am Coll Nutr.* 2002;21(2):120-7.

[162] Rolls BJ, Roe LS, Meengs JS. Salad and satiety: energy density and portion size of a first-course salad affect energy intake at lunch. *J Am Diet Assoc.* 2004;104(10):1570-6.

[163] Bell EA, Roe LS, Rolls BJ. Sensory-specific satiety is affected more by volume than by energy content of a liquid food. *Physiol Behav.* 2003;78(4-5):593-600.

[164] Rolls BJ, Bell EA, Thorwart ML. Water incorporated into a food but not served with a food decreases energy intake in lean women. *Am J Clin Nutr.* 1999;70(4):448-55.

[165] Rolls BJ, Bell EA, Waugh BA. Increasing the volume of a food by incorporating air affects satiety in men. *Am J Clin Nutr.* 2000;72(2):361-8.

[166] Anderson DA, Williamson DA, Johnson WG, Grieve CO. Estimation of food intake: effects of the unit of estimation. *Eat Weight Disord.* 1999;4(1):6-9.

[167] Guthrie HA. Selection and quantification of typical food portions by young adults. *J Am Diet Assoc.* 1984;84(12):1440-4.

[168] Diliberti N, Bordi PL, Conklin MT, Roe LS, Rolls BJ. Increased portion size leads to increased energy intake in a restaurant meal. *Obes Res*. 2004;12(3):562-8.

[169] Rolls BJ, Roe LS, Meengs JS, Wall DE. Increasing the portion size of a sandwich increases energy intake. *J Am Diet Assoc*. 2004;104(3):367-72.

[170] Kral TV, Roe LS, Rolls BJ. Combined effects of energy density and portion size on energy intake in women. *Am J Clin Nutr*. 2004;79(6):962-8.

[171] Rolls BJ, Roe LS, Kral TV, Meengs JS, Wall DE. Increasing the portion size of a packaged snack increases energy intake in men and women. *Appetite*. 2004;42(1):63-9.

[172] Katz DL, Gonzalez MH. *The Way to Eat*. Naperville, Illinois: Sourcebooks. Jacobson/ estle, Etc; 2002.

In: Weight Loss, Exercise and Health Research
Editor: Carrie P. Saylor, pp. 29-48

ISBN 1-60021-077-5
© 2006 Nova Science Publishers, Inc.

Chapter 2

INHIBITORS OF FATTY ACID SYNTHASE FROM PLANTS AND THEIR EFFECTS ON WEIGHT CONTROL

Wei-Xi Tian

Department of Biology, Graduate School of Chinese Academy of Sciences.
Beijing, China 100049

1 BACKGROUND

1.1 Obesity Has Been A Perilous Factor that Obviously Threatens Human Health

Obesity sweeps all over the world presently at an astonishing speed. The rate of the disease ascends in both the developed and developing countries. According to a report in 1998 from the world Health organization, it can be estimated that about 250 million adults are obese all the world, and that at least 500 million adults are overweighed[1]. About 2%-7% annual medical expenses of the developed countries are used for obesity by conservative estimation[2].

At present, the most obvious diseases that imperil human life and health have pertinence with obesity. It has been known that diabetes II is related to obesity. Artheriosclerosis and thrombosis has concernful affiliation with abundance of fat, and they may result in apoplexy, parapoplexy and coronary heart disease [3-5]. The newest report was that mortality from cancer is related to overweight or obesity. Calle et al. prospectively investigated more than 900 thousand U.S. adults who were free of cancer at enrollment in 1982, there were 57145 deaths from cancer during 16 years. It was found that the increased body-mass index in 1982 was associated with increase death rates for all cancer[6]. The effect of obesity is serious to health, economy and social psychology.

People try to understand the mechanism of obesity all along. In the ninetieth of last century, the positional cloning of obese gene was a significant advance[7]. Much work on obese gene and leptin has been done up to now[8, 9]. The discovery and cloning of obese gene make progress in explaining obesity at a molecular level.

But obesity is a complex multi-factor decompensate disease[2]. A single gene mutation cannot be regarded as the cause of prevalence of obesity. In recent years, lots of hormones related to regulation of appetite and body weight are depicted in experimental models[10-12]. However, essential obesity results from breakage of the balance between food intake and energy-consumption.

1.2 Fatty Acid Synthase (FAS) was Found as a Potential Therapeutic Target for Obesity

In 2000, Loftus et al. reported a new significant progress. In mice by intraperitoneal injection of C75 that is a synthetic inhibitor of FAS, Loftus and his colleagues observed profound weight loss in a dose-dependent manner. The weight loss persisted for a duration that is increased with dose. No obvious toxicity exhibited, and mice regained weight after the treatment was stopped[13]. C75-induced weight loss was due primarily to inhibition of feeding. It is plausible that C75 does not influence normal metabolism although it reduced food intake of rats by comparison of treatment with fasting and intraperitoneal administration of C75. Hungriness induces the expression of hypothalamic Neuropeptide Y (NPY) to promote feeding[14]. Northern blot analysis of hypothalamic tissue indicated that NPY mRNA lever in C75-treated mice were even lower than those in fed control mice, even though the C75-treated mice had not eaten. Loftus et al. pretreated mice with either TOFA, an inhibitor of acetyl-CoA carboxylase, or vehicle by ICV injection and examined the ability of an intraperitoneal injection of C75 to inhibit feeding. TOFA largely restored food intake in C75-treated mice, supporting the hypothesis that malonyl CoA mediated feeding inhibition and the inhibitor of FAS did not inhibit feeding directly. Therefore, FAS may represent an important link in feeding regulation, and it may be a potential therapeutic target for obesity[13].

1.3 Relationship Between Level of Body Fat and Activity of FAS

We previously reported that the FAS activity of fowls was highly related to their fat level. The average abdomen fat per kilogram of duck and chicken was 61.7 and 16.6g respectively. Correspondingly, the FAS activity per gram of liver for duck and chicken were 567.1 units and 87.8 units respectively. The studies on different ages of the same species also shows that the abdomen fat level of chicken was positively correlated with FAS activity[15]. Tian supposed that it may be an effective way to control the body weight by adjusting FAS activity.

1.4 Searching of FAS Inhibitors with High Activity and Low Toxicity

To confirm the validity that FAS is a therapeutic target for obesity, more effective FAS inhibitors are needed. More and more inhibitors with high activity and low toxicity are valuable for application. Cerulenin was the first reported FAS inhibitor, it is the exclusively known FAS inhibitor in the last century[16]. But it is chemically unstable, and is worthless for medical application. C75 is a synthetic and chemically stable inhibitor of FAS, it reacts on the ketoacyl shynthase in FAS like cerulenin dose, but without apparent toxicity[17]. In the past several years C75 is the first choice as FAS inhibitor in scientific studies, but the disadvantage of C75 is that a large dosage of C75 is needed for peripheral injection, therefore resulting in some side-effects[18].

It is shown that the study on FAS inhibitors is in initial strings. Searching more inhibitors with high inhibitory ability is the most important work at present.

2 INHIBITION TO FAS AND EFFECTS AN CONTROL OF BODY WEIGHT AND FOOD INTAKE BY TEA EXTRACTS AND THEIR COMPONENTS

2.1 History and Components of Tea

Tea tree (*camellia sinensis*) is a plant of Theaceae. It was produced in Yunnan of China. In "Huayang chorography, Ba chorography", it was recorded that tea tree was cropped in Bashu country (in the south-west of China) before 3000 years. In the Han dynasty before 2000 years, the effects for health care of tea leaf had been studied. Before 1000 years (Tang dynasty) production of tea leaf had spread all over south China. In this time tea leaf and the drinking method diffused to the world from China.

Tea polyphenols and theins are the major active components in green tea. Several catechins including epigallocatechin gallate (EGCG), epicatechin gallate (ECG), epigallocatechin (EGC), epicatechin (EC), catechin (C) are the major members of tea polyphenol, They are contain 9-13%, 3-6%, 3-6%, 1-3% and less than 1% of dry weight of tea leaf respectively[19]. In the manufacture of green tea leaf steaming is needed. In the steaming process, tea polyphenol oxidase was inactivated by heating and therefore keeping the polyphenols in a non-oxidative state. In the manufacture of black tea leaf most of polyphenols are oxide-polymerized to theaflavin and thearobingin in the fermentation.

2.2 Inhibition to FAS by Tea Extracts

2.1.1 We found that tea extracts inhibited FAS potently. The inhibition of FAS by green tea extracts included reversible and irreversible inhibition. The optimal extraction solvent for the FAS inhibitors existing in green tea were about 50% ethanol. The solvent could extract most FAS inhibitors components during 100 min at room temperature (Figure 1)[20].

The Long Jing green tea extract by 50% ethanol shows potent reversible inhibition of FAS with IC_{50} value of 12.2μg/ml, which is 37μg tea leaf. Long Jing tea is the most famous green tea in China, it was produced in ZheJiang province, eastern China. As a control, The IC_{50} of cerulenin was reported to by 20μg/ml[16]. The IC_{50} showed the concentration of inhibitor that inhibited 50% activity of enzyme. It is an index for inhibitory ability, the lower IC_{50}, the higher ability. Thus the FAS inhibitory ability of Long Jing tea extract is higher than that of cerulenin, even the later is a pure compound and the former is a mixer.

The extract also shows time-dependent irreversible inactivation of FAS. 0.37mg/ml the tea extracts could make about 87% of FAS to inactivate during 60 minutes.

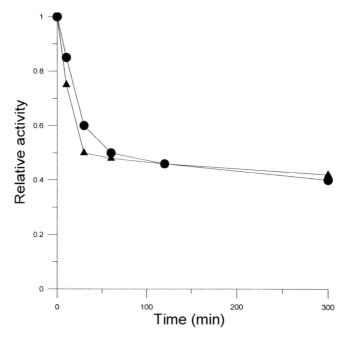

Figure 1. Determination of optimal time for extraction of tea. The relative activity of FAS with extraction of tea was assayed, the extracting temperature was 25℃ （●）, 80℃ （▲□

Is effective enough for extracting FAS inhibitors from green tea leaf the general method with boiling water? We simulated the method. 2 grams Long Jing green tea leaf was put in 200 ml boiling water. The extract solution was checked for FAS inhibition in the incubation time interval of 10, 20, 30, 60, 300 and 600 minutes respectively. It was found that the inhibitory activity of the solution did not change obviously after 10 minutes. While the extract solution was put out at 30 minutes, then same value of boiling water was put in, after 30 minutes incubation the new extract solution still exhibited high inhibitory activity. But contrast with the tea extract by 50% ethanol the total extraction efficiency of two times of boiling water extract was only 26% [20]. It is shown that the general method for tea drink with boiling water does not obtain the main part of active component for FAS inhibition.

2.2.2 Different solvents with various polarities to extract the black tea were tested. The results showed that 50% ethanol was the optimal extraction solvent for the FAS inhibition, which is similar with the extracting of green tea. The measurement of IC_{50} showed that 2 main kinds of black teas in China exhibited stronger inhibitory ability on FAS than that of green tea. One of them is Keemun black tea produced in Auhui province of east China with IC_{50} value of 14μg and the other is Dian black tea produced in Yunnan province in the southwest China.

Black tea extracts also exhibited time-dependent irreversible inactivation on FAS. 0.5mg tea leaf/ml of Keemun black tea inactivated 80% FAS activity during 56 minutes.

The most general method with boiling water is not the optimum method to produce high FAS inhibition for black tea too. Only 10 to 23% of effective inhibitors of FAS were extracted out from black tea leaf by boiling water for 10 to 720 minutes, while the 50% ethanol was as controlling solvent for extracting.

2.2.3 The extracts with 50% ethanol from 18 different kinds of teas in China show different inhibitory activity to FAS. The maximum difference of their IC_{50} is more than 10-folds. These IC_{50} are shown in Figure 2. Among them, two kinds of black tea exhibited maximum inhibitory ability with IC_{50} value of 14mg tea leaf/ml for Keemun black tea and 12µg tea leaf/ml for Dian black tea and Lu'anguapian green tea shows the weakest ability with IC_{50} value of 130 µg tea leaf/ml. The Long Jing green tea shows good inhibitory ability on FAS with IC_{50} value of 37 µg tea leaf/ml. The best green teas for inhibition on FAS are Jingshan Maofeng and Suzhou green tea. The IC_{50} is 28µg tea leaf/ml.

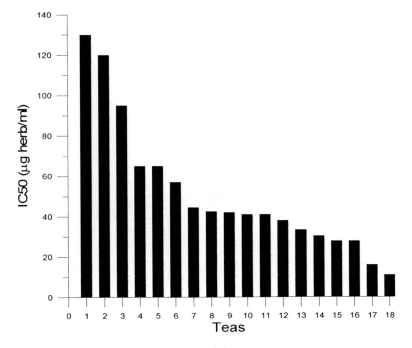

Figure 2. Reversible inhibitions of different kinds of teas[20].

2.3 THE EFFECTS OF TEA EXTRACTS ON BODY WEIGHT AND FOOD INTAKE OF MICE OR RATS

Is there pertinence between the effect on weight reducing and inhibition of FAS by tea? The effects of two green teas were tested by oral intubation to mice with tea extracts for 10 days. One tea was Jingshan Maofeng green tea produced in Jiangsu province of China with IC_{50} value of 28µg tea leaf/ml, and another was Lu'anguapian green tea produced in Anhui province of China which shows the weakest ability with IC_{50} value of 130 µg tea leaf/ml. The result showed that the mean body weight of mice decreased 9.1% and 3.0% by Jingshan Mafeng tea extracts and Lu'anguapian tea extracts respectively. In the same testing the mean body weight of control mice increased 1%. By the covariance analysis, the body weight of mice treated with Jingshan Mafeng tea extracts was reduced significantly, but that with

Lu'anguapian tea extracts did not (see Figure 3A). In the other hand, treatment with both above tea extracts reduced food intake of mice, but the results of Jingshan Mafeng tea extracts was more obvious (see Figure 3B)[20].

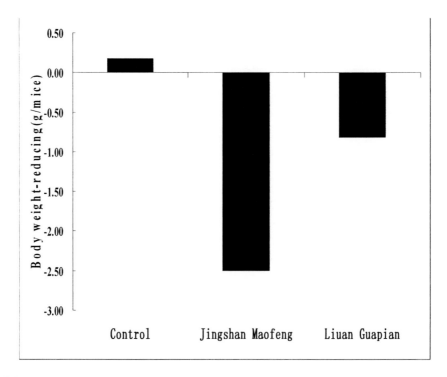

Figure 3A

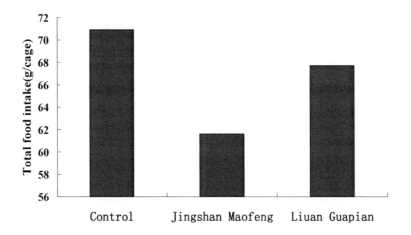

Figure 3B The effects on the body weight and food intake by Jingshan Maofeng and Liuan Guapian. (A)The effect on the body weight change during 10 days (B) The effect on the total food intake during 10 days

The body weight of rats dosed with extracts of Keemun black tea decreased substantially in 10 days. Mean values of body weight change of the dosed group and control group showed significantly difference (P<0.01). The mean body weight decreased approximately 18.7g (6%). (Fig 4A)

The average food intake of dosed group also significantly decreased in 10 days with approximately 13%. (Fig 4B)

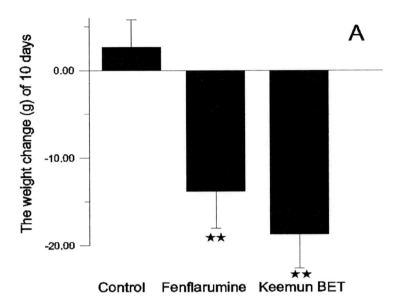

Figure 4A

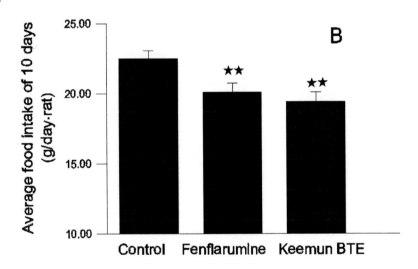

Figure 4B.The effects on the body weight and food intake by Keemun BTE and fenfluramine. The results are expressed as means ±s.e. of 10 SD rats [28].(A)The effect on the body weight during 10 days (B) The effect on the average food intake during 10 days □□, P<0.01vs. Control group, n=10.

The decrease of body weight is consistent with that of food intake for both green tea and black tea. Also the results are consistent with those with the known FAS inhibitors C75 and cerulenin. The difference in reduction of body weight and food intake are consistent with those of inhibitory ability to FAS for two kinds of green tea, which suggested that the weight-reducing effects of green tea are related to the FAS inhibition. Also the result provides a new evidence for the inference that FAS may be a therapeutic target for obesity. Of course, more evidences are needed to confirm the validity of the target.

If the target validity is confirmed, the inhibitory ability to FAS would standard the choice of tea for weight-control purpose. It should be noteworthy that the general method for drinking tea with boiling water may need some change for the weight-reducing purpose.

3 INHIBITION TO FAS BY SOME MEDICINAL HERBS

3.1 Determination of the Inhibition to FAS by Some Medicinal Herbs in the Weight-Reducing Prescriptions

3.1.1 Historically, Chinese medical herbs gained much practical experience for the control of body weight. More than two thousand years ago, herbalist physicians began to understand and treat obesity, and since that time more than one hundred Chinese medical herbs have been used for weight-reducing. Understanding their physiological and biochemical mechanisms is important for the application of herbs in weight control.

Many Chinese medical herbs have utilized prescriptions for the purpose of fat-reduction[21]. It is likely that these herbs may involve many physiological and biochemical mechanisms that are not yet clear. We might naturally come to wonder, is there any relationship between their weight-reducing effects and inhibition of FAS?

3.1.2 Over thirty herbs among weight-reducing prescriptions have been investigated for their inhibitory ability on FAS. It was found that FAS inhibitors are ubiquitous in these herbs. Extracts from 18 herbs exhibited reversible or irreversible inhibition on FAS, and extracts from 10 herbs strongly inhibited FAS. Among them both reversible and irreversible inhibition on FAS by 7 herbs were very strong. Which includes rhubarb root, parasitic loranthus, licorice root, tuber fleece flower root, ginkgo leaf, galangal root and tuber fleece flower stem[22]. The result suggests that they contain potent inhibitors of FAS, and that the weight reducing property of some Chinese herbal medicines may be related to their ability to inhibit FAS.

These 7 herbs were extracted with different solvents of various polarities from water to petroleum ether. The effective components from ginkgo leaf dissolve in the solvents with relatively weaker polarity, while stronger polarity solvents were suitable for extracting rhubarb root. For the other 5 herbs 40% to 60% ethanol is the optimum extracting solvent (Table 1)[22, 23]

The traditional index of inhibitory ability, half-inhibition concentration IC_{50}, was obtained from the curves of remaining activity of inhibited enzyme versus concentration of inhibitor. The IC_{50} values of the above 7 herbs extracted with their optimal solvents are listed in Table 1. The concentration of μg herbs/ml refers to the initial herb weight contained in 1ml FAS assay solution. The results showed that the extracts of raw tuber fleeceflower root, parasitic loranthus and galangal root exhibited the most potent inhibition on FAS. Their IC_{50} values of 2 μg dried herb /ml showed that their inhibitory abilities were one order of magnitude higher than those of green and black tea leaf, and are also one order of magnitude higher than the abilities of pure cerulenin. Considering the IC_{50} values of these herbs were measured in crude extracts level, the effective components in these herbs should have more inhibitory ability on FAS.

Table 1. Inhibitory effect of different extracting solvents[22]

Solvent	20%Ethanol	50%Ethanol	40%Ethanol	40%Ethanol	Acetone	50%Ethanol	40%Ethanol
	Rhubarb	Parasitic	Licorice	Tuber	Ginkgo	Tuber	Galangal
Herbs	root	loranthus	root	fleeceflower	leaf	fleeceflower	root
				root		stem	
IC50 (µg herb/ml)	180	2	180	2	19	2	2

3.1.3 Figure 5 shows the time course of irreversible inactivation after mixing FAS with the extracts of 5 herbs and green tea leaf. 0.12mg/ml C75 solution was used as control. Considering the effective components are generally less than 5% of dry weight of herb, the actual concentrations of the effective of these herbs were less than or close to that of C75. In the plots it was found that an initial rapid decrease of FAS activity was followed by a long slow decrease of enzyme activity for both C75 and these herbs, although their inhibitory reactions are different. In this analysis, the inactivation of FAS by extracts of tuber fleece flower root, parasitic loranthus, ginkgo leaf and licorice root were faster than that of C75, and that of green tea leaf was similar to that of C75, only that of rhubarb root was weaker.

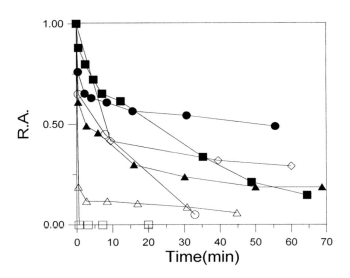

Figure 5. Time course of slow-binding inhibition on FAS with extracts of herbs and C75.The herb (or C75) and its concentration in reaction was (●) 4 mg rhubarb root/ml, (▲)4 mg licorice root/ml, (■) 1.61 mg green tea leaf/ml, (○) 2.5 mg ginkgo leaf/ml, (□) 1.5 mg parasitic loranthus /ml, (˝) 0.83 mg tuber fleeceflower root /ml, (□) 0.12 mg C75/ml, respectively.

3.2 The Weight-Reducing Test in Rats and Mice

To detect the weight-reducing effect by herbs that inhibit FAS more strongly or weakly, oral intubation tests of rats with herb's extracts for 20 days were processed twice. In the first test, 7 herbs were used, distilled water was the control and an effective chemical fat-reducing drug fenfluramine was as positive control. The body weight of each rat was measured daily. On the second test two herbs, parasitic loranthus and tuber fleeceflower root were tested repeatedly, which reduced body weight most obviously in the first test. The controls were same with the first test, and the measurement of daily food intake was added.

The body weight change, average daily food intake and statistical result of each group of rat during the weight reducing test are listed in Table 2. Statistical analysis of the data revealed that the reduction of body weight and food intake by parasitic loranthus, tuber fleeceflower root and fenfluramine were significant [22].

Table 2. Body weight change, average daily food intake and statistical result of each group of rat during the weight reducing test[22]

Group	Herbs	Average weight change		Average daily food intake		IC_{50} **
		(gram/rat)	p value of t-test	(gram/rat)	p value of t-test	(µg/ml)
1	control 1	5.35				
2	fenflarumine	-5.35	0.014			
3	Rhubarb root	9.7	0.391			180
4	Parasitic loranthus	-9.85	0.002			2
5	Safflower	7.35	0.453			>500
6	Chrysanthemum flower	1.85	0.258			>500
7	Licorice root	2.1	0.347			180
8	Ginkgo leaf	3.6	0.694			19
10	Roast tuber fleeceflower root	-12	0.003			2
11	control 2	7.55		23.6		
12	fenflarumine	-8.05	0.043	21.6	0.016	
13	Parasitic loranthus	-8.15	0.019	20.1	0.003	2
14	Roast tuber fleeceflower root	-8.05	0.023	21.5	0.046	2

Analysis of the results shows that a positive correlation between the effect of weight reduction and FAS inhibitory ability of these herbs. 7 herbs in this test could be divided into two groups according to their IC_{50} values. One group ($IC_{50} \geq 180$µg/ml), consisting of rhubarb root, safflower, chrysanthemum and licoride root, had no obvious effect on weight reducing. Another group ($IC_{50} < 20$µg/ml), including parasitic loranthus, tuber fleeceflower root and ginkgo leaf, lowered body weight on rats except ginkgo leaf. It is suggested that the inhibition of FAS produced by these herbs may be an important action leading to weight reduction. The only exception is ginkgo leaf that produced no weight reducing effect, possibly because of its low solubility in polar solvent.

The results in second test showed that the reduction of body weight and food intake by parasitic loranthus or tuber fleeceflower root occurred concurrently. These results are consistent with those found with other FAS inhibitors, including C75, cerulenin, EGCG and extract of green tea or black tea.

The similar result was displayed in the oral intubation test of mice. Extracts of parasitic loranthus, tuber fleece flower root or stem, green tea leaf or black tea leaf reduced significantly body weight and food intake of mice by oral administration of the extracts during the 20 days testing.

3.3 The Wide Sources of Medicinal Herb Parasitic Loranthus

As we penetrated with parasitic loranthus, it was found that the original plants for this herb are complicated with a wide distribution among different genera in the family *Loranthaceae* and *Viscaece*. Our recent results indicate that the plant extracts from most of the family *Loranthacea* shows potent FAS inhibition both reversibly and irreversibly, whereas those from *Viscum L.* of the family Viscaceae, to the contrary, exhibited almost no inhibition on FAS with an extremely high IC_{50} values [24].

3.4 Different Inhibitory Characters of these Extracts of Herbs

The aforementioned medical herb extracts and tea extracts all showed strong inhibition on FAS, but from the inhibition kinetics, it was found that their inhibitory characters were different. Table 3 lists the inhibition types of extracts of tuber fleeceflower root, parasitic loranthus, galangal root, ginkgo leaf, Keemun black tea leaf and Long Jing green tea leaf to three different substrates acetyl CoA, malonyl CoA and NADPH, and showed that their characters are distinct, which suggests that the FAS inhibitors containing in these medical herbs or teas mostly not the same constitutes, and there may exist different kinds of compounds with different inhibitory mechanisms. All these phenomena are beneficial to understanding the inhibition mechanism of FAS, providing evidence for FAS as a weight loss target and developing new inhibitors.

Table 3. Inhibition types of extracts of different herbs

Substrates	Acetyl-CoA	Malonyl-CoA	NADPH
Herbs			
Tuber fleeceflower root	un	com	non+com
Parasitic loranthus	com	non	non+com
Galangal root	non	un	un
Ginkgo leaf	non	com	non+com
Keemun black tea	non	non	non+com
Longjing green tea	non+com	un	non+com

com: competitive, un: uncompetitive, non: noncompetitive, non+com: mixed of non and com

4. INHIBITION TO FAS BY POLYPHENOLS

4.1 Inhibitory Ability of Polyphenols and Analysis

As mentioned above, the main polyphenols existing in green tea are such gallated catechins as EGCG, ECG and CG, as well as, those ungallated chtechins like EGC, EC, C (Fig. 6). We discover that EGCG is a FAS inhibitor with IC_{50} value of 52μM in 2001[25]. To elucidate the structure-activity relationship of the inhibitory effects of tea polyphenols, we investigated the inhibition kinetics of the major catechins and analogues. Ungallated catechins did not show obvious inhibition to FAS. IC_{50} of EGC EC and C are >3.0, 3.8 and 1.6mM respectively, and they do not show any irreversible inactivation on FAS. Another gallated catechin, ECG was also found as a potent inhibitor of FAS with IC_{50} value of 42μM[26].

EGCG and ECG are two major gallated catechins in green tea. But in furthers study it was found that inhibitory ability of Long Jing green tea extracts was much more potent than that of EGCG plus ECG. We found that (-)-epicatechin gallate (CG) was a more potent FAS inhibitor with IC_{50} value of 3.4μM. This compound has much smaller quantity in green tea but inhibit FAS much stronger than EGCG and ECG[27].

All the three gallated catechins showed similar potent irreversible inactivation on FAS. Furthermore, the analogues of galloyl moiety without the catechin skeleton such as propyl gallate also showed obvious inactivation on FAS. The gallated catechins inactive FAS following saturation kinetics, for that the inhibitor reversibly associates on FAS first, it subsequently chemically modifies some essential group in the enzyme resulting in the irreversible loss of enzyme activity. But the analogue propyl gallate inactivate FAS with a simple second-order reaction[26].

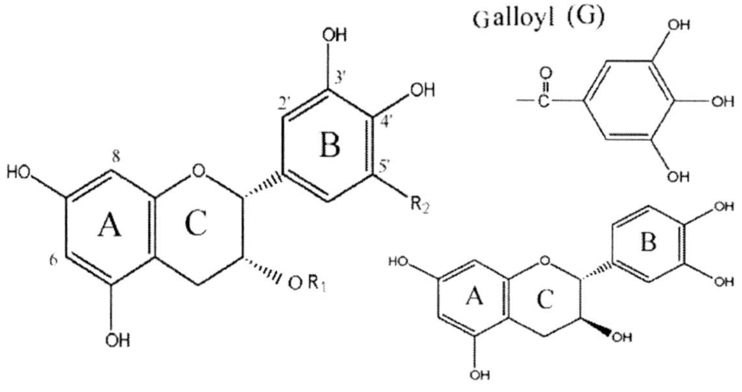

Figure 6. Structures of major tea polyphenols

	R1	R2
(-)-epicatechin (EC)	H	H
(-)-epigallocatechin (EGC)	H	OH
(-)-epicatechin gallate (ECG)	G	H
(-)-epigallocatechin gallate (EGCG)	G	OH

The gallated catechins EGCG and ECG have lower gap energies between the HOMO and the LUMO than those without galloyl moiety. The carbon atom of the galloyl moiety of gallated catechins have a mulliken positive charge 2 to 3 folds that of carbon atoms at other sites. (Table 4) The results suggest that carbon atoms of the galloyl moiety of EGCG and ECG have higher susceptibility toward a nucleophilic attack than those of other catechins. It is possible that EGCG and ECG can act on electronegative site of FAS more easily than ungallated catechins.

We also found phenolic hydroxyl groups have some influence on FAS activity. The phenolic groups on the B ring and galloyl moiety of catechin may be involved in the reversible inhibition. The carbon atom of the ester bond of gallated catechins is involved in irreversible inactivation. The lower gap energies of gallated catechins indicate a higher susceptibility toward a nueleophilic attack, which are consistent with the inactivation abilities of green tea catechins[26].

Table 4. The calculation results of catechins and analogues of the gallate group[26]

Chemicals	HOMO (eV)	LUMO (eV)	H-L gap (eV)	Mulliken charge on carbon atoms
The catechins				
EC	-0.2	0.0129	0.213	0.230-0.300
EGC	-0.209	0.00214	0.211	0.230-0.300
ECG	-0.207	-0.0486	0.158	0.708
EGCG	-0.205	-0.0354	0.17	0.679
The gallate analogues				
Propyl gallate	-0.212	-0.0325	0.18	0.705
Propyl p-hydroxylbenzoate	-0.23	-0.0319	0.198	0.699

4.2 Inhibition to FAS by Theaflavins

In the manufacture of black tea, most of gallated catechins undergo oxidative polymerization during the fermentation. But the inhibitory ability was still kept even increased in some black tea. Therefore, the theaflavins, which is major product of fermentation of tea leaf, were checked for FAS inhibition. The IC_{50} value of theaflavins was 1.27μg/ml[28] that is much lower than those of EGCG and cerulenin which were reported as 24μg/ml and 20μg/ml respectively[25, 16].

Theaflavins also showed strong irreversible inhibition, 19 μg/ml of theaflavins can inactivate 80% of FAS activity at 120min[28], but this extent of inhibition may need as much as 150 μg/ml of EGCG. This indicates that the inhibitory ability of theaflavins is one order of magnitude stronger than that of gallated chatechins, which could probably explain the relatively stronger inhibitory ability of black tea than green tea. Interestingly, Keemun black tea showed a slightly more potent ability in weight loss and food intake reduction on rats than green tea, and this result displays a better prospect for application of black tea.

The irreversible inactivation of FAS by theaflavins was slowed by NADPH. The result suggested that this inactivation may be related to NADPH binding site on the p-ketoacyl reductase domain of FAS[28].

The plot of inactivation rate constant k_{obs} vs concentration of theaflavins showed a hyperbola and the double reciprocal plot was a straight-line. This result showed saturation kinetics and suggested that inactivation of FAS by theaflavins is a affinity labeling reaction involving two steps as equation(1)

$$E + I \xleftrightarrow{K_s} E - I \xrightarrow{k} KI \tag{1}$$

The observed first order rate constant k_{obs} is shown as equation (2):

$$k_{obs} = \frac{k[I]}{K_s[I]} \tag{2}$$

The plot $1/k_{obs}$ vs. $1/[I]$ [Fig 7B] is linear and is fitted to equation (3)

$$\frac{1}{k_{obs}} = \frac{K_s}{K[I]} + \frac{1}{k} \tag{3}$$

K_s of 29.2 µg/ml and k of 0.035min^{-1} for inactivation of FAS by theaflavins were calculated from this plot.

The inhibition kinetics measurement showed that the inhibition patterns of black tea extract to each substrate of FAS were the same as those of theaflavins. This result indicates that theaflavins is the major FAS inhibitor in the extract of black tea.

4.3 Inhibitory Ability to FAS by Flavonoids and the Structure-Activity Analysis

Parasitic loranthus, galangal root and ginkgo leaf, that all potently inhibit FAS, contain a lot of flavonoids. The inhibitory effects of 13 flavonoids on FAS were investigated, and 9 of them were found to inhibit FAS with IC$_{50}$ values ranging from 2 to 112 μM. The results are listed in Table 5[29].

Comparing the inhibitory ability of galangin (IC$_{50}$>100 μM), kempferol (IC$_{50}$=10.38±0.67 μM), quercetin (IC$_{50}$=4.29±0.34 μM), Morin (IC$_{50}$=2.33±0.09 μM) and myricetin (IC$_{50}$27.18±0.24 μM), their structural differences lie in the number of hydroxyl groups in the B ring, varying from none to three morin and quercetin with two hydroxyl groups in the B ring exhibited most potent inhibitory ability, and galangin without hydroxyl in the B ring only showed a little activity. Thus, the hydroxyl groups in the B ring are very important for the inhibition of FAS. On the contrary, the presence of 3-hydroxyl group in the C ring and 5-hydroxyl group in A ring were not indispensable to activity[29].

The flavanone (dihydroflavone) derivatives such as ($\pm$) Taxifolin (IC_{50}=41.16$\pm$0.59 μM) and hesperetin (IC_{50}=68.86$\pm$4.49 μM) are weaker FAS inhibitors than the flavone. The result shows that the 2, 3 double bond contributed to activity. Compared with the flavanone the flavanol derivatives nearly no FAS inhibitory ability which indicated that the absence of the 4-carbonyl group was disadvantageous to FAS inhibitory ability of the flavonoids[29].

Table 5. Inhibitory abilities of flavonoids on FAS

[b] the IC50 values are the means $\pm$ SD for three experiments.

[c] galangin is poorly soluble in reaction mixture. About 20% of FAS overall reaction was inhibited in the presence of 100 μM galangin.

[d] n.i is no inhibition□IC_{50}□1 mM□.

[e] G is glucose.

Flavonoid	Class	IC_{50}[b] (μM)	Derivative
Morin	Flavone	2.33±0.09	3,5,7,2',4'-OH
Luteolin	Flavone	2.52±0.10	5,7,3',4'-OH
Quercetin	Flavone	4.29±0.34	3,5,7,3',4'-OH
Kaempferol	Flavone	10.38±0.67	3,5,7, 4'-OH
Fisetin	Flavone	18.78±0.49	3,7,2',4'-OH
Myricetin	Flavone	27.18±0.24	3,5,7,3',4',5'-OH
Baicalein	Flavone	111.69±2.29	5,6,7-OH
Galangin[c]	Flavone	□100	3,5,7-OH
Flavone	Flavone	n.i.[d]	no
Flavonol	Flavone	n.i.	3-OH
Rutin	Flavone-3-Gly	n.i.	5,7,3',4'-OH, 3-G-G[e]
($\pm$)-Taxifolin	Flavanone	41.16±0.59	3,5,7,3',4'-OH
Hesperetin	Flavanone	68.86±4.49	5,7,3' –OH, 4'-OCH$_3$

Three different kind of flavonoids, morin, luteolin and taxifolin showed same inhibitory mode. They inhibit FAS competitively with acetyl CoA.

The result suggests that these flavonoids may combine on the transacylase domain of FAS. On the contrary, gallated catechins inhibit FAS competitively with NADPH, which should be mainly related to the ketoacyl reductase domain of FAS.

It is assumed that the structure of A ring with 7-hydroxyl group and B ring with 4'-hydroxyl group, in which the two rings lie in the same plane, is necessary for inhibiting transacylase activity in FAS, while the structure of B ring and galloyl moiety, in which the two rings are nonconjugatedly connected, is essential for inhibition of ketoacyl reductase activity in FAS.

5. PROSPECT AND PROBLEMS

5.1 Application—How Far We are?

Our studies showed that a variety of FAS inhibitors with strong activity existed among different plants, the inhibitory ability of the active compounds in parasitic loranthus, tuber fleeceflower, galangal root and black tea was at least 10-folds stronger than that of C75, and this potency has already reached the qualification of application. Furthermore, animal experiments have also exhibited that, the extracts of parasitic loranthus, tuber fleeceflower, black tea and green tea were effective in weight loss and food intake reduction via oral intubation. More importantly, they are safe in application. Both black tea and green tea are prevalent beverage on the world scale; Tuber fleeceflower root wine has long been used for the treatment of white-hair disease. Parasitic loranthus has been used to replenish liver and to prevent miscarriage for hundreds of years in China. The crude extracts of these plants or the active components extracted from them are plausible to exhibit a better application prospect than the chemically-synthesized inhibitors.

However, two main problems need resolving before taking account into application. The first and most important one should be that the effectiveness of FAS as a weight loss target still needs to be validated. There is only five years since the proposal of this idea; this short duration and the paucity of effective inhibitors hamper the validation of the effectiveness. Secondly, the potent inhibitors with clear structure and inhibition mechanism are far from abundant. Recently, we have only discovered theaflavin and CG from black tea and green tea respectively. In accordance with the oral animal experiments, the daily dosage for the typically known inhibitors, for instance, C75 and EGCG would be used as high as 10g to actualize the weight-reducing effects, which is apparently too high. The inhibitory capacity of extracts of parasitic loranthus, tuber fleece flower, galangal root and so on is potent enough for this, but their active compounds are not clear yet. Due to the imperfectness of modern scientific quality standard for herbal medicines which are influenced by producing areas, season and climates or else, hardly can it be widely accepted by public without understanding the effective compounds and reaction mechanisms. Therefore, plant-sourced FAS inhibitors with high capacity but low toxicity would predicatively obtain far-ranging application.

5.2 Research Presumption on the Effectiveness of FAS as a Weight Loss Target

Currently an important qualification to corroborate the target-effectiveness of FAS is to possess various inhibitors with a large range of inhibitory capacity. Except for their different capacity, the same or similar inhibition properties of these materials would be of great advantage. So far, our group mainly focuses in investigation this area.

We have obtained two main kinds of inhibitors, including plant extracts and some specific-type compounds. The plant extracts are referred to two kinds of materials, that is, different kinds of green tea and black tea with different inhibitory activity on FAS; medicinal herb parasitic loranthus with its plants sourced from different family or genera which showed obvious distinction in FAS inhibition. Firstly, all tea samples originate from the same plant *Camellia Sinensis*, however, they showed different inhibitory effects. And the chemical constituents from different green tea and from different black tea are mostly similar, except for the different structures of polyphenols between them. Another striking result exhibited that the stronger inhibitor Jingshan Maofeng green tea showed a better weight loss and food intake effects than the relatively weaker inhibitor Lu'an guapian green tea. Secondly, the most advantage of parasitic loranthus as a good candidate for validity research lies in its great range of inhibitory capacity, for instance, the inhibition of genus *Taxillus* from family *Loranthaceae* was three order of magnitude stronger than that of geunus *Viscum* from family *Viscaceae*. However, the shortage of parasitic loranthus is the complicated relation of its plants in taxonomy. Moreover, another plant extracts we are studying right now can also be a good example for this research.

Another possible candidates for exploring the validity of FAS as a target is the polyphenols, including flavonoids, catechins and other polyphenols like theaflavins and resveratrol. As the aforementioned results, great difference exists in reversible and irreversible inhibition among polyphenols. According to the structure-activity analysis of the flavonoids and catechins, we are in process of exploring new compounds and reconstructing the known compounds in order to obtain FAS inhibitors with high activity and low toxicity.

Taking into account the above analysis, we have possessed plenty of materials to explore the effectiveness of FAS as a weight loss target.

The related studies contain:

1. Animal experiments of weight loss and food intake reduction

Rats and mice, or fowl (as their FAS are rich in liver, which is beneficial to accurately assay the FAS activity) are used by oral intubations or injection to observe the influence of different materials on body weight and food consumption, change of FAS activity, or even change of body fat. Then the correlation between inhibitory capacity on FAS and weight loss effects, as well as between FAS activity *in vivo* and weight loss effects are analyzed. The high relation can be good evidence for the effectiveness of FAS as a target.

2. Public prevention studies

As tea is widely used as a common beverage, flavonoids and catechins are also applied as nontoxic drugs or health products, therefore, public prevention studies by oral administration can be indubitably carried on. It can be evaluated from the studies whether there is correlation between inhibitory capacity on FAS and weight reducing effects, thereby directly validating the effectiveness of FAS as a target.

3. Epidemiological investigation

Due to the prevalence of drinking tea in China and the regional difference among tea in FAS inhibition, we can survey on the body weight of groups of people with different habits on drinking local tea, including heavy drinkers, normal drinkers and seldom drinkers. And it can be analyzed the relationship between weight reducing effects of drinking tea and their inhibitory capacity on FAS, thereby conforming the effectiveness of FAS as a target, and furthermore providing some instructive suggestion on the application of tea industry.

5.3 POSSIBLE VALUES FROM ENERGY METABOLISM ANALYSIS OF FAS AND THE WEIGHT-REDUCING EFFECT STUDIES OF FAS INHIBITORS

For the weight-reducing mechanism of FAS inhibitors, Loftus et al have proposed a reasonable interpretation on the molecular level: inhibiting FAS results in the accumulation of substrate malonyl CoA, which blocks the expression of hypothalamic NPY, therefore reducing appetite, causing the decrease in food consumption and body weight in animal experiments. However, can this be the exclusive reason for weight reduction? As previously described in 1.3, we discovered that high correlation existed between body fat level of fowl and their liver FAS activity. Here the distinction of FAS activity is not a short-term change, so it cannot be explained by the above process mediated by malonyl CoA. Hereby we suggest another approach, that is, the whole process is related to the balance of energy metabolism. The energy metabolism analysis shows that after primary catabolism, carbohydrate, fat and most amino acids lead to the production of acetyl CoA, which is the starting substance of citric acid circulation and fat synthesis. Acetyl CoA acts as a key point for energy metabolism, it collects most of the energy substances and transforms them into energy or fat, and there should be a balance point between energy-producing and fat-producing. When FAS exhibits a lower activity, the approach of fat-producing is not smooth enough, therefore the balance point will favor the energy-producing approach. As the energy substances produce less fat, the entire fat level would relatively decline after a period of accumulation. Relative evidence as reported showed that injection of C75 increased the metabolic level and enhanced the body energy. Admittedly, this idea needs more evidence to substantiate the validity, however, if as suggested, FAS inhibitors can display dual effects of lowering food intake and increasing body energy.

In conclusion, obesity is a multi-factor decompensate disease, so comprehensive therapy might be more effective than single-factors intervention. Recently the cocktail therapy of "diet control +exercise +anti-obesity drug" is proposed. So FAS inhibitors could be one of the optimal candidates for anti-obesity drug among it. As described previously, FAS inhibitors can control appetite, which is beneficial to those obese people with a good appetite. On the other hand, FAS inhibitors might also help shift energy metabolism balance toward energy-producing, thereby transforming most of the energy substances into energy, which may promote exercises, change the terrible habits of sloth for those obese people. As a result, FAS inhibitors shows dual effects in anti-obesity: in short-term effects, inhibiting FAS may lower expression of NPY mediated by malonyl CoA, thereby reducing food intake and body weight; in long-term effects, inhibiting FAS might possibly favor the energy-producing direction and reduce the accumulation of fat, and hold the maintenance of sufficient energy under the circumstances of decreasing the ingestion of energy substances. So FAS inhibitors might be promising and favorable in the application of anti-obesity therapy, and what is more, FAS inhibitors from plants might be of the greatest value.

ACKNOWLEDGEMENT

Hereby the author gratefully appreciates Yan Wang, Binghui Li and Liangwei Zhong for completing this article. Xuan Wang, Lichun Li, Binghui Li, Yatao Du, Wenping Xiao, Rui Zhang, Yan Wang, Xiaodong Wu and Chuanchu Chen are devoted in the research work related in this paper.

REFERENCES:

[1]   Bray GA. Contemporary Diagnosis and management of obesity. Newtown, Pa.: *Handbooks in Health Care*. 1998

[2]   Seidell J C. The impact of obesity on health status: some implication for health care cost. *Int J Obesity*, 1996,19(6):S13-S16

[3]   Must A, Spadano J, Coakley EH, et al., The Disease Burden Associated With Overweight and Obesity. *J Am Med Assoc*,1999, 282(16):1523~1529

[4]   Lew E A. Mortality and weight: insured lives and the American Cancer Study. *Annals of Intern. Med*,1985,103:1024~1029

[5]   Hubert H B. The importance of obesity in the development of coronary risk factors and disease: the epidemiological evidence. *Annu Rev Public Health*, 1986,7:493~502

[6]   Calle E E, Rodriguez C, Walker-Thurmond K, Thun M J. Overweight, Obesity, and Mortality from Cancer in a Prospectively Studied Cohort of U.S. Adults. *N Engl J Med*. 2003, 348 (17) :1625-1838

[7]   Zhang Y, Proenca R, Maffei M, et al. Positional cloning of the mouse obese gene and its human homologue. *Nature*, 1994,372(6505):425~432

[8]   Friedman J M, Halaas J L. Leptin and the regulation of body weight in mammals. *Nature*, 1998,395 (6704):763~770

[9]   Ahima R S, Prabakaran D, Mantzoros C, et al. Role of leptin in the neuroendocrine response to fasting. *Nature*, 1996,382 (6588):250~252

[10]   Bouchard C. Inhibition of food intake by inhibitors of fatty acid synthase. *N Engl J Med*,2000, 343 (25) :1888~1889

[11]   Chagnon Y C, Pérusse L, Weisnagel S J, et al., The human obesity gene map: the 1999 update. *Obesity Res*,2000,8:89~117

[12]   Schwartz M W, Woods S C, Porte D Jr, et al. Central nervous system control of food intake. *Nature*, 2000, 404(6778): 661~667

[13]   Loftus T M, Jaworsky D E, Frehywot G L, et al. Reduced food intake and body weight in mice treated with fatty acid synthase inhibitors. *Science*, 2000,288(30):2379~2381

[14]   O'Shea D, Morgan DG, Meeran K, et al. Neuropeptide Y induced feeding in the rat is mediated by a novel receptor. *Endocrinology*, 1997, 138(1):196~202

[15]   Li M, Yan S, Tian W X, et al. Factors influencing the levels of fatty acid synthase complex activity in fowl. *Biochemistry and Molecular Biology International*, 1999,47(1):63-69

[16]   Vance D., Goldberg I., Mitsuhashi O., Bloch K., Inhibition of fatty acid synthatase by the antibiotic cerulenin. *Biochemical and Biophysical Research Communications* 1972,48(3), 649-655.

[17] Kuhajda F P, Pizer E S, Li J N, et al. Synthesis and antitumor activity of an inhibitor of fatty acid synthase. *Proc Natl Acad Sci USA*, 2000,97(7):3450-3454

[18] Clegg D J, Wortman M D, Benoit S C et al. Comparison of central and peripheral administration of C75 on food intake, body weight and conditioned aversion. *Diabetes*. 2002,51:3196-3201

[19] Coxon D T, Holmes A, Olis W D, Vora V C, Grant M S, Tee J L. Flavanol digallates in green tea leaf. *Tetrahedron*, 1972, 28:2819-2826

[20] Zhang Rui, Xiao Wen-ping, Tian Wei-xi. Inhibitory effects of green tea extract on fatty acid synthase. *Journal of Yunnan University*, 2004, 26, 6A: 42-47 (in Chinese)

[21] Xie Y M, Wong W L, Reducing fat with traditional Chinese medicine. *Symposium International Conference of Weight Reducing in Beijing*. 2000, P132

[22] Tian W X, Li L C, Wu X D, Chen C C. Weight reducing by Chinese medicinal herbs may be related to inhibition of fatty acid synthase. *Life Science* 2004, 74: 2389-2399

[23] Li B H and Tian W X. Presence of Fatty Acid Synthase Inhibitors in the Rhizome of Alpinia officinarum Hance. *Journal of Enzyme Inhibition and Medicinal Chamistry*, 2003, 18(4): 349-356

[24] Wang Y, Zhang S Y, Ma X F, Tian W X. Potent inhibition of fatty acid synthase by parasitic loranthus [*Taxillus chinenesis* (DC.) Danser] and its constituent avicularin. *Journal of Enzyme Inhibition and Medicinal Chemistry*, 2006, 21(1): 87-93

[25] Wang X and Tian W X. Green Tea Epigallocatechin Gallate: A Natural Inhibitor of Fatty-Acid Synthase. *Biochmical and Biophysical Research Communications* 2001, 288: 1200-1206

[26] Wang X, Song K S, Guo Q X, Tian W X. The galloyl moiety of green tea catechins is critical structural feature to inhibit fatty-acid synthase. *Biochemical Pharmacology* 2003, 66: 2039-2047

[27] Zhang R, Xiao W P, Wang X, Wu X D, Tian W X. Novel Inhibitors of Fatty Acid Synthase from Green Tea with High Activity and New Reacting Site. *Biotechnology and Applied Biochemistry*, 2006, 43: 1-7

[28] Du Y T, Wang X, Wu X D, Tian W X. Keemun black tea extract contains potent fatty acid synthase inhibitor and reduces food intake and body weight of rats via oral intubation. *Journal of Enzyme Inhibition and Medicinal Chemistry*, 2005, 20, 4: 349-356

[29] Li B H and Tian W X. Inhibitory Effects of Flavonoids on Animal Fatty Acid Synthase. *Journal of Biochemistry* 2004, 135 (1): 85-91

In: Weight Loss, Exercise and Health Research
Editor: Carrie P. Saylor, pp. 49-58

ISBN 1-60021-077-5

Chapter 3

GALLSTONES FOLLOWING WEIGHT LOSS AND RECOMMENDATIONS FOR THEIR PREVENTION

G.S. Mijnhout[1], M.E. Craanen[2] and Y. M. Smulders[1]

Departments of Internal Medicine[1] and Gastroenterology[2],
VU University Medical Centre, Amsterdam, The Netherlands.

ABSTRACT

Obesity is an increasing health problem. As a consequence, many people attempt to lose weight by dieting or participation in weight loss programs. Weight loss is associated with an increased risk of gallstone formation: the incidence is 10-40%, of which 30-40% becomes symptomatic. This leads to substantial morbidity (cholecystitis, choledocholithiasis, biliary pancreatitis) and expensive treatments (hospital admission, endoscopic retrograde cholangiopancreatography, cholecystectomy). Weight reduction and fasting lead to bile lithogenicity through four mechanisms: biliary cholesterol oversaturation due to mobilisation of peripheral fat, increased production of mucine by the gallbladder, 40% increase of bile calcium concentration, and reduction of gallbladder motility. Risk factors for gallstone formation during weight reduction are: rate of weight loss > 1.5 kg/week, total weight loss > 25% of pre-existing weight, very low calorie (< 600 kcal/day) and low fat (< 2 g/day) diets and weight loss following bariatric surgery. Preventive measures include limiting the rate of weight loss to less than 1.5 kg per week, and providing a fat intake of at least 7 g/day. Randomized controlled trials have shown that ursodeoxycholic acid (600 mg daily) is effective for prevention of gallstones (risk reduction 25%). Aspirin is less effective than ursodeoxycholic acid; non-steroidal anti-inflammatory drugs (NSAIDs) have not proven effective. Prophylaxis with ursodeoxycholic acid should be considered in obese patients (BMI > 30 kg/m2) in whom the expected weight loss is rapid or difficult to control, for example after bariatric surgery.

INTRODUCTION

Obesity is an increasing public health problem. Both obesity and weight loss are associated with an increased risk of developing gallstones. Ten to 40% of patients develop *de novo* gall-stones during rapid weight reduction. New-onset gallstones become symptomatic in 30 tot 40% of cases [1-3], leading to substantial morbidity (cholecystitis, choledocholithiasis, biliairy pancreatitis) and costs (hospital admission, endoscopic retrograde cholangiopan-creatography (ERCP), cholecystectomy). These aforementioned procedures are not without complications. Prevention of gallstone formation during rapid weight loss may substantially decrease morbidity and save costs. The clinical cases below illustrate the risk of symptomatic gallstones during weight reduction. This chapter reviews the risk factors for gallstone development during rapid weight reduction and the available strategies for prevention.

CASE 1

Patient A, a 27-year-old woman, was admitted to our Internal Medicine department because of severe pain in the upper abdomen. She had morbid obesity (weight 137 kg, length 1.79 m, BMI 43 kg/m^2) and, independently from any weight loss program, lost 13 kg over a period of 5 weeks on a diet. Otherwise she was healthy. The laboratory findings revealed elevated liver enzymes (bilirubin 54 μmol/l, alkaline phosphatase 89 U/l, gamma-GT 571 U/l, ASAT 262 U/l, ALAT 402 U/l) and elevated amylase (1262 U/l). Abdominal ultrasound showed cholecystolithiasis without dilation of bile ducts. Because the pancreas could not be visualized on ultrasound, an abdominal CT scan was performed, which showed edema of the pancreas. The day after admission, bilirubin and amylase levels had normalised. The diagnosis of a mild biliary pancreatitis due to a passed gallstone was made, and the patient was scheduled for laparoscopic cholecystectomy. However, a few days later she became febrile; abdominal CT now showed a severe pancreatitis with several fluid collections in the upper abdomen compatible with pseudocysts. She was treated conservatively and slowly made it to a full recovery. Elective cholecystectomy was performed four months later and was uneventful.

CASE 2

Patient B, a 32-year-old woman, had no medical history. Because of her overweight (weight 77 kg, length 167 cm, BMI 27.6 kg/m^2, with predominant trunk obesity) she went for a 'slimming holiday' to a south-European country. With a diet consisting of just fruit juice, in combination with an activity program, she lost 9 kg in 3 weeks. Two weeks after return, she developed colic pains and progressive jaundice. Abdominal ultrasound showed cholecystolithiasis and dilation of the common bile duct. An ERCP was performed, during which a gallstone was removed from the common bile duct. Subsequently she underwent an uncomplicated open-procedure cholecystectomy. Some years later she again attends a 'weight reduction holiday' organized by the same organisation. It strikes her that, in contrast to the first time, the morning portion of fruit juice is supplemented with 3 table-spoons of olive oil.

OBESITY AND INCIDENCE OF GALLSTONES

Obesity is associated with an increased risk of developing gallstones [1, 4]. In obesity, the activity of hydroxymethyl coenzyme A-reductase (HMG CoA reductase) is increased. This leads to an increased synthesis of cholesterol by the liver and supersaturation of the bile with cholesterol. The relative proportion of bile acids and phospholipids decreases. Compared to people of normal weight, gallbladder contractility is decreased and gallbladder volume is increased [5]. This contributes to bile stasis and predisposes to cholesterol stone formation. The risk of gallstones is strongly correlated with BMI [1]. A body weight exceeding 120% of ideal weight is associated with a 2-3 times increased risk of gallstones, a doubling of ideal weight (morbid obesity) is associated with an 8 times increased risk [6]. In women, estrogens and pregnancy also have a role in the pathogenesis.

BILE CHANGES DURING WEIGHT REDUCTION

During weight reduction and fasting, lithogenic bile can develop through a number of mechanisms [5, 7]. Due to mobilisation of peripheral fat stores, cholesterol saturation of bile increases, influencing the relative proportions of cholesterol, bile acids and phospholipids. In addition, the gallbladder produces 18 times more mucin, a glycoprotein, leading to formation of a mucin-gel-matrix ('sludge') [8]. Furthermore, there is a 40% increase in bile calcium concentration [8] and a substantial decrease of gallbladder contractility due to reduced caloric intake (particularly in the form of fat) [9]. Together, these factors lead to a decreased nucleation time, i.e. an increased tendency to form cholesterol crystals.

RAPID WEIGHT REDUCTION

Rapid weight reduction occurs during very low calorie diets, after placement of a gastric balloon and after bariatric surgery (gastric bypass, biliodigestive anastomosis according to Scopinaro or laparoscopic band gastroplasty: LapBand procedure). During very low calorie diets (< 600 kcal/day) the incidence of new gallstones on ultrasound is 11-28% [10-12]. After bariatric surgery, the incidence has been reported to be as high as 36%, probably because the rate of weight loss is higher [2, 13]. After gastric bypass operations, interruption of the enterohepatic circulation, resulting in depletion of bile acids, is an additional predisposing factor for gallstone formation. Gallstones may develop within 4 to 8 weeks after the start of a diet. The mean time is 76 days (range 42-133) [10]. In the eighties, it was common practice to perform a prophylactic cholecystectomy in patients undergoing bariatric surgery for obesity [14], but the benefit in terms of prevention of symptomatic gallstones has never been determined.

RISK FACTORS FOR GALLSTONE DEVELOPMENT DURING WEIGHT LOSS

The amount of weight loss is an important risk factor: reduction of more than 25% of initial body weight is associated with an increased risk of 22% [4]. Also the rate of weight loss has a role [10]: weight loss exceeding 1.5 kg per week is associated with an exponential rise of gallstone risk [15] (figure 1). A study including 47153 female nurses showed that substantial variation in weight ('weight cycling') was associated with an increased risk of gallstones (relative risk 1.2-1.7 for light and severe cyclers, respectively) [16].

In the beginning of the nineties, the disadvantages of very low calorie and low fat (< 2 g fat per day) diets were discovered. A fat intake below 2 g/day decreases gallbladder emptying by 50% [9], leading to an increased risk of gallstones [9, 17]. The threshold for complete gallbladder contraction is at > 7 g fat a day [18]. The commonly used meal substitute Modifast® is a very low calorie diet (500 kcal/day) with a supply of 6.9 g fat a day. Table 1 shows practical recommendations for prevention of gallstones, intended for obese patients who attend a weight reduction program.

Tabel 1. Recommendations for prevention of gallstones during weight reduction.

DIET
1. Provide a fat intake of at least 7 g per day.
2. Avoid long overnight fasting periods; do not skip breakfast.
3. Use a diet rich in fibres.
WEIGHT LOSS
1. Maintain the rate of weight loss at less than 1.5 kg per week.
2. Keep the total weight loss below 25% of preexistent weight in 6 months.
MEDICAL PREVENTION
1. Prophylactic use of ursodeoxycholic acid (dose 600 mg/day) should be considered in obese patients with BMI > 30:   * in whom rapid weight loss (> 1.5 kg per week) in a short period (4-6 months) is expected, for example after bariatric surgery.   * who cannot adhere to the above-mentioned preventive measures regarding diet and rate of weight loss.
2. Aspirin is less effective than ursodeoxycholic acid. NSAIDs are not proven effective.

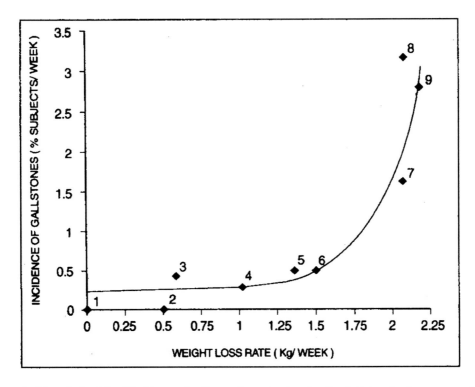

Figure 1. The relationship of incidence of gallstone formation to rate of weight loss in obese persons based upon published studies. Each point represents one observation group, including 17-68 patients (total, 388 patients). This figure has been reproduced from reference 15, with kind permission of the author and the publisher, Elsevier Science.

ROLE OF DRUGS IN THE PREVENTION OF GALLSTONES DURING WEIGHT LOSS

Aspirin and NSAIDs

Aspirin and NSAIDs decrease mucin secretion by the gallbladder through inhibition of prostaglandin synthesis [19]. The result is less sludge formation [8]. In a controlled clinical trial, aspirin decreased the incidence of echographic gallstones and sludge during rapid weight reduction by 41% [20]. For Ibuprofen, such an effect could not be demonstrated [3, 21], but the results were confounded by a high loss of patients, poor compliance with the diet and short follow-up (table 2).

URSODEOXYCHOLIC ACID

Ursodeoxycholic acid is a bile acid that naturally exists in bile. It improves the solubility of cholesterol in bile and decreases bile cholesterol secretion. Originally, ursodeoxycholic acid was extracted from bile of bears (ursos). It was discovered that ice bears never developed

Tabel 2. Randomized controlled trials on the benefit of usodeoxycholic acid for prevention of gallstones during weight reduction in patients with (morbid) obesity

Study (reference)	Year	N	BMI (before intervention)	Rate of weight loss (kg per week)	Intervention	Weight loss (% of baseline)	Follow-up	Incidence of gallstones (%)			Level of evidence*
								Placebo	Ursodeoxy-cholic acid (mg/dag)	Aspirin/ Ibuprofen	
Broomfield (20)	1989	68	Unknown; mean weight = 103.2 kg	2.3	520 kcal diet	22%	4 months	22%	1200mg: 0%	9% (A)	1b
Worobetz (22)	1993	29	Unknown; mean weight = 144.4 kg	2.0	vertical-band gastroplasty	19%	3 months	43%	1000mg: 0%	n.a.	1b
Sugerman (13)	1995	233	49.4	1.4	gastric bypass	24%	6 months	32%	300mg: 13% 600mg: 2% 1200mg: 6%	n.a.	1b
Shiffman (10)	1995	788	44.2	1.5	520 kcal diet	19%	4 months	28%	300mg: 8% 600mg: 3% 1200mg: 2%	n.a.	1b
Marks (21)	1996	47	36.6	1.0	520 kcal diet	9.5%	3 months	0%	1200mg: 0%	0% (I)	2b
Wudel (3)	2002	41	Unknown; mean weight = 158.6 kg	1.0	gastric bypass	28%	12 months	64%	600mg: 47%	93% (I)	2b
Miller (23)	2003	152	44.0	1.0 2.1	adjustable gastric banding vertical banded gastroplasty	20% 40%	24 months	30%	500mg: 8%	n.a.	1b

* Level of evidence, Centre for Evidence-Based Medicine of the National Health Service Research and Development, 1999. *Http://cebm.jr2.ox.ac.uk/docs/ levels.html.*

gallstones, despite the fact that they fast during the winter because of food scarcity. The bile of these bears turned out to contain a high concentration of ursodeoxycholic acid. Despite the fact that there are still 247 bear farms in China, where bile is extracted from around 7000 living bears for traditional Chinese medicine [22, 23], nowadays ursodeoxycholic acid is mainly produced synthetically (Ursochol®, Ursofalk®).

The benefit of ursodeoxycholic acid was demonstrated in 5 of 7 randomized controlled trials [3, 10, 13, 20, 24, 25]. Patients with morbid obesity were treated with ursodeoxycholic acid (dose varying from 300 to 1200 mg/day) or placebo during weight reduction induced by a diet or bariatric surgery. Patients with preexistent gallstones on ultrasound were excluded. During 3-24 months follow-up, the development of gallstones was examined by ultrasound. Table 2 summarises the results of these randomized trials. The optimal dose of ursodeoxycholic acid appears to be 600 mg/day [10, 13]. The higher dose of 1200 mg/day proved to be less effective because of non-compliance due to side-effects [13]. In high-risk patients undergoing gastric bypass surgery, ursodeoxycholic acid was moderately effective in one study (risk reduction 27%) [3]. Another study demonstrated that ursodeoxycholic acid is cost-effective for prevention of gallstones in patients with morbid obesity [26], based on the two most important clinical trials [10, 13]. In the United States, ursodeoxycholic acid is approved for this indication by the Food and Drug Administration (FDA) since 1996 [27].

INDICATIONS FOR URSODEOXYCHOLIC ACID

Although ursodeoxycholic acid is also effective if total weight loss is < 25% of baseline weight [10, 13, 20, 24, 25], the absolute risk of gallstones in patients losing weight 'according to the rules' is limited and prophylaxis may not be cost-effective in this group. In our opinion, ursodeoxycholic acid should be considered selectively in patients with morbid obesity, if it is expected that the weight loss will be rapid (> 1.5 kg /week) or difficult to control, for example after bariatric surgery.

OTHER POTENTIALLY EFFECTIVE TREATMENTS

Orlistat (Xenical®), an intestinal lipase inhibitor used for induction of weight loss, may also have a protective effect on weight-loss induced changes in biliary lipid composition. Orlistat seems to preserve bile acid and phospholipid secretion during weight reduction [28]. This effect may be mediated by a specific effect on lipid metabolism in the intestine. However, a recent study shows that orlistat significantly impairs gallbladder motility through decreased cholecystokinin release [29]. In one randomised trial, fish oil (n-3) polyunsaturated fatty acids (11.3 g/day) were able to prevent the decrease of cholesterol nucleation time during rapid weight loss [30]. The impact of this observation on prevention of cholesterol gallstones has not yet been determined. A diet rich in fibres may help prevent gallstone development through the induction of bile acid synthesis [31]. Statins would theoretically be effective through inhibition of HMG-CoA reductase, resulting in a lower cholesterol concentration of bile. Human studies are not available, but a recent animal model showed no prophylactic effect of simvastatin in dogs on a lithogenic diet [32].

CHOLECYSTECTOMY DURING LAPAROSCOPIC BARIATRIC SURGERY

In patients undergoing bariatric surgery, routine preoperative ultrasound examination offers the opportunity to detect pre-existing gallstones. If gallstones are diagnosed, simultaneous cholecystectomy should be considered. Whether or not routine cholecystectomy is advisable during bariatric surgery, cannot be derived from the literature. In a recent study [33], gallstones were detected by intra-operative ultrasound in 14% of patients undergoing laparoscopic gastric bypass surgery for morbid obesity. During follow-up, 7% of patients without stones developed symptomatic gallstone disease within 6 months (under treatment with ursodeoxycholic acid!), requiring cholecystectomy.

CONCLUSION

Not only obesity, but weight reduction too carries health risks. Weight reduction diets should therefore aim at gradual moderate weight loss (about 10% of preexistent weight in 6 months [34]) using a healthy, balanced, and energy-limited diet in combination with physical exercise. Under these circumstances, the risk of gallstones is small. However, with very low calorie 'crash' diets, after bariatric surgery and malabsorption-inducing operations, the risk of gallstones is substantial and medical supervision required. In these situations, ursodeoxycholic acid is a cost-effective treatment for the prevention of gallstones.

REFERENCES

[1]   Erlinger S. Gallstones in obesity and weight loss. *Gastroenterol Hepatol* 2000;12:1347-52.
[2]   Shiffman ML, Sugerman HJ, Kellum JM, Brewer WH, Moore EW. Gallstone formation after rapid weight loss: a prospective study in patients undergoing gastric bypass surgery for treatment of morbid obesity. *Am J Gastroenterol* 1991;86:1000-5.
[3]   Wudel LJ, Wright JK, Debelak JP, Allos TM, Shyr Y, Chapman WC. Prevention of gall-stone formation in morbidly obese patients undergoing rapid weight loss: results of a rando-mized controlled pilot study. *J Surg Res* 2002;102:50-56.
[4]   Everhart JE. Contributions of obesity and weight loss to gallstone disease. *Ann Intern Med* 1993;119:1029-35.
[5]   Marzio L, Capone F, Neri M, Mezzetti A, de Angelis C, Cuccurullo F. Gallbladder kinetics in obese patients. Effect of a regular meal and low-calorie meal. *Dig Dis Sci* 1988;33:4-9.
[6]   Maclure KM, Hayes KC, Colditz GA, Manson JE, Willett WC. Weight, diet and the risks of symptomatic gallstones in middle-aged women. *N Engl J Med* 1989;321:563-9.
[7]   Reuben A, Qureshi Y, Murphy GM, Dowling RH. Effect of obesity and weight reduction on biliary cholesterol saturation and the response to chenodeoxycholic acid. *Eur J Clin Invest* 1985;16:133-42.

[8]   Shiffman ML, Sugerman HJ, Kellum JM, Moore EW. Changes in gallbladder bile compo-sition following gallstone formation and weight reduction. *Gastroenterology* 1992;103:214-221.

[9]   Gebhard RL, Prigge WF, Ansel HJ, Schlasner L, Ketover SR, Sande D et al. The role of gallbladder emptying in gallstone formation during diet-induced rapid weight loss. *Hepatology* 1996;24:544-8.

[10] Shiffman ML, Kaplan GD, Brinkman-Kaplan V, Vickers FF. Prophylaxis against gallstone formation with ursodeoxycholic acid in patients participating in a very-low-calorie diet program. *Ann Intern Med* 1995;122:899-905.

[11] Yang H, Petersen GM, Roth MP, Schoenfield LJ, Marks JW. Risk factors for gallstone formation during rapid loss of weight. *Dig Dis Sci* 1992;37:912-8.

[12] Liddle RA, Goldstein RB, Saxton J. Gallstone formation during weight-reduction dieting. *Arch Intern Med* 1989;149:1750-3.

[13] Sugerman HJ, Brewer WH, Shiffman ML, Brolin RE, Fobi MAL, Linner JH et al. A multicenter, placebo-controlled, randomised, double-blind, prospective trial of prophylactic ursodiol for the prevention of gallstone formation following gastric-bypass-induced rapid weight loss. *Am J Surg* 1995;169:91-7.

[14] Schmidt JH, Hocking MP, Rout WR, Woodward ER. The case for prophylactic cholecys-tectomy concomitant with gastric restriction for morbid obesity. *Am Surg* 1988;54:269-72.

[15] Weinsier RL, Wilson LJ, Lee J. Medically safe rate of weight loss for the treatment of obesity: a guideline based on risk of gallstone formation. *Am J Med* 1995;98:115-7.

[16] Syngal S, Coakley EH, Willett WC, Byers T, Williamson DF, Colditz GA. Long-term weight patterns and risks for cholecystectomy in women. *Ann Intern Med* 1999;130:471-7.

[17] Festi D, Colecchia A, Orsini M, Sangermano A, Sottili S, Simoni P et al. Gallbladder motility and gallstone formation in obese patients following very low calorie diets. Use it (fat) to lose it (well). *Int J Obes Relat Metab Disord* 1998;22:592-600.

[18] Kalfarentzos F, Spiliotis J, Chalmoukis A, Vagenas C, Vagenakis A. Gallbladder contraction after hormonal manipulations in normal subjects and patients under total parenteral nutrition. *J Am Coll Nutr* 1992;11:17-20.

[19] Marks JW, Bonorris GG, Schoenfield LJ. Roles of deoxycholate and arachidonate in pathogenesis of cholesterol gallstones in obese patients during rapid loss of weight. *Dig Dis Sci* 1991;36:957-60.

[20] Broomfield PH, Chopra R, Sheinbaum RC, Bonorris GG, Silverman A, Schoenfield LJ et al. Effects of ursodeoxycholic acid and aspirin on the formation of lithogenic bile and gallstones during loss of weight. *N Engl J Med* 1988;319:1567-72.

[21] Marks JW, Bonorris GG, Schoenfield LJ. Effects of ursodiol or ibuprofen on contraction of gallbladder and bile among obese patients during weight loss. *Dig Dis Sci* 1996;41:242-9.

[22] World Society for the protection of Animals. The trade in Bear Bile. *http://www.animalsvoice.com/PAGES/invest/bear.html.*

[23] MacDonald AC, Williams CN. Studies of bile lipids and bile acids of wild North American black bears in Nova Scotia, showing a high content of ursodeoxycholic acid. *J Surg Res* 1985; 38:173-9.

[24] Worobetz LJ, Inglis FG, Shaffer EA. The effect of ursodeoxycholic acid therapy on gall-stone formation in the morbidly obese during rapid weight loss. *Am J Gastroenterol* 1993;88: 1705-10.

[25] Miller K, Hell E, Lang B, Lengauer E. Gallstone formation prophylaxis after gastric restrictive procedures for weight loss. *Ann Surg* 2003;238:697-702.

[26] Shoheiber O, Biskupiak JE, Nash DB. Estimation of the cost savings resulting from the use of ursodiol for the prevention of gallstones in obese patients undergoing rapid weight reduction. *Int J Obesity* 1997;21:1038-45.

[27] U.S. Food and Drug Administration, Drug and Device Product Approvals for March 1996, 19-594, suppl-016. *http://www.fda.gov/cder/da/ddpa396.htm*.

[28] Trouillot TE, Pace DG, McKinley C, Cockey L, Zhi J, Häeussler J et al. Orlistat maintains biliary lipid composition and hepatobiliary function in obese subjects undergoing moderate weight loss. *Am J Gastroenterol* 2001;96:1888-94.

[29] Mathus-Vliegen EM, van Ierland-van Leeuwen ML, Terpstra A. Lipase inhibition by orlistat: effects on gallbladder kinetics and cholecystokinin release in obesity. *Aliment Pharmacol Ther* 2004;19:601-11.

[30] Méndez-Sánchez N, González V, Aguayo P, Sánchez JM, Tanimoto MA, Elizondo J et al. Fish oil (n-3) polyunsaturated fatty acids beneficially affect biliary cholesterol nucleation time in obese women losing weight. *J Nutr* 2001;131:2300-3.

[31] Moran S, Uribe M, Prado ME, de la Mora G, Munoz RM, Perez MF et al. Effects of fiber administration in the prevention of gallstones in obese patients on a reducing diet. *A clinical trial. Rev Gastroenterol Mex* 1997;62:266-72.

[32] Davis KG, Wertin TM, Schriver JP. The use of simvastatin for the prevention of gallstones in the lithogenic prairie dog model. *Obes Surg* 2003;13:865-8.

[33] Villegas L, Schneider B, Provost D, Chang C, Scott D, Sims T et al. Is routine cholecystectomy required during laparoscopic gastric bypass? *Obes Surg* 2004;14:206-11.

[34] Seidell JC, Visscher TLS. Voeding en gezondheid – obesitas. *Ned Tijdschr Geneeskd* 2003;147:281-286

In: Weight Loss, Exercise and Health Research
Editor: Carrie P. Saylor, pp. 59-75
ISBN 1-60021-077-5
© 2006 Nova Science Publishers, Inc.

Chapter 4

INDEPENDENT AND INTERACTIVE EFFECTS OF BODY MASS AND WEIGHT CHANGE ON SKELETAL HEALTH – A REVIEW AND POPULATION-BASED STUDY

Joonas Sirola[1,5,*], *Marjo Tuppurainen*[1,2] *Jukka S. Jurvelin*[3] *and Heikki Kröger*[1,4]

[1]University of Kuopio, Bone and Cartilage Research Unit (BCRU), Kuopio, Finland
[2]Department of Obstetrics and Gynaecology, [3]Department of Clinical Physiology and Nuclear Medicine, [4]Department of Surgery, Kuopio University Hospital Kuopio, Finland
[5]Mikkeli Central Hospital, Department of Surgery / Ortopaedics, Finland

ABSTRACT

Introduction

Low body mass and weight loss are strong independent risk-factors for low bone mineral density (BMD) (osteoporosis) and bone loss among postmenopausal women. Although this relationship has fairly convincingly been demonstrated in recent studies the underlying contribution of fat tissue related estrogen production, bone effects of leptin, role of nutritional and mechanical factors remain to be resolved. The present study reviews the recent findings on effects of body mass and weight loss on skeletal health in early postmenopause. Furthermore, it accompanies these findings with new unpublished research results on independent and interactive effects of body mass and weight change on bone loss in a prospective population based Osteoporosis Risk Factor and Prevention (OSTPRE) -study.

---

[*] Correspondence to: Dr. Joonas Sirola, MD, PhD,Bone and Cartilage Research Unit (BCRU),University of Kuopio, Mediteknia building,P.O. Box 1627, 70211,KUOPIO, FINLAND,Tel. +358-50-355 59 38 Fax. +358-17-162 940,e-mail: joonas.sirola@uku.fi

Subjects and Methods

For the present study, the study population, 954 early postmenopausal women, was selected from a random sample (n=2025) of the OSTPRE study cohort (n=13 100) in Kuopio, Finland. Dual X-ray absorptiometry (DXA) bone mineral density (BMD; g/cm^2) at the lumbar spine (LS) and femoral neck (FN), and body mass (kg), were measured at baseline in 1989–91 and repeated at five-year follow-up in 1994–97. Women were divided into tertiles based on their baseline body mass: under 63 kg, 63-72 kg and over 72 kg.

Results

Weight loss and low BMI were associated with higher bone loss, low BMD and increased risk of osteoporosis. Weight loss during the follow-up significantly predicted greater bone loss rate in FN in all baseline tertiles (p<0.02 in regression model). In LS, the women in the lowest tertile had significant negative relationship between bone loss and weight loss (p=0.031) but not in other tertiles (p=NS). This effect was independent of adjustments for age, use of HRT, calcium intake and other potential confounders. There were no differences between absolute body mass change values (kg) and percent change of body mass. The interaction analysis (regression model) showed significant interaction for bone loss between weight loss and baseline weight in LS (p=0.022) but not in FN (p=NS). This effect was also not affected by any adjustments.

Conclusion

In conclusion, body mass and weight change are the most important life-style determinants of postmenopausal bone density and rate of bone loss. According to present prospective study, weight change affects bone loss independently of start point body mass in FN but not in LS. This most likely represents differences in the structure of bone tissue in these areas and may suggest independent pathogenesis for weight change induced bone density changes.

INTRODUCTION

Osteoporosis and associated low trauma energy fractures are major cause of morbidity, disability and increased medical care costs among the elderly (Lindsay 1992, Cooper et al. 1992, Cooper and Melton III 1996). Osteoporosis affects approximately 30 % of the postmenopausal population and the estimated lifetime risk for an osteoporotic fracture in a 50-year woman is about 40 % (Melton III et al 1992, Kanis et al. 1993, WHO 1994, Gullberg et al. 1997). The prevalence of the most devastating complication of osteoporosis, hip fractures, is expected to rise world-wide by over 200 percent by the year 2050 in the female population (Gullberg et al. 1997).

Ovarian dysfunction and accompanying decline in estrogen levels during menopausal transition has been considered as the most important and inevitable determinant of bone loss leading to osteoporotic bone density (Hansen et al. 1991, Pouilles et al. 1993, Kröger et al. 1994, Ensrud et al. 1995, Prior et al. 1998, Ahlborg et al. 2001, Sirola 2003a). In addition, many other environmental and life-style related factors also contribute to menopausal bone loss (Kröger et al. 1994, Burger et al. 1998, Hannan et al. 2000, Sirola 2003a, Sirola 2003b) although role of only few factors is well established. One such determinant is the relationship between fatness and weight loss with high BMD and increased bone loss, respectively (Brot et al. 1997, Burger et al. 1998, Nguyen et al. 1998, Yoshimura et al. 1998, Hannan et al. 2000, Sirola et al 2003b). However, the exact pathophysiological mechanisms underlying the relationship between bone health and body mass are not completely clear. Contribution of fat tissue derived estrogens, leptins, nutritional factors and mechanical stress to weight change related postmenopausal bone mass changes have been suggested (Coin et al. 2000, Blain et al. 2001, Jensen et al. 2001, Nelson and Bulun 2001, Blain et al. 2002)

Although the association of weight and weight change with BMD and bone loss has previously been clearly recognised, the interaction between these two determinants has not been properly established. Ensrud et al. have reported results on postmenopausal women concluding that weight loss increases the risk of bone loss and hip fractures irrespective of current weight or weight loss intention (Ensrud et al. 2003). Large prospective population-based studies investigating possible interaction between weight and weight change are thus sparse.

For the purposes of this chapter a short review on recent findings on effects of body mass and its changes on bone health is presented. In addition, this chapter presents new unpublished results on the interaction between weight and weight change on postmenopausal bone loss on a random population-based sample of 954 early postmenopausal women derived from the prospective Osteoporosis Risk Factor and Prevention (OSTPRE) –study, Finland.

REVIEW

The present review is limited to clinical and observational human subject studies in postmenopausal women unless otherwise stated along the text reference.

The Strong Association of Body Mass and Weight Change with Osteoporosis

High body mass and weight increase are associated with the maintenance of BMD and reduced bone loss whereas thinness and weight loss lead to low BMD and enhanced bone loss in postmenopausal women (Brot et al. 1997, Burger et al. 1998, Nguyen et al. 1998, Yoshimura et al. 1998, Hannan et al. 2000, Sirola 2003b). The effect of weight loss induced bone loss has been suggested to be independent of current weight or intention to lose weight (Ensrud et al. 2003). In addition, high body mass has been demonstrated to be a strong independent predictor of postmenopausal hip and other frailty fractures (Ensrud et al. 1997a, Huopio et al. 2000, Margolis et al. 2000). Furthermore, weight loss increases and weight increase decreases the risk of hip and other osteoporotic fractures (Langlois et al. 1996, Ensrud et al. 1997b). Body mass and weight change has also been suggested to correlate with levels of bone biochemical markers, although not constantly (Ravn et al. 1999, Rico et al. 2002, Papakitsou et al. 2004).

Body mass may be useful in directing patients to axial bone density measurements and it has been suggested that weight and age are superior risk factors in differentiating osteoporotic women from normal bone density population (Wildner et al. 2003). Accordingly, body mass and related parameters have become clinically valuable and have been included as major determinants in recently developed screening tools for primary diagnosis of osteoporosis (Michaelsson et al. 1996, Weinstein and Ullery 2000, Cadarette et al. 2001).

Underlying Pathophysiology: Current Knowledge

The effects of body weight on skeletal health may partly be linked with fat tissue related estrogen production which is well known bone antiresorptive agent and also widely used therapeutic agent for treatment of osteoporosis (National Osteoporosis Foundation 1998, Nelson and Bulun 2001). Fat mass, rather than fat free mass, has been suggested to be correlated positively with bone mass and negatively with bone loss (Chen et al. 1997, Coin et al. 2000, Blain et al. 2004). According to Chen et al., however, lean mass may be correlated better with BMD than fat mass, while bone mass changes are more strongly correlated with fat mass (Chen et al. 1997). Furthermore, it has been suggested that in weight bearing bone sites the adiposity is not as relevant factor in determining bone mass as in non-weight bearing regions (Glauber et al. 1995). Hence, some studies have favoured the theory that high mechanical load itself may lead to bone strengthening via mobility induced weight-bearing stress (Harris and Dawson-Hughes 1996, Jensen et al 2001). In cellular level this theory has been suggested to be mediated through mechanical strain sensory function of osteocytes ("mechanostat") introduced by early work of Frost et al. (Frost et al. 1987) and supported in later experimental studies (Lanyon 1993, Rodan 1997). Some recent observational studies have also indirectly investigated the relationship between fat tissue related estrogen production and body mass suggesting that weight and weight loss induced bone mass changes are partly dependent on the use of HRT (Cifuentes et al. 2003, Sirola et al. 2003b, MacDonald et al. 2004).

The effects of fat mass regulating hormone, leptin, on bone health has also been recently speculated. However, the results on relationship between leptin and bone are not constant (Thomas 2003, Hamrick 2004). Although the relationship between leptin and BMD has been favoured in some studies (Pasco et al. 2001, Yamauchi et al. 2001, Blain et al 2002) other studies oppose it (Blum et al. 2003, Roux et al. 2003). Analogously, the correlation of leptin levels with bone biochemical markers has not supported bone related effects in some studies (Goulding et al. 1998, Shaarawy et al. 2003) while other studies have suggested the opposite (Blain et al. 2002). The potential mechanism by which leptin could exert its bone effects has been suggested to involve both direct osteogenic properties (Steppan et al. 2000, Cornish et al. 2002) and central hypothalamic-relay pathways (Ducy et al. 2000, Karsenty 2001) in experimental animal models.

The heavier population has higher nutritional intake, and demand, and may thus consume more calcium and other bone preserving products, including proteins. Accordingly, it has been suggested that undernutrition may play an important role in poor bone health among underweight elderly women (Coin et al. 2000). Cifuentes et al. recently performed a randomized controlled trial, in which they observed weight loss induced activation of PTH-calcitriol axis (Cifuentes et al. 2004) which was proposed to be a substantial underlying mechanism for weight loss induced bone mass changes. Hypothetically, declining PTH levels of weight losers would lead to increase in renal loss of calcium as observed in earlier studies (Atkinson et al. 1978, Andersen et al. 1988). In addition, it has been suggested that calcium may prevent weight loss induced bone loss (Ricci et al. 1998, Jensen et al. 2001), although mechanical stimuli was proposed to be the leading etiological mechanism for weight loss induced bone loss itself according to Jensen et al. (Jensen et al. 2001). The protective effects of calcium on weight loss induced bone loss may be mediated through PTH-calcitriol axis function (Jensen et al. 2001).

Part of the observed BMD changes related to weight alterations may be due to methodological difficulties encountered in the measurement techniques adopted to deal with body compositional factors, most importantly fat tissue (Bolotin 1998, Bolotin et al. 2001). As the DXA technique uses the soft tissue density as its reference for bone density measurements, the unequal distribution of fat mass changes around and inside bones may result in significant errors in bone loss estimates (Bolotin et al. 2001). It has been estimated, that inaccuracies as high as over 20 % could be anticipated clinically (Bolotin et al. 2001). However, the magnitude of possible methodological difficulties should be interpreted in the light of studies on osteoporotic fractures which are independent of any such measurement error. Also, it has been speculated that the possible errors in axial bone density measurements due to body compositional factors could be effectively corrected in serial DXA measurements (Blake et al. 2000).

To summarize, although the relationship between body mass, weight change and bone metabolism is clearly recognized, the underlying pathophysiology is not yet perfectly understood and the exact contribution of each suggested mechanism still needs further research.

The Clinical Paradigm of Body Mass Versus Osteoporosis

The relationship between weight control and osteoporosis is clinically problematic as large weight and a weight increase can protect from bone loss (Brot et al. 1997, Nguyen et al. 1998, Yoshimura et al. 1998) but, at the same time, overweight is a significant risk factor for increased cardiovascular mortality and morbidity especially in the postmenopausal age group (Srinivasan et al. 1996, Rea et al. 2001). Accordingly, a significant weight increase or overweight should naturally not be encouraged despite its positive bone effects but, on the other hand, significant weight loss should either not be recommended at the time of menopause, especially in women with normal body weight. Also, women that lose weight should receive special attention in osteoporosis risk assessment. In future studies, it would be worthwhile to investigate the risk-benefit ratio of body mass and its changes in comparative light of mortalities and morbidities from combined skeletal and cardiovascular aspects in order to achieve proper consensus. In addition, therapies that would effectively prevent weight loss related bone loss need further research and should receive attention in clinical practice (Jensen et al. 2001, Sirola et al. 2003b, Cifuentes et al. 2004).

MATERIALS AND METHODS

Osteoporosis Risk Factor and Prevention (OSTPRE) -study is a population-based 3-level prospective cohort study which investigates genetic and acquired factors associated with fractures, falls, bone mineral density (BMD) and bone loss in peri- and postmenopausal women (Honkanen et al. 1991). It was established in 1989 and is still ongoing.

Study Population

The study population was formed from the prospective Kuopio Osteoporosis Risk Factor and Prevention (OSTPRE) study cohort. The OSTPRE cohort was established in 1989 by selecting all women born in 1932–1941 and resident in Kuopio Province, Finland (n=14 220). The baseline postal inquiry, including questions about health disorders, medication, use of HRT, gynaecological history, nutritional habits, calcium intake, physical activity, alcohol consumption, smoking habits, and anthropometric information was sent to these women at baseline in 1989. The five-year questionnaire was sent in 1994 to the 13 100 women who responded at baseline (Honkanen et al. 1991).

Of the respondents to the baseline inquiry, 11 055 (84.4%) were willing to undergo dual X-ray absorptiometry (DXA). A random sample of 2362 women was selected for densitometry, of whom 2025 actually underwent baseline densitometry during 1989–91. The questionnaire information was updated individually at the time of bone densitometry. A total of 1551 women of the 1873 who actually underwent both baseline (1989–91) and five-year (1994–97) measurements had serial valid measurements for both the lumbar spine and femoral neck (no osteoarthritis, scoliosis or other bone deformities). For this study, the following groups were successively excluded: 1) hysterectomized women (for whom it was impossible to define menopausal status) and bilaterally ovariectomized women (n=445), 2) premenopausal women (n=152). Thus, the final study population consisted of 954 women (beginning of menopause either before (postmenopausal) or during (perimenopausal) the study) aged 48 to 59 years at baseline densitometry. The beginning of menopause was defined as 12 months' amenorrhea (World Health Organization 1994) and its duration varied from 1 week to 26 years among the 954 women at five-year measurement. The duration of follow-up among these women varied from 3.8 to 7.9 years (mean 5.8 years).

Weight (kg) was measured at the baseline and five-year densitometries. Women were categorized into tertiles according to baseline weight, body mass index (BMI) and weight change. Weight tertiles were: 1.<63 kg (n=338) 2. 63-72 kg (n=302) 3. >72 kg (n=314). BMI tertiles were: 1.<24 kg/m^2 (n=234) 2. 24-28 kg/m^2 (n=391) 3. >28 kg/m^2 (n=279). Weight change tertiles were: 1. <1.5 % 2. 1.5-6.5 % 3. >6.5 %. Simultaneously, grip strength was measured with a hand-held dynamometer (Martin Vigorimeter, Germany) and taken to be the mean of three measurements. The calcium intake of each participant was calculated according to self-reported ingestion of dairy products and reported as the mean of two measurements (baseline, five-year follow-up). The amount of nutritional calcium ingested was approximated at 120 mg/dl for fluid milk products (milk, sour milk, yoghurt, etc.) and 87 mg/slice for cheese. Also the calcium intake has been validated by a food diary which has been described in detail previously (Sirola et al. 2003c).

Bone Mass Measurements

The bone mineral densities of lumbar spine (L2-L4), left femoral neck, Ward's triangle and trochanter major were determined using dual X-ray absorptiometry (DXA) (Lunar DPX, Madison, Wisconsin, USA). The measurements were carried out in Kuopio University Hospital by specially trained personnel. Quality standards were tested daily. The short term reproducibility of this method has been shown to be 0.9 % for lumbar spine and 1.5 % for femoral neck BMD measurements (Kröger et al. 1992). The long-term reproducibility (CV) of the DXA instrument for BMD during the study period, as determined by regular phantom measurements, was 0.4 % (Komulainen et al. 1998).

Statistical Methods

Statistical analyses were carried out using the Statistical Package for Social Sciences (SPSS 9.0, SPSS Inc., Chicago, Illinois, USA) for Windows. The annual BMD changes at both measurement site were calculated according to the following formula: [(BMD at the 5-year follow-up - BMD at baseline) / duration of follow-up] and reported as percentage of baseline BMD. Weight change was computed as differences of follow-up and baseline body mass and computed as percentage of baseline weight in addition to actual values. Body mass index (BMI) was computed according to formula: $Weight (kg)/Height (m)^2$. For multinomial regression model BMD was categorised according to WHO osteoporosis definition (n in baseline/follow-up): >-1 SD normal (n=663/n=551), -2.5 to -1 SD osteopenia (n=271/n=363) and <-2.5 SD osteoporosis (n=19/n=34) in femoral neck and >-1 SD normal (n=529/n=442), -2.5 to -1 SD osteopenia (n=350/n=386) and <-2.5 SD osteoporosis (n=75/n=126) in lumbar spine. Adjustment for age, baseline weight, baseline height, baseline BMD, calcium intake, use of HRT, duration of menopause, grip strength, physical activity level and bone-affecting diseases/medication (yes/no) was used when appropriate (reported in the text). In the regression models adjustment variables were entered simultaneously with the dependent variables in the same model. In the interaction linear regression the interactive term [baseline weight x weight change] was entered simultaneously to regression model with both of the dependent variables and adjustment variables. The selection of bone-affecting diseases/medication (used in adjustments) has been described previously by Kröger *et al* (Kröger et al. 1998). Diseases were: renal disease, liver disease, insulin-dependent diabetes, malignancies, rheumatoid arthritis, endocrine abnormalities (parathyroid/thyroid glands, adrenals), malabsorption (including lactose malabsorption), total/partial gastrectomy, postovariectomy status, premenopausal amenorrhoea, alcoholism and long-term immobilisation. Medication included: corticosteroids, diuretics, cytotoxic drugs, anticonvulsive drugs, anabolic steroids, calcitonin, bisphosphonates and vitamin D.

RESULTS

Table 1 describes the characteristics of the present study population according to baseline weight tertiles. In the present population, heavier population was taller, had higher BMD, used more frequently HRT, used less alcohol and had higher grip strength/physical activity level (p<0.05). These differences were taken into consideration as adjustment variables among other potential confounders. The contribution of weight and weight change to peri- and postmenopausal bone loss among other risk factors for bone loss has been reported in the same population previously (Sirola et al. 2003a, 2003b)

Table 1. Baseline and follow-up characteristics of the study population
Baseline weight tertiles*

Characteristic	1st (n=338)	2nd (n=302)	3rd (n=314)	Total (n=954)	Sig.
A. Continuous variables (SD)					
Duration of follow-up (years)	5.8 (0.5)	5.8 (0.4)	5.8 (0.4)	5.8 (0.5)	
Age (years)	53.6 (2.8)	53.7 (2.9	53.5 (2.8)	53.6 (2.8)	
Years postmenopausal **	7.9 (4.3)	7.7 (4.5)	7.8 (4.3)	7.8 (4.4)	
Height (cm)	159.1(5.0)	161.5(4.7)	163.0(5.0)	161.1(5.2)	††
Weight change (kg)	2.7 (4.0)	3.0 (4.8)	3.1 (6.2)	2.9 (5.1)	
Grip strength (kPA)	60.5 (16.1)	63.9 (14.9)	62.9 (17.4)	62.4 (16.2)	†
Mean calcium intake (mg/day) §	778 (316)	778 (301)	823 (330)	793 (316)	
Baseline LS BMD (g/cm^2)	1.06 (0.15)	1.11 (0.15)	1.17 (0.15)	1.11 (0.16)	††
Baseline FN BMD (g/cm^2)	0.86 (0.11)	0.92 (0.11)	0.99 (0.12)	0.92 (0.12)	††
B.Distribution of category variables (%)					
Use of HRT during follow-up					††
No	53.6	54.3	68.8	58.8	
Occasional (<90%)	31.7	35.8	26.4	31.2	
Continuous (≥90%)	14.8	9.9	4.8	10.0	
Fracture history at baseline	21.8	19.8	22.1	21.3	
Alcohol >1 drink/week at baseline	38.2	34.7	28.7	33.9	†
Current smoker at baseline	10.9	8.6	8.9	9.5	
High overall physical activity level §§	30.8	37.3	31.0	32.9	†
No bone affecting disease/medication	35.5	40.7	34.7	36.9	

*   Weight tertiles: 1st<63 kg, 2nd 63-72 kg, 3rd >72 kg. ** at five-year (second) measurement.
§   mean of baseline and five-year (second) measurements.
§§   women divided into three categories based on combined physical activity at work and leisure (low/moderate/high).
†† p<0.001 † p<0.05

Figure 1 represents the association of BMI and bone mass as well as the relationship of weight change to bone loss. In all, 172 women (18 %) lost weight during follow-up (mean -3.7 kg / -5.1% of baseline weight). Baseline BMD was observed significantly higher in both femoral neck and lumbar spine regions in second (p<0.001) and third (p<0.001) baseline BMI tertiles in comparison to first BMI tertile. Identical relationship between BMI and BMD was also observed in the follow-up measurement (data not shown). In addition, women in lowest weight change tertile had significantly lower bone loss rate in comparison to the other two tertiles in both lumbar spine (p<0.05) and femoral neck (p<0.001)(Figure 1). In weight losers annual bone loss rate was (LS/FN) 0.6% / 0.8% in comparison to 0.4% / 0.5% in weight gainers (p<0.014 / p<0.001). Furthermore, the annual bone loss rate was –0.4% / -0.7% (LS) and -0.7 % / -1.0% (FN) in women losing under/over 5 percent of baseline weight. All statistically significant differences in the above mentioned results remained significant after the adjustments for potential confounders.

Table 2 represents the multinomial regression model for identification of osteoporosis (World Health Organization (WHO) classification) according to BMI. The RR in separating both normal bone density and osteopenic women from osteoporotic women was significant in both lumbar spine and femoral neck (RR 1.09-1.77, p<0.05). There were no differences in this effect concerning the baseline and follow-up measurements representing different age groups (Table 2).

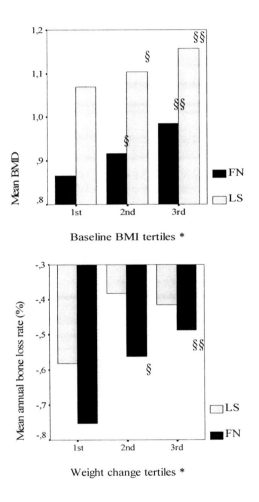

Figure 1. Body mass index (BMI)*, weight change* and their association with of low BMD and increased bone loss in the present study population (n=954).*) Baseline BMI tertiles: 1st <24 kg/m², 2nd 24-28 kg/m², 3rd >28 kg/m². Weight change tertiles: 1st < 1.5 %, 2nd 1.5 – 6.5 %, 3rd > 6.5 % .§ p<0.05, §§ p<0.001 in comparison to the first tertile.

Table 3 represents the independent and interactive effects of body mass and weight change on bone loss in a linear regression model. In femoral neck there was a significant relationship between weight change and bone loss rate in all baseline body mass tertiles (p<0.05). In lumbar spine this positive relationship was significant only in the first tertile in contrast to second and third tertiles (p=NS). These results remained unchanged after the adjustments. Also, the results did not change in percent weight change values of baseline weight. Table 3 also shows the linear regression interaction model in which there was a significant interaction between baseline weight and weight change in lumbar spine bone loss ($p > 0.05$) but not in femoral neck bone loss (p=NS) independent of any adjustments.

Table 2. Multinomial logistic regression model[a]: risk of osteoporosis[b] according to BMI in lumbar spine and femoral neck.

A. Baseline measurement

Group[b]	Area	Intercept	Standard error	Significance (p-value)	RR (95 % CI)
Normal	FN	0.54	0.10	p<0.001	1.71(1.41-2.07)
	LS	0.19	0.04	p<0.001	1.21(1.12-1.30)
Osteopenia	FN	0.32	0.10	p<0.001	1.37(1.13-1.66)
	LS	0.09	0.04	p=0.025	1.09(1.01-1.18)

B. Follow-up measurement

Group[b]	Area	Intercept	Standard error	Significance (p-value)	RR (95 % CI)
Normal	FN	0.36	0.07	p<0.001	1.44(1.26-1.64)
	LS	0.22	0.03	p<0.001	1.24(1.17-1.32)
Osteopenia	FN	0.19	0.07	p=0.004	1.21(1.06-1.37)
	LS	0.12	0.03	p<0.001	1.13(1.06-1.20)

a) Three category grouping variable[b]: normal BMD, osteopenia and osteoporosis. Reference group: osteoporosis. Dependent variable: body mass index (BMI) in baseline (*A*) and in follow-up measurement (*B*).

b) WHO classification (*see Materials and methods, Statistical methods*).

Table 3. Effects of weight and weight change on bone loss: independent and interactive linear regression models (n=954).

A. Effect of weight change according to start point weight*

Tertile*	Site	Coefficient	Standard error	T	Significance (p-value)
1st	Lumbar spine	0.032	0.015	2.169	0.031
	Femoral neck	0.029	0.012	2.384	0.018
2nd	Lumbar spine	0.006	0.012	0.462	0.644
	Femoral neck	0.024	0.010	2.344	0.020
3rd	Lumbar spine	0.007	0.010	0.781	0.436
	Femoral neck	0.030	0.008	3.651	<0.001

B. Analysis of interaction**

Site	Coefficient	Standard error	T	Significance (p-value)
Lumbar spine	-0.001	0.0004	-2.30	0.022
Femoral neck	-0.0000052	0.0003	-0.02	0.988

* Baseline weight tertiles: 1st<63 kg, 2nd 63-72 kg, 3rd >72 kg.

** Analysis of interaction. The equations describe the coefficients of term of interaction [baseline weight x weight change] in a linear regression model including: 1. the term of interaction 2. baseline weight 3. weight change during the follow-up 4. adjustment variables (*see Materials and methods, Statistical methods*), entered simultaneously.

CONCLUSION

The present study evaluated the effects of body mass and its changes as well as their interaction on bone mineral density and bone loss among postmenopausal women in a prospective population based study. It was suggested that while body mass and its changes inevitably are strong independent predictors of bone loss there might be unique interactions between these two factors. However, the interaction was found to depend on the measured bone site: in femoral neck weight loss predicted bone loss irrespective of start point weight whereas in lumbar spine such independency was not observed.

The strengths of our study were its prospective population-based nature, large base population and long-term follow-up period. Bone mass and weight measurements were performed under supervision of trained personnel suppressing occasional confounders due to measurement errors. Furthermore, the follow-up interval was equal between the study groups. The study population was randomly selected following that selection bias was unlikely to have occurred. Finally, comprehensive adjustment, including a variety of bone-affecting diseases, was used in the analyses.

In epidemiological studies the possibility of uncontrolled confounding is present. One source of confounding may be that the majority of the approximately 18 percent of weight losers lost less than 10% of their baseline weight, making it difficult to reliably determine bone loss rate in more significant weight-losers. In addition, in present study the initial reason for weight loss was not known but adjusting for bone affecting diseases and medications made bias due to pathologic conditions unlikely. Also, the possibility of fat tissue related measurement error of axial DXA measurements was present and not accurately determined in the present sample. Finally, the study population, although randomly selected, presented a relatively small part of the original OSTPRE cohort. These limitations can only be avoided in randomized controlled trials.

The present study confirmed the indisputable role of body mass and weight loss as major determinant of bone mass and bone loss in accordance with other population based estimates (Brot et al. 1997, Burger et al. 1998, Nguyen et al. 1998, Yoshimura et al. 1998, Hannan et al. 2000, Sirola 2003b). In addition, the present study was in accordance with previous findings on superiority of differentiation of osteoporotic women according to body mass (Wildner et al. 2003). The present study was not aimed at investigating the actual underlying pathophysiology of body mass change related bone mass changes and no biochemical samples were collected. However, the previous findings on the same population strongly, although indirectly, suggest that fat and soft-tissue mass dependent estrogen production (Nelson and Bulun 2001) is a substantially important mechanism (Sirola et al. 2003b). The other possible underlying mechanisms are thoroughly discussed in the review part of this chapter. Overall, the observed effects between body mass, weight change and bone mass changes have important clinical implications. Normal and underweight women should receive special attention with regards osteoporosis screening and women with weight loss intention, or involuntary weight loss, might benefit from follow-up bone density measurements.

Previously Ensrud et al. have suggested the independent role of weight loss on bone loss (Ensrud et al. 2003). Present study suggested that this independency may be limited to femoral neck. This effect may be due to different structure of these bony areas. The composition of bones varies, in terms of cortical and trabecular areas, and thus the response to e.g. hormonal factors also differ as trabecular bone in lumbar spine is more metabolically active in comparison to predominant metabolically inert cortical bone in femoral neck. In addition mechanical load is likely to affect femoral areas more in comparison to lumbar regions. In a previous study it has been suggested that there are differences in the effects of lean mass and fat mass (or adiposity) regarding weight bearing and non weight-bearing skeletal sites (Glauber et al. 1995) which could well explain the observed differences between spinal and femoral bone loss in the present study. Glauber speculated that in non-weight bearing sites the association between weight loss and bone loss may be driven by metabolic factors in contrast to weight bearing sites, such as femoral neck (Glauber et al. 1995). Hypothetically, mechanical factors could predominate in the association between bone mineral density and body mass focusing on cortical bone, i.e. femoral neck, whereas weight loss may affect through estrogen, PTH-calcitriol and/or leptin dependent pathways concentrating on trabecular compartment i.e. lumbar spine. This hypothesis would be in accordance with the present findings as weight loss independently predicted bone loss in inert cortical bone of femoral neck, possibly driven by diminished mechanical load. While the present study was unable to investigate the exact contribution of these factors it should receive further interest in future studies.

In conclusion, the results of the present study suggest, in the light of previously published data, that weight loss affects bone loss independently of start point weight in femoral neck but not in lumbar spine. This difference is probably caused by different composition of these sites in terms of trabecular and cortical bone. Accordingly, weight loss may affect bone loss trough independent metabolic pathway in addition to mechanical load. Future research on this issue is needed and essential.

ACKNOWLEDGEMENTS

This study has received financial support from The Finnish Medical Foundation, Emil Aaltonen Foundation and Academy of Finland.

REFERENCES

[1]   Lindsay R. The growing problem of osteoporosis. *Osteoporosis Int* 1992;2:267-268
[2]   Cooper C, Campion G, Melton LJ. Hip fractures in the elderly: a worldwide projection. *Osteoporos Int* 1992;2:285-9
[3]   Cooper C, Melton LJ III. Magnitude and impact of osteoporosis and fractures. In: *Osteoporosis*. Edit. Marcus R, Feldman D, Kelsey J, San Diego: Academic Press, Inc.,1996;419-31
[4]   Melton LJ III, Chrichilles E, Cooper C, Lane A, Riggs L. Perspective. How many women have osteoporosis ? *J Bone Res* 1992;7:1005-1010
[5]   Kanis JA. The incidence of hip fracture in Europe. *Osteoporosis Int* 1993;suppl 1:S10-S15.
[6]   WHO. Assessment of osteoporotic fracture risk and its role in screening for postmenopausal osteoporosis. *WHO Technical Report Series*, Geneva 1994.

[7]   Gullberg B, Johnell O, Kanis JA. World-wide projections for hip-fracture. *Osteoporosis Int* 1997;7(5):407-13

[8]   Hansen MA, Overgaard K, Riis BJ, Christiansen C. Role of peak bone mass and bone loss in postmenopausal osteoporosis: 12 year study. *Br Med J* 1991;303:961-964

[9]   Pouilles JM, Tremollieres F, Ribot C The effects of menopause on longitudinal bone loss from the spine. *Calcif Tissue Int* 1993;52:340-343

[10] Kröger H, Tuppurainen M, Honkanen R, Alhava E, Saarikoski S. Bone mineral density and risk factors for osteoporosis-a population based study of 1600 perimenopausal women. *Calcif Tissue Int* 1994;55:1-7

[11] Ensrud KE, Palermo L, Black DM, Cauley J, Jergas M, Orwoll ES, Nevitt MC, Fox KM, Cummings SR. Hip and calcaneal bone loss increase with advancing age: longitudinal results from the study of osteoporotic fractures. *J Bone Miner Res* 1995;10:1778-1787

[12] Prior JC. Perimenopause: the complex endocrinology of the menopausal transition. *Endoc Res* 1998;19(4):397-428

[13] Ahlborg HG, Johnell O, Nilsson BE, Jeppson S, Rannevik G, Karlsson MK. Bone loss in relation to menopause: a prospective study during 16 years. *Bone* 2001;28:327-31

[14] Sirola J, Kröger H, Honkanen R, Jurvelin JS, Sandini L, Tuppurainen M, Saarikoski S. Factors affecting bone loss around menopause in women without HRT: a prospective population based cohort study. *Maturitas* 2003a; 45: 159-167

[15] Kröger H, Tuppurainen M, Honkanen R, Alhava E, Saarikoski S. Bone mineral density and risk factors for osteoporosis – a population-based study of 1600 perimenopausal women. *Calcif Tissue Int* 1994;55:1-7.

[16] Burger H, de Laet CE, van Daele PL, Weel AE, Witteman JC, Hofman A, Pols HA. Risk factors for increased bone loss in an elderly population: the Rotterdam Study. *Am J Epidemiol* 1998;147:871-9

[17] Hannan MT, Felson DT, Dawson-Hughes B, Tucker KL, Cupples LA, Wilson PW, Kiel DP. Risk factors for longitudinal bone loss in elderly men and women: the Framingham osteoporosis study. *J Bone Miner Res* 2000;15:710-720.

[18] Sirola J, Kröger H, Honkanen R, Sandini L, Tuppurainen M, Jurvelin JS, Saarikoski S. Risk factors associated with peri- and postmenopausal bone loss - does HRT prevent weight loss- related bone loss? *Osteoporosis Int* 2003b; 14: 27-33.

[19] Brot C, Jensen LB, Sorensen OH. Bone mass and risk factors for bone loss in perimenopausal Danish women. *J Intern Med* 1997;242(6):505-11

[20] Nguyen TV, Sambrook PN, Eisman JA. Bone loss, physical activity, and weight change in elderly women: the Dubbo Osteoporosis Epidemiology Study. *J Bone Miner Res* 1998;13:1458-146

[21] Yoshimura N, Hashimoto T, Morioka S, Sakata K, Kasamatsu T, Cooper C. Determinants of bone loss in a rural Japanese community, the Taiji Study. *Osteoporosis Int* 1998;8(6):604-10.

[22] Coin A, Sergi G, Beninca P, Lupoli L, Cinti G, Ferrara L, Benedetti G, Tomasi G, Pisent C, Enzi G. Bone mineral density and body composition in underweight and normal elderly subjects. *Osteoporos Int* 2000;11(12):1043-50

[23] Blain H, Vuillemin A, Teissier A, Hanesse B, Guillemin F, Jeandel C. Influence of muscle strength and body weight and composition on regional bone mineral density in healthy women aged 60 and older. *Gerontology* 2001;47(4):207-12.

[24] Jensen LB, Kollerup G, Quaade F, Sorensen OH. Bone mineral changes in obese women during moderate weight loss with and without calcium supplementation. *J Bone Miner Res* 2001;16(1):141-7

[25] Nelson LR, Bulun SE. Estrogen production and action. *J Am Acad Dermatol* 2001; 5(Suppl 3): 116-24

[26] Blain H, Vuillemin A, Guillemin F, Durant R, Hanesse B, de Talance N, Doucet B, Jeandel C. Serum leptin level is a predictor of bone mineral density in postmenopausal women. *J Clin Endocrinol Metab* 2002;87(3):1030-5

[27] Ensrud KE, Ewing SK, Stone KL, Cauley JA, Bowman JP, Cummings SR. Intentional and unintentional weight loss increase bone loss and hipfracture risk in older women. *J Am Geriatr Soc* 2003:51(12);1740-7.

[28] Ensrud KE, Lipschutz RC, Cauley JA, Seeley D, Nevitt MC, Scott J, Orwoll ES, Genant HK, Cummings SR. Body size and hip fracture risk in older women: a prospective study. Study of Osteoporotis Fractures Research Group. *Am J Med* 1997a;103(4):274-80

[29] Huopio J, Kröger H, Honkanen R, Saarikoski S, Alhava E. Risk factors for perimenopausal fractures: a prospective study. *Osteoporos Int* 2000;11(3):219-27

[30] Margolis KL, Ensrud KE, Schreiner PJ, Tabor HK. Body size and risk for clinical fractures in older women. Study of Osteoporotic Fractures Study Group. *Ann Intern Med* 2000;133(2):123-7

[31] Langlois JA, Harris T, Looker AC, Madans J. Weight change between age 50 years and old age is associated with risk of hip fracture in white women aged 67 years and older. *Arch Intern Med* 1996;156(9):989-94

[32] Ensrud KE, Cauley JA, Lipschutz RC, Cummings SR. Weight change and fractures in older women. Study of Osteoporotic Fractures Research Group. *Arch Intern Med* 1997b;157(8):857-63

[33] Ravn P, Cizza G, Bjarnason NH, Thompson D, Daley M, Wasnich RD, McClung M, Hosking D, Yates AJ, Christiansen C. Low body mass index is an important risk factor for low bone mass and increased bone loss in early postmenopausal women. Early Postmenopausal Intervention Cohort (EPIC) study group. *J Bone Miner Res* 1999;14(9):1622-7

[34] Rico H, Arribas I, Casanova FJ, Duce AM, Hernandez ER, Cortes-Prieto J. Bone mass, bone metabolism, gonadal status and body mass index. *Osteoporos Int* 2002;13(5):379-87

[35] Papakitsou EF, Margioris AN, Dretakis KE, Trovas G, Zoras U, Lyritis G, Dretakis EK, Stergiopoulos K. Body mass index (BMI) and parameters of bone formation and resorption in postmenopausal women. *Maturitas* 2004;47(3):185-93

[36] Wildner M, Peters A, Raghuvanshi VS, Hohnloser J, Soebert U. Superiority of age and weight as variables in predicting osteoporosis in postmenopausal white women. *Osteoporos Int* 2003;14(11):950-6

[37] Michaelsson K, Bergström R, Mallmin H, Holmberg L, Wolk A, Ljunghall S. Screening for osteopenia and osteoporosis: selection by body composition. *Osteoporos Int* 1996;6:120-126

[38] Weinstein L, Ullery B. Identification of at-risk women for osteoporosis screening. *Am J Obstet Gynecol* 2000;183:547-549

[39] Cadarette SM, Jaglal SB, Murray TM, McIsaac WJ, Joseph L, Brown JP. Evaluation of decision rules for referring women for bone densitometry by dual-energy x-ray absorptiometry. *JAMA* 2001;286:57-63

[40] National Osteoporosis Foundation. Osteoporosis: review of the evidence for prevention, diagnosis, and treatment and cost-effectiveness analysis-status report. *Osteoporosis Int* 1998;8 (suppl 4):S1-S88

[41] Chen Z, Lohman TG, Stini WA, Ritenbaugh C, Aickin M. Fat or lean tissue mass: which one is the major determinant of bone mineral mass in healthy postmenopausal women ? *J Bone Miner Res* 1997;12(1):144-51

[42] Blain H, Carrire I, Favier F, Jeandel C, Papoz L. Body weight change since menopause and percentage body mass are predictors of subsequent bone mineral density change of the proximal femur in women aged 75 years and older: results of a 5 year propective study. *Calcif Tissue Int* 2004;75:32-39

[43] Glauber HS, Vollmer WM, Nevitt MC, Ensrud KE, Orwoll ES. Body weight versus body fat distribution, adiposity, and frame size as predictors of bone density. *J Clin Endocrinol Metab* 1995;80(4):1118-23

[44] Harris SS, Dawson-Hughes B. Weight, body composition, and bone density in postmenopausal women. *Calcif Tissue Int* 1996;59(6):428-32

[45] Frost HM. Bone "mass" and the "mechanostat": a proposal. *Anat Rec* 1987;219:1-9

[46] Lanyon LE. Osteocytes, strain detection, bone modelling and remodelling. *Calcif tissue Int* 1993;53:S102-7

[47] Rodan GA. Bone mass homeostasis and bisphosphonate action. *Bone* 1997;20:1-4

[48] Cifuentes M, Johnson MA, Lewis RD, Heymsfield SB, Chowdhury HA, Modelsky CM, Shapses SA. Bone turnover and body weight relationships differ in normal-weight compared with heavier postmenopausal women. *Osteoporos Int* 2003;14(2):116-22

[49] MacDonald HM, New SA, Cambell MK, Reid DM. Influence of weight and weight change on bone loss in perimenopausal and early postmenopausal Scottish women. *Osteoporos Int* 2004;DOI 10.1007/s00198-004-1657-7

[50] Thomas T. Leptin:a potential mediator for protective effects of fat mass on bone tissue. *Joint Bone Spine* 2003;70(1):18-21

[51] Hamrick MW. Leptin, bone mass, and the thrifty phenotype. *J Bone Miner Res* 2004;19(10):1607-11

[52] Jensen LB, Kollerup G, Quaade F, Sorensen OH. Bone minerals changes in obese women during moderate weight loss with and without calcium supplementation. J Bone Miner Res 2001; 16(1):141-7

[53] Pasco J, hentry M, Kotowicz M, Collier G, Ball M, Ugoni A, Nicholson G. Serum leptin levels are associated with bone mass in nonobese women. *J Clin Endocrinol Metab* 2001;86:1884-1887

[54] Yamauchi M, Sugimoto T, Yamaguchi T, Nakaoka D, Kanzawa M, Yano S, Ozuru R, Sugishita T, Chihara K. Plasma leptin concentrations are associated with bone mineral density and the presence of vertebral fractures in postmenopausal women. *Clin Endocrinol* 2001; 55(3): 341-7

[55] Blain H, Vuillemin A, Guillemin F, Durant R, Hanesse B, de Talance N, Doucet B, Jeandel C. Serum leptin is a predictor of bone mineral density in postmenopausal women. *J Clin Endocrinol Metab* 2002;87:1030-5

[56] Blum M, Harris S, Must A, Naumova E, Phillips S, Rand W, Dawson-Hughes B. Leptin, body composition, and bone mineral density in postmenopausal women. *Calcif Tissue Int* 2003;73:27-32

[57] Roux C, Arabi A, Porcher R, Garner P. Serum leptin as a determinant of bone resorption in healthy postmenopausal women. *Bone* 2003;33:847-52

[58] Goulding A, taylor RW. Plasma leptin values in relation to bone mass and density and to dynamic biochemical markers of bone resorption and formation in postmenopausal women. *Calcif tissue Int* 1998;63(6):456-8

[59] Shaarawy M, Abassi AF, Hassan H, Salem ME. Relationship between serum leptin concentrations and bone mineral density as well as biochemical markers of bone turnover in women with postmenopausal osteoporosis. *Sertil Steril* 2003;79(4):919-24

[60] Steppan C, Crawford T, Chidsey-Frink K, Ke H, Swick A. Leptin is a potent stimulator of bone growth in ob/ob mice. *Regul Pept* 2000;92:73-8

[61] Cornish J, Callon K, bava U, Lin C, Naot D, Hill B, Grey A, Broom N, Myers D, Nicholson G, Reid I. Leptin directly regulates bone cell function in vitro and reduces bone fragility in vivo. *J Endocrinol* 2002;175:405-15

[62] Ducy P, Amling M, Takeda S, Priemel M, Schilling A, Beil F, Shen J, Vinson C, Rueger J, Karsenty G. Leptin inhibits bone formation through a hypothalamic relay: a central control of bone mass. *Cell* 2000;100:197-207

[63] Karsenty G. Leptin controls bone formation through a hypothalamic relay. *Recen Prog Horm Res* 2001;56:401-15

[64] Cifuentes M, Riedt CS, Brolin RE, Field MP, Sherrel RM, Shapses SA. Weight loss and calcium intake influence calcium absorption in overweight postmenopausal women. *Am J Clin Nutr* 2004;80(1):123-30

[65] Atkinson R, Dahms W, Bray G, Schwarz A. Parathyroid hormone levels in obesity. *Miner Electrolyte Metab* 1978;1:315-20

[66] Andersen T, McNair P, Hyldstrup L, Fogh-Andersen N, Nielsen T, Astrup A, Transbol I. Secondary hyperparathyroidism of morbid obesity regresses during weight reduction. *Metabolism* 1988;37:425-8

[67] Ricci TA, Chowdhury HA, Heymsfield SB, Stahl T, Pierson RN jr, Shapses SA. Calcium supplementation suppresses bone turnover during weight reduction in postmenopausal women. *J Bone Miner Res* 1998;13:1045-1050

[68] Bolotin HH. A new perspective on the causal influence of soft tissue composition on DXA-measured in vivo bone mineral density. *J Bone Miner Res* 1998;13:1739-1746

[69] Bolotin HH, Sievänen H, Grashuis JL, Kuiper JW, Jarvinen TL. Inaccuracies inherent in patient-specific dual-energy X-ray absorptiometry bone mineral density measurements: comprehensive phantom-based evaluation. *J Bone Miner Res* 2001;16:417-26

[70] Blake GM, Herd RJ, Patel R, Fogelman I. The effect of weight change on total body dual-energy X-ray absorptiometry: results from a clinical trial. *Osteoporos Int* 2000;11(10):832-9

[71] Srinivasan SR, Bao W, Wattigney WA, Berenson GS. Adolescent overweight is associated with adult overweight and related cardiovascular risk factors: the Bogalusa Heart Study. *Metabolism* 1996;45(2):235-40

[72] Rea TD, Heckbert SR, Kaplan RC, Psaty BM, Smith NL, Lemaitre RN, Lin D.Body mass index and the risk of recurrent coronary events following acute myocardial infarction. *Am J Cardiol* 2001;88(5):467-72.

[73] Honkanen R, Tuppurainen M, Alhava E, Saarikoski S. Kuopio Osteoporosis Risk Factor and Prevention Study. Baseline postal inquiry in 1989. Publications of the University of Kuopio, Community Health, Statistics and Reviews 3/1991; *Kuopio* 1991.

[74] Sirola J, Kröger H, Honkanen R, Jurvelin JS, Sandini L, Tuppurainen M, Saarikoski S. Smoking may impair the bone protective effects of nutritional calcium- a population based approach. *J Bone Miner Res* 2003c; 18: 1036-1043

[75] WHO Scientific Group. Research on the menopause in the 1990's. *A report of the WHO Scientific Group*. World Health Organisation, Geneva, Switzerland. 1996;866:1-79.

[76] Kröger H, Heikkinen J, Laitinen K, Kotaniemi A. Dual-energy X-ray absorptiometry in normal women: a cross-sectional study of 717 Finnish volunteers. *Osteoporosis Int* 1992;2(3):135-140.

[77] Komulainen MH, Kröger H, Tuppurainen MT, Heikkinen A-M, Alhava E, Honkanen R, Saarikoski S. HRT and vit D in prevention of non-vertebral fractures in postmenopausal women; a 5 year randomised trial. *Maturitas* 1998;31:45-54

In: Weight Loss, Exercise and Health Research
Editor: Carrie P. Saylor, pp. 71-97

ISBN 1-60021-077-5
© 2006 Nova Science Publishers, Inc.

Chapter 5

A SIGNAL DETECTION APPROACH TO GROUPING PARTICIPANTS FOR TAILORED WORK-SITE WEIGHT-LOSS PROGRAMS

Akihito Hagihara[1]

Department of Health Services Management and Policy, Graduate School of Medicine,
Kyushu University, 3-1-1 Maidashi, Higashi-ku, Fukuoka, 812-8582, Japan

ABSTRACT

Although numerous work-site obesity prevention programs have been widely promoted thus far, majority of them have been unsuccessful. Problems of the previous programs are as follows. (1) Programs have a high rate of attrition. (2) Participants find it very difficult to maintain the decreased weight. (3) Many participants feel that the programs are not fit for them. These problems imply that it is necessary to develop effective work-site programs that match the type of intervention to the participants and offer the necessary support. In this article, I will introduce a new approach to grouping participants for tailored work-site weight loss programs. Specifically, based upon the signal detection analysis, higher-order interaction of the causal factors of obesity are analyzed.

The subjects were male, white-collar workers (20 to 64 years of age), in Osaka, Japan. Since conventional methods, such as regression analysis or analysis of variance, cannot deal with the interaction of many variables, signal detection analysis by Kraemer was used to identify the higher-order interaction of multiple predictors of obesity.

Out of 15 independent variables, a higher-order interaction consisting of 8 significant variables was identified. Consequently, the subjects were categorized into nine subgroups. It was revealed that the obesity of two groups of workers, 40 or more years old with a high degree of obesity, had different causes: one was related to working conditions, and one was related to smoking cessation. For the other terminal groups, further factors related to obesity were revealed.

---

[1] Address for correspondence: Akihito Hagihara, DMSc, MPH, Department of Health Services Management and Policy, Kyushu University Graduate School of Medicine, Higashi-ku, Fukuoka, 812-8582, Japan, E-mail: hagihara@hsmp.med.kyushu-u.ac.jp

Although the applicability of the findings is limited, the methodology using signal detection analysis might be applicable to other weight loss programs as a way of facilitating the matching of the type of intervention and the target group. To verify the efficacy of this approach to grouping participants for tailored work-site weight loss programs, an intervention study for weight loss will be necessary.

Keywords: work-site, weight loss, programs, signal detection analysis

I.   INTRODUCTION

The conditions of being obese or overweight are rapidly spreading global health problems. A recent survey estimated that one in every two adults in the USA is either overweight or obese, which represents an increase in 25% over the last three decades [Flegal et al., 1998]. In the UK, the prevalence of obesity has more than doubled between 1980 and 1993, a trend that is similar for both men and women of all age groups [Pirozzo et al., 2003]. Being obese or overweight contributes to an ever-increasing disease burden. Excessive body weight is related to an increased risk of heart disease [Nubert et al., 1983], non-insulin-dependent diabetes mellitus [US Department of Health, Education and Welfare, 1975; Kannel et al., 1979; Garfinkle, 1985], hypertension [Stamler et al., 1978; Garrison et al., 1987], colorectal, prostate, breast, and endometrial cancer [Garfinkle, 1985], and osteoarthritis [Bray, 1985]. Although genetic susceptibility plays a role [Perusse and Bouchard, 2000], more important factors are thought to be the widespread reduction in physical activity and the availability of affordable energy-dense food, especially fatty foods. Thus the prevention and treatment of obesity often requires a reduction of fatty-food intake and increased physical activity. It is of general concern to determine how to help weight-loss program participants acquire these preferable health behaviors. Before discussing the signal detection approach to grouping participants for tailored intervention programs, previous findings concerning weight loss intervention are summarized in the next section.

WEIGHT-LOSS INTERVENTION FOCUSED ON PHYSICAL ACTIVITY AND FATTY FOODS

Several problems have been reported with intervention programs geared toward increasing the level of physical activity or decreasing the intake of fatty foods. Findings regarding increased physical activity are not consistent. Some studies have reported that a large amount of physical activity predicts a smaller weight change (less increase in weight), implying that physical activity is effective in preventing weight gain [Klesges et al., 1992; Owens et al., 1992; Haapanen et al., 1997]. Klesges and colleagues [1992] also reported that high baseline physical activity was associated with lower weight gain at a later point in time, although Haapanen et al. [1997] found that this correlation held only for men, not for women. In contrast, other studies have reported that a large amount of vigorous physical activity at baseline was associated with greater weight gain at a later point in time [Klesges et al., 1992; Bild et al., 1996]. The Bangkok Consensus Meeting in 2002 issued the following guidelines

[Saris et al., 2003]: (1) At least 30 minutes of physical activity of moderate intensity per day are important for reducing the risks of a number of chronic diseases, including diabetes and coronary heart disease. (2) To prevent weight gain or regain, 60-90 minutes of physical activity pre day are required. The guidelines also emphasized, however, that since the social environment can present barriers to regularly obtaining the recommended level of physical activity, political actions will be required. These guidelines indicate that engaging in regular physical activity is a complex problem with implications ranging from health sciences to politics.

Findings are also inconsistent for weight-loss intervention programs focused on reducing the intake of fatty foods. The most recent review [Avenell et al., 2004] reported that low-fat diets resulted in significant weight loss up to 36 months, and that blood pressure, blood lipids after fasting, and plasma glucose improved with low-fat diets after 12 months. The study concluded that little evidence supports the use of diets other than low-fat diets for weight reduction. On the other hand, a systematic review of randomized controlled trials to evaluate the effectiveness of low-fat diets in achieving sustained weight loss found no significant difference between low-fat diets and other weight-reducing diets in terms of sustained weight loss [Pirozzo et al., 2003]. Although differences between these two studies, such as the length of intervention, nationality of participants, key words, and types of database used, must be taken into consideration, it appears that interventions geared at reducing fatty food intake are not always effective in reducing weight.

Work-Site Weight-Reduction Intervention Programs

To reach a wider range of participants, the workplace has been considered a potentially effective place for obesity prevention. Merits include easy access to a large audience, a high level of participation, cost-effectiveness, the potential for social support from colleagues or management [Jeffery, 1993], and the potential for cost recovery by companies through lower health-care expenditures [Fielding, 1990]. In addition, it is believed that work-site programs ultimately contribute to increased productivity, increased employee morale and job commitment, and reduced employee absenteeism and turnover [Sapolsky, 1981; Weinstein, 1983; Foshee et al., 1986].

Obesity prevention programs at the work site can be categorized into three groups: (1) behavior modification programs [Anderson et al., 1993], (2) hybrid programs [Lasater et al., 1991], and (3) self-help programs [Cameron et al., 1990]. The results of work-site weight-loss programs have not been very impressive [Dishman et al., 1998]. The largest problem is the high attrition rate of participants [Fielding, 1990]. Dropout rates from work-site weight-loss programs have been reported to range from 0.5 to 80% [Jeffery et al., 1993] and are greater than those of non-work-site programs [Fielding, 1990]. These high attrition rates make work-site programs less cost-effective [Jeffery, 1995]. The second-largest problem is that participants in work-site programs do not maintain their decreased body weights over the long term [Battle and Brownell, 1996; Hennrikus and Jeffery, 1996]. In addition, a history of previous participation in a weight-loss program has been shown to be positively related to an increase in body weight in later years, although this finding is not limited to work-site programs [Hennrikus and Jeffery, 1996; Shah et al., 1993; French et al., 1994]. In summary, work-site obesity prevention programs are largely ineffective, given that an adequate conceptual model has not been devised, a high rate of attrition is always observed, and participants find it very difficult to maintain their decreased weight [Battle and Brownell,1996].

EFFICACY OF TAILORED INTERVENTION

As indicated, numerous problems have been identified with weight-loss intervention programs that increase physical activity or decrease dietary fat intake. In addition, although the workplace should be an effective place for obesity prevention, the effects of work-site weight-loss interventions are limited. However, tailoring programs for participants may be an effective way to overcome the problems discussed above. In tailored interventions, the types of intervention and necessary support are matched to the participants, which can thus render intervention programs more effective, with lower attrition rates. Theoretically, tailored interventions should have the greatest advantage when there is significant variability within the target population in the key determinants of an intended outcome [Kreuter and Wray, 2003]. These determinants may include such factors as knowledge, beliefs, and behaviors. Because determinants of behaviors like altering dietary fat consumption, increasing physical activity, and ceasing tobacco use vary widely among adult subjects, the process of tailoring should make more messages more relevant to more people than would targeted messages [Kreuter et al., 1999; Kreuter and Wray, 2003].

How does tailoring work? According to the elaboration likelihood model (ELM), people are more likely to actively and thoughtfully process information when they are motivated and able to do so [Petty and Cacioppo, 1981]. The perceived personal relevance of the message is one of the most important determinants of motivation. The ELM is based upon the premise that people can be active information processors, i.e., considering messages carefully, relating them to other information they have encountered, and comparing them to their own past experience, when they are motivated and able [Cook and Flay, 1978; Petty, 1977]. It has also been verified that messages processed in the "elaborated" fashion tend to be retained for a longer time and are more likely to lead to enduring attitude and behavior changes [Cook and Flay, 1978; Petty, 1977].

Concomitantly, studies have reported associations between tailoring and participant satisfaction [Dale et al., 1999; Leighl et al., 2001], and between participant satisfaction and reduced dropout rates from programs [Steel et al., 2000; Ziguras and Stuart, 2000]. Thus, it is hypothesized that tailoring programs leads to increased participant satisfaction, which results in a lower dropout rate and more effective intervention.

TRANSTHEORETICAL MODEL

Weight-loss interventions based upon Prochaska's Transtheoretical Model (TM) are typical examples of tailored interventions [Prochaska et al, 1995]. According to the TM, the process of behavior change is conceptualized as a passage through a series of distinct stages (Fig. 1). The earliest stage of change is "precontemplation". In this stage, individuals are unaware of their health problems and do not intend to make any changes to their lifestyle (e.g., quitting smoking, doing more physical exercise, decreasing fatty food intake). The second stage is "contemplation", in which individuals become aware of their problems. Although they are seriously thinking of solving their problems, they have not yet made a commitment to take action. The third stage is "preparation". Individuals in this stage have decided to take action, and are preparing to change their lifestyles. The fourth and fifth stages are "action" and "maintenance". The stages are distinguished by increasingly more definitive and stable behavioral and cognitive changes that overcome or replace the problem behaviors [Prochaska et al., 1995; Prochaska and DiClemente, 1984, DiClemente et al., 1991].

According to the TM, different therapeutic interventions that depend upon the stage of change of a participant are more effective than a uniform intervention for all participants [Sutton et al., 2003; Prochaska et al., 1988; Ruggiero et al., 1997]. Other studies have reported that such tailoring of intervention leads to enhanced patient progress and a more effective use of therapeutic resources [Prochaska et al., 1993; Velicer et al., 1999]. It is obvious that an accurate assessment of the stage of change is a prerequisite to effective tailoring of intervention. However, potential problems in the accurate assessment of the stage of change have been raised. With respect to dietary behaviors, (1) participants may be unable to remember or unwilling to report their intake accurately, (2) participants may misunderstand global labels such as "low-fat diet", and (3) participants may lack knowledge of the nutrient content of their diet [Bull et al., 2001; Sternfield et al., 1999; Masse et al., 1998; Eyler et al., 1998]. To increase the accuracy of assessing the stage of change, Sutton et al. [2003] used a multi-item algorithm for weight loss-related behaviors, which they concluded was a better guide for matching treatment to stage.

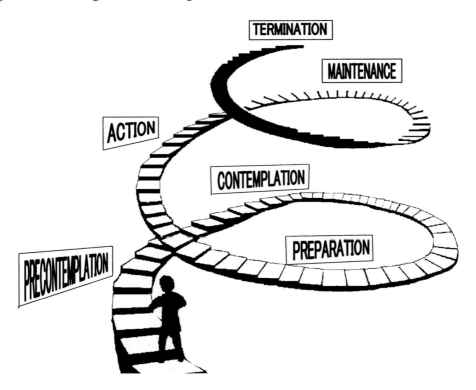

Figure 1. Prochaska's "stages of change", modified from Prochaska et al. [1995, p49].

II.   TAILORED WORK-SITE INTERVENTIONS BASED UPON A SIGNAL DETECTION APPROACH (SDA)

Background and Aim of the Study

The effects of weight-loss intervention programs focused upon physical activity and fatty foods are limited, although tailored interventions seem to be a promising approach to improve their efficacy. It is imperative for tailored interventions to accurately assess the stage of change of participants, and multiple factors may need to be considered for the accurate assessment of the stage of change. Currently, however, no effective methodology for considering multiple factors simultaneously has been established.

In light of these considerations, a tailored work-site intervention based upon a signal detection approach (SDA) may be effective. In such programs, identification of groups with shared causal risk factors for obesity is a prerequisite. To this end, it is necessary to analyze the higher-order interactions of causal factors, including personal attributes, personal health practices, and working conditions, which are thought to contribute to the incidence of obesity among employees. In other words, the causes of obesity vary for groups of people, as defined by lifestyle and working conditions. For example, excessive alcohol consumption may be a cause of obesity among middle-aged workers who have quit smoking, while it may not be a cause among younger workers who have quit smoking. If we can identify participants based on the higher-order interactions of multiple variables related to obesity, we can facilitate matching them with types of intervention and necessary support, and thus develop more effective programs with lower attrition rates. In studying obesity, multiple regression analysis and analysis of variance (ANOVA) conventionally use the degree of obesity as the dependent variable, and potential factors as independent variables. However, these methods are not useful in dealing with the higher-order interaction of variables. The practical number of factors is limited to three or four in an ANOVA, above which the cell size becomes very small and the interpretation of higher-order interactions becomes very confusing. When higher-order interactions of variables are evaluated within the framework of multiple regression analysis, there is usually a problem with multi-colinearity, and the interpretation of the interaction is again very confusing.

To tailor weight-loss programs, we need to identify subgroups with shared causal risk factors for the incidence of obesity by analyzing higher-order interactions of causal factors of obesity. There are 32,767 ($=_{15}C_1 + _{15}C_2 + \ldots + _{15}C_{14} + _{15}C_{15}$) possible combinations of the 15 variables in Table 1. Conventional methods cannot deal with this many possible combinations of variables. In addition, since a simple "prescription" to prevent obesity is needed, the importance of identifying easily described predictors of obesity has come to be recognized recently [French et al., 1994; Kahn et al., 1997]. There are several other statistical methods, including discriminant analysis, cluster analysis, and structural equation modeling. These analyses try to summarize information based on a key parameter, such as the discriminant score, association measure, or latent variable. However, these statistical methods do not necessarily produce objective, easily described predictors of obesity. Nor do they explain how the higher-order interaction of independent variables affects the incidence of obesity. Since signal detection analysis recursively reveals the strongest interaction of factors among groups based upon the largest chi-square statistics, subgroups with a shared causal risk for obesity are eventually produced. Thus, signal detection analysis produces information useful for tailored work-site intervention.

If we can analyze how lifestyle or work environment factors selectively interact to affect the incidence of obesity using easily described predictors, the following useful results are expected. (1) Based on a group of people isolated by predictors of obesity, we can facilitate matching the type of intervention and the necessary support. (2) Consequently, we can develop more effective intervention programs with low attrition rates. To our knowledge, no studies have evaluated how higher-order interaction factors interact to produce obesity. Therefore, in this study, we use the signal detection analysis approach advocated by Kraemer [Kraemer, 1988; Kraemer, 1992; Winkleby et al., 1994] to isolate subjects with multiple predictors of obesity as a prerequisite for developing tailored work-site weight loss programs. In the analysis, variables concerning personal health practices and working conditions are described in a simple manner. We then explore the complex interactions of personal health practices or working conditions and obesity, which otherwise might not be fully revealed.

METHODS

Subjects

The subjects of this study were Japanese male white-collar workers (20 to 64 years of age) who worked at the head office of one of Japan's leading steel companies in Osaka, Japan. Since the Japanese Labor Act mandates an annual health check for company employees, the company's occupational health workers were able to make use of this opportunity and collect data concerning personal health practices, working conditions, work stresses, and anthropometric measures (e.g., body weight and height). Relevant data were collected from 405 (87.1%) of all the male subjects (n = 465) during their annual health check in July 1997 using a self-administered questionnaire to evaluate personal health practices, work stress, and personal attributes. The analysis used the 398 responses that had no missing data.

Variables

The body mass index (BMI) (weight[kg]/height[m]^2) was used as the dependent variable. Obesity was defined as a BMI $\geq$ 24, the criterion advocated for Japanese male adults [Kataoka, 1989]. The rest of the variables in Table 1 were independent variables. The personal health practices numbered 5, 6, 7, 8, 11, 12, and 13 in Table 1 have been shown to be related to the physical health status of Japanese people [Morimoto, 1991]. In order to cover a wider range of potential predictors of obesity, in addition to these fundamental variables, Table 1 includes variables concerning age (No. 1), position in the office (No. 2), lifestyle (No. 3), marital status (No. 4), diet (Nos. 9 and 10), and working conditions (Nos. 14 and 15). In particular, this study used the subjective psychological stressors for working conditions, "job demand" and "decision latitude", advocated by Karasek [Karasek and Theorell, 1990; Tarumi et al, 1993]. "Job demand" is a measure of the degree of job demand (Cronbach's α = 0.80), and "decision latitude" is a measure of the degree of decision authority and skill discretion (Cronbach's α = 0.71). The score for job demand ranged between 1 and 3, and a higher score indicated a higher job demand. The score for decision latitude ranged between 1 and 6, and a higher score indicated more decision latitude. According to the methods of Karasek, a decision latitude score equal to or higher than the mean was regarded as a high decision latitude, while a job demand score equal to or higher than the mean was regarded as a high job demand [Karasek and Theorell, 1990; Tarumi et al, 1993]. According to Karasek's model, job strain is measured by the combination of job demand and decision latitude. However, job demand and decision latitude were individually used as a work stress measure in the present study.

Statistical Procedures

In order to examine how the individual personal health practices and working conditions listed in Table 1 interact to lead to obesity in male workers, the signal detection analysis method of Kraemer was used [Kraemer, 1988; Kraemer, 1992; Winkleby et al., 1994]. Signal detection analysis has been performed as a form of recursive partitioning, and has provided useful results, especially when many interactions are expected [Kraemer, 1988]. We are indebted to Kraemer for the model, which focuses on the parameters of *sensitivity* and *specificity*. Briefly, *sensitivity* is defined as the probability of obesity (BMI $\geq$ 24) among individuals with unfavorable personal health practices or working conditions [Morimoto, 1991; Karasek and Theorell, 1990; Tarumi et al., 1993; Minkler, 1999]. *Specificity* is defined as the probability of non-obesity (BMI < 24) among those without those unfavorable personal health practices or working conditions. The selection of a variable significantly related to obesity should be based on a measure that includes both *sensitivity* and *specificity*. Kraemer advocates that such an optimal measure approximates the chi-square distribution whose degree of freedom (*df*) is one [Kraemer, 1988; Kraemer, 1992; Winkleby et al., 1994].

$$\chi^2 = n \times [(SE-Q)/Q'] \times [(SP-Q')/Q] \ (df = 1)$$

where, n = sample size, SE = sensitivity, SP = specificity, Q = (the number of "obesity" cases) / n, Q' = 1-Q.

This signal detection parameter is equivalent to the chi-square statistics (*df* = 1), which means that the subjects are categorized into a 2 × 2 table consisting of dependent and independent variables. When the parameter reports the largest chi-square value (*df* = 1), the variable and its cutoff point in the equation is the best predictor of obesity. Since the chi-square value is largest, this variable and its cutoff point divide the population into two subgroups that are mutually and exclusively discriminated from each other.

Therefore, the dependent variable (obesity) and the independent variables in Table 1 were entered into the model along with minimal and maximal values and intermediate cutoff points. As shown in Table 1, the variables had one to seven cutoff points. For example, "lifestyle" (living alone, living with someone), "decision latitude" ($\geq$mean, <mean), and "job demand" ($\geq$mean, <mean) have one cutoff point. "Smoking" has two cutoff points (current smokers, ex-smokers, never-smokers); "marital status" (married, single, separated, divorced)

and "sleeping hours" ($\leqq 5h$, 6h, 7h, 8h) have three cutoff points; and "physical exercise" (none, less than twice per month, once per week, twice per week, three times per week or more often) and "working hours" ($\leqq 8h$, 9h, 10h, 11h, 12h or longer) have four cutoff points. Finally, "age" has 7 cutoff points, every fifth year between 20 and 64 years.

With respect to the probability of obesity (BMI$\geqq$ 24), based upon the largest chi-square measure, the algorithm for the signal detection model checked every variable in Table 1 and the possible cutoff points to determine the optimally efficient variable and its cutoff point. After the signal detection algorithm selects the first optimally efficient variable along with its cutoff point, which is the largest chi-square value, the signal detection program begins to look for the next optimally efficient variable and its cutoff point separately in each of the newly divided subgroups. This procedure is repeated separately for all the remaining variables until one of the following happens [Winkleby, 1994]: (1) no further predictors exist in a newly formed subgroup, (2) no more significant variables are detected at a level of $p < 0.05$, or (3) the number of subjects in the newly divided group becomes too small ($n \leqq 10$).

In summary, based upon the probability of obesity (BMI$\geqq$ 24), we used this method and the personal health practices, work stress variables, and personal attribute variables listed in Table 1 to divide the study population into subgroups that were maximally discriminated from each other and mutually exclusive.

To facilitate interpretation of the results obtained in this study, a profile of each group identified by the signal detection analysis is provided. Specifically, after a whole population was categorized into several subgroups by signal detection analysis, newly divided subgroups were compared in terms of study variables. Categorical or continuous variables were compared by the chi-square test or one-way ANOVA.

RESULTS

Table 1 lists the prevalence of the personal health practices, work stress variables, and personal attribute variables for all the subjects. The mean age of the subjects was 40.96 ($\pm$ 9.33) years, and the mean daily number of working hours was 9.47 ($\pm$ 1.33) hours.

Figure 2 shows the results of an optimally efficient algorithm for identifying distinct subgroups of the subjects (n = 398) based on the probability of obesity. As shown in the figure, 37.4% were obese (BMI$\geqq$ 24). The optimally efficient variable that distinguished between those who were obese and those who were not was the age of the subjects ["age", $x^2 = 8,60$ ($p - 0.003$)]. Of the workers aged 40 or older, 43.6% were obese, while only 29.2% of those younger than 40 were obese. Next, we focused exclusively on detecting the optimally

Table 1. Profiles of the subjects (n = 398)

	Number of categories (number of cutoff points)	
(Independent variables)		
1. Age (mean ± SD) (yr.)	8 (7)	40.96 ± 9.33
2. Work status in office	4 (3)	
Staff member /lower level manager		190 (47.7%)
Middle/upper level manager		208 (52.3%)
3. Lifestyle	2 (1)	
Lives alone		118 (29.7%)
Lives with someone		280 (70.4%)
4. Marital status	4 (3)	
Married		313 (78.7%)
Single/separated/divorced		85 (21.4%)
5. Physical exercise	5 (4)	
None/less than twice per month		260 (65.3%)
Once/ twice/ three times per week or more often		138 (34.7%)
6. Smoking	3 (2)	
Current smoker		172 (43.2%)
Ex-smoker		79 (19.8%)
Never smoked		147 (36.9%)
7. Breakfast	3 (2)	
Every morning		319 (80.2%)
Sometimes does not eat		79 (19.8%)
8. Nutritional balance of meals	3 (2)	
Attentive		149 (37.4%)
Somewhat attentive/never attentive		249 (62.6%)
9. Frequent intake of salty foods	2 (1)	
Yes		170 (42.7%)
No		228 (57.3%)
10. Frequent intake of vegetables or fruit	2 (1)	
Yes		313 (78.6%)
No		85 (21.4%)
11. Alcohol consumption	3 (2)	
Almost everyday/4 or 5 days per week		224 (56.3%)
2 or 3 days per week or less		174 (43.7%)
12. Sleeping hours	4 (3)	
7h/8h		164 (41.2%)
5h or less/6h		234 (58.8%)
13. Working hours (mean ± SD) (min.)	5 (4)	9.47±1.33
14. Decision latitude	2 (1)	2.12±0.67
15. Job demand	2 (1)	1.41±1.43
(Dependent variables)		
16. BMI (mean ± SD)		23.41±2.91

efficient variable among workers at least 40 years old that distinguished between those who were obese and those who were not. The subject's position in the company ("work status") was the best predictor (χ^2=6.99, p = 0.01). This variable divided the group into two groups: one consisting of upper and middle level managers and the other of lower level managers and staff members; 60.9% of the former and 39.2% of the latter were obese. The optimally efficient variable that distinguished between those who were obese and those who were not in the group consisting of upper and middle level managers was the intake of vegetables and fruit ("vegetable and fruit intake") (p = 0.02). This variable divided the group into two groups: those who ate vegetables and fruit frequently (Group 1) and those who did not (Group 4). In Group 1, 73.3% of the workers were obese (BM I$\geq$ 24). In Group 4, 37.5% of the workers were obese (BMI$\geq$ 24).

Among lower level managers and staff members who were 40 or more years old, the optimally efficient variable that distinguished between those who were obese and those who were not was the number of sleeping hours ("sleeping hours") (χ^2=4.43, p = 0.04). This variable divided the group into two groups: those who slept for 7 or 8 hours (Group 6) and those who slept for 6 hours or less. In Group 6, 31.5% of the workers were obese (BMI$\geq$ 24). Among lower level managers and staff members who were at least 40 years of age and slept 6 hours or less, the optimally efficient variable that distinguished between those who were obese and those who were not was decision latitude ("decision latitude") (χ^2=6.22, p = 0.01). This variable divided the group into those with low decision latitude (Group 7) and those with high decision latitude. Finally, within the high decision latitude group, the best predictor was smoking status ("smoking") (χ^2=5.17, p = 0.02). This variable divided the group into two groups: those who were current smokers (Group 3) and those who were ex-smokers or had never smoked (Group 2). In Groups 2, 3, and 7, the prevalence of obesity (BMI$\geq$ 24) was 69.7, 39.1, and 30.6%, respectively.

Among workers younger than 40, the optimally efficient variable that distinguished between those who were obese and those who were not was nutritional balance ("nutritional balance") (χ^2=5.89, p = 0.02). This variable divided the group into two groups: those with a nutritionally balanced diet and those with a diet that was not nutritionally balanced (Group 5). As shown in Fig. 2, of those who ate a nutritionally balanced diet, the optimally efficient variable that distinguished between those who were obese and those who were not was alcohol consumption ("alcohol consumption", p = 0.03). This variable divided the group into two: those who consumed alcohol at least 4 days per week (Group 8) and those who consumed alcohol less than 4 days per week (Group 9). In Groups 5, 8, and 9, the prevalence of obesity (BMI$\geq$ 24) was 35.9, 30.0, and 8.6%, respectively.

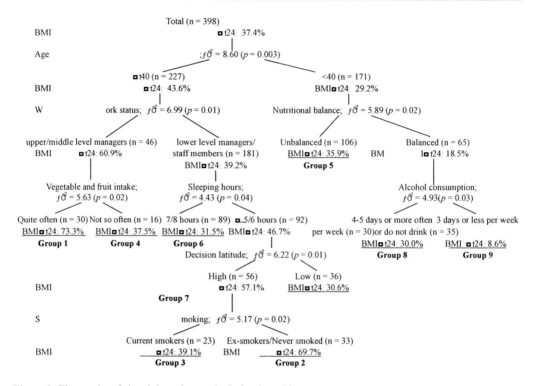

Figure 2. The results of signal detection analysis for the subjects.

Table 2 presents the profiles of the subgroups identified by the signal detection analysis. The terminal groups in Table 2 are numbered in order of descending prevalence of obesity (BMI$\geq$ 24). The mean BMI of the terminal groups only exceeded the criteria value (BMI$\geq$ 24) in three groups (Groups 1, 2, and 3). Although the workers in Group 1 experienced more work stress (i.e., 93.3% had a high job demand; 53.3% had a high decision latitude) compared with the other terminal groups, they tended to have favorable personal health practices, except for "smoking" (36.7%) and "nutritional balance" (36.7%). The mean BMI of the workers in Group 2 was highest among the nine terminal groups (mean = 25.19). The most notable characteristic of this group was that none of the workers smoked: 85.6% were ex-smokers and 14.4% had never smoked. The workers in Group 3 were smokers, and consumed the largest amount of alcohol among the nine terminal groups (252.35 mg of ethanol per week). Their personal health practices seem to be negatively influenced by their heavy drinking. Compared with the rest of the groups, they were more likely to eat nutritionally unbalanced meals (69.6%) and salty foods, typically salty snacks with a drink (60.9%). In addition, only 34.8% of those in Group 3 exercised regularly.

DISCUSSION

In this study, we used the novel method of signal detection analysis. In the following sections, subtitled (1) Characteristics of signal detection analysis and interpretation of the

Table 2 Profiles of nine terminal groups divided by signal detection analysis (n = 398)

	Group1	Group2	Group3	Group4	Group5	Group6	Group7	Group8	Group9	p
1. Age (mean ± SD) (yr.)	49.80±6.21	47.64±4.94	47.09±3.63	47.63±4.83	31.33±4.24	48.30±5.25	47.03±3.43	32.33±6.21	31.69±3.42	0.001
2. Work status in office Upper/middle level managers (%)	100.0	0.0	0.0	100.0	82.1	0.0	0.0	90.0	85.7	0.001
3. Life style Living with someone (%)	93.3	78.8	60.9	75.0	44.3	86.5	80.6	80.0	65.7	0.001
4. Marital status Married (%)	93.3	97.0	91.3	93.8	46.2	95.5	94.4	83.3	65.7	0.001
5. Physical exercise in a week Once/twice/three times or more (%)	60.0	42.4	34.8	37.5	27.4	37.1	44.4	20.0	22.9	0.017
6. Smoking Ex-smoker/never smoked (%)	36.7	100.0	0.0	43.8	52.8	55.1	77.8	63.3	68.6	0.001
7. Breakfast Every morning (%)	83.3	87.9	78.3	87.5	58.5	91.0	94.4	90.0	82.9	0.001
8. Nutritional balance of meals (i.e. excessive meat) Balanced (%)	36.7	45.5	30.4	6.3	0.0	39.3	41.7	100.0	100.0	0.001
9. Frequent intake of salty foods (i.e. salty snack with a drink) Yes (%)	36.7	33.3	60.9	62.5	42.5	44.9	47.2	50.0	20.0	0.045
10. Frequent intake of vegetable or fruits Yes (%)	100.0	93.9	73.9	0.0	61.3	93.3	77.8	93.3	88.6	0.001
11. Alcohol consumption 4-5 days or more often per week	63.3	66.7	69.6	68.8	36.8	65.2	80.6	100.0	0.0	0.001
12. Quantity of ethanol consumed per week (Mean) (mg)	148.3	161.6	252.4	182.6	103.1	182.8	214.5	143.1	51.6	0.001
13. Sleeping hours 7/8 hours (%)	40.0	0.0	0.0	6.3	33.0	100.0	0.0	60.0	25.7	0.001
14. Working hours (Mean ± SD)	9.15±1.38	9.20±1.22	9.61±1.41	10.06±1.57	9.75±1.22	8.92±1.19	9.29±1.07	9.93±1.30	9.94±1.65	0.0001
15. Decision latitude High* (%)	53.3	100.0	100.0	68.8	51.9	61.8	0.0	66.7	60.0	0.001
16. Job demand High** (%)	93.3	75.8	65.2	87.5	62.3	77.5	80.6	63.3	71.4	0.018

Table 2. Profiles of nine terminal groups divided by signal detection analysis (n = 398) - Continued

	Group1	Group2	Group3	Group4	Group5	Group6	Group7	Group8	Group9	p
17. BMI										
≧ 24 (%)	73.3	69.7	39.1	37.5	35.9	31.5	30.6	30.0	8.6	0.001
18. BMI										
(Mean ± SD)	24.48±2.20	25.19±3.10	24.14±1.98	23.20±2.59	23.54±3.11	22.84±3.24	23.20±2.24	22.81±2.89	22.17±1.77	0.0002

*: Score is 2.12 or higher.
**: Score is 1.41 or higher.

One-way ANOVA was used for the continuous variables (nos. 1, 12, 14, and 18) and the chi-square test for the remaining categorical variables.

findings, and (2) Application of the findings to tailored work-site programs, we discuss the important findings of this study and their practical implications.

(1) Characteristics of signal detection analysis and interpretation of the findings

Although signal detection analysis is an analytic technique, this approach can provide information far beyond mere description. The higher-order interaction of predictors revealed in this study implies that the significant variables cause obesity in the group of employees with the specific preceding significant factors. For example, frequent intake of vegetables and fruit is a cause of obesity only for upper and middle level managers who are at least 40 years old, and not for employees younger than 40 (Fig. 2). Except for "age", which is a very significant predictor, the other significant predictors in Fig. 2 contribute to the incidence of obesity only in specific groups of subjects. Therefore, these variables might not be detected as significant within the framework of a multiple regression analysis or ANOVA based on the total sample.

The significant predictors of obesity identified in our study were generally in line with previous findings. It is widely recognized that body weight tends to increase with age in men until the age of at least 55 [Brownell, 1986]. Concomitantly, age was the most significant predictor of obesity among these workers, and 40 years of age was identified as the optimally efficient cutoff point (Fig. 2). Among workers at least 40 years of age, work position was closely related to obesity ($p = 0.01$). Although this study did not examine the work done by upper, middle, and lower level managers and staff members, it is widely recognized that the higher the rank of managers, the more opportunities they have to eat and drink during business-related functions [Hagihara et al., 2000]. We believe that this finding is related to the style of doing business in Japan, but this needs to be verified by future studies. This finding has an important implication for work-site obesity prevention programs for workers in Groups 1 and 4, since their work environment is the true causative agent of obesity, and should be regarded as the logical point of intervention [Battle and Brownell, 1996; Brownell, 1986; Jeffery, 1995]. Therefore, if we can successfully identify problems embedded in the working conditions of upper and middle level managers after evaluating their work, intervention to improve the problems associated with their work habits would be much more efficient than the implementation of conventional weight loss programs. To this end, more studies are required to evaluate the nature of their work, and this is a topic for future study. As for vegetable and fruit intake, those who eat large amounts of fruit and vegetables are more likely to be obese (Fig. 2). There are two possibilities for this finding. First, there could be a confounding effect within the assessed variables because of the hierarchical analysis. Second, this is due to confounding factors that are not assessed, such as that the subjects are trying to lose weight, or that there are unassessed socio-economic factors having an impact here. In order to evaluate the first possibility, multiple regression analysis with BMI as a dependent variable and the independent variables in Table 1, except for Nos. 1 and 2, was performed only among upper/middle level managers (n = 46). However, no independent variables were significant, implying that "vegetable and fruit intake" did not function as a surrogate for another true causal factor. In order to evaluate the second possibility, further studies are necessary.

As for mental health status, although the degree of depression is positively associated with weight gain [Gerace and George, 1996], the association between stress and weight gain is unclear [Ferreira et al., 1995]. Concerning the relationship between smoking status and obesity, many studies have reported that quitting smoking cigarettes leads to an increase in weight [Gerace and George, 1996; Seidell, 1995]. Among lower level managers younger than 40, sleeping hours, decision latitude, and smoking status were significantly related to obesity (Fig. 2). The workers in Groups 3 and 7 consumed more alcohol than workers in the other groups (252.35 and 214.50 mg, respectively) (Table 2). This study identified specific higher-order interactions of these variables, and the process leading to obesity. Quitting cigarettes was only significantly related to weight gain for the workers in Group 2, who had high decision latitude or little mental stress, and relatively few sleeping hours (Fig. 2).

The findings concerning an association between alcohol consumption and weight gain are not consistent, and the relationship between these two factors is unclear [Kahn et al., 1997; Seidell, 1995]. According to our findings, the workers in Group 3 were all smokers, and had unfavorable eating habits, such as nutritionally unbalanced meals and lots of salty foods, together with little physical exercise (Table 2). This indicates that unsatisfactory dietary or physical exercise habits, induced by heavy drinking, might be the cause of weight gain by the workers in Group 3.

Among workers younger than 40 years, nutritional balance and alcohol consumption were predictors of obesity. Here again, the dietary and physical exercise habits induced by heavy drinking might also be a cause of weight gain (Table 2).

(2) Application of the findings to tailored work-site programs

The major problems with work-site programs, that is, high attrition and maintaining decreased weight [Dishman et al., 1998; Jeffery et al., 1993; Jeffery, 1995; Battle and Brownell, 1996; Hennrikus and Jeffery, 1996; Shah et al., 1993; French et al., 1994], seem to result from the way work-site programs are run. Weight loss programs conducted within work-site settings are typically the same for all of the workers voluntarily participating in the programs, and these programs do not take into account the working conditions or lifestyles of the participants. If, for example, a participant exercises regularly, it seems obvious that intervention focused on increased physical exercise would result in the participant dropping out of the program. Intervention emphasizing diet would similarly lead to a high rate of attrition among participants with adequate eating habits. In this regard, some researchers have pointed out that previous work-site programs have not identified the most suitable individuals to target [Jeffery, 1995].

Higher-order interactions of multiple predictors of obesity among white-collar workers were analyzed by signal detection analysis. We also used readily described behaviors as potential predictors of obesity. As hypothesized previously, tailoring programs is supposed to lead to a lower dropout rate from programs via increased participant satisfaction. Concomitantly, previous studies have reported that tailoring the intervention is very effective for improving adherence to programs [Basler, 1995; Fukuda et al., 1996a; Fukuda et al., 1996b].

This study identified eight predictors of obesity. Based on this finding, we isolated three groups of subjects who need obesity prevention intervention. Due to their high prevalence of obesity, when every group cannot be treated because of limited resources, Groups 1, 2, and 4 should be prioritized. Specifically, since the work environment seems to be a causative agent of obesity in Groups 1 and 4 [Battle and Brownell, 1996; Brownell, 1986; Jeffery, 1995], evaluation of their work should be given the first priority in work-site intervention. As for the workers in Group 2, they had quit smoking and felt less work stress; it is very likely that quitting smoking triggered the appetites of most of these workers, formerly suppressed by smoking [Gerace and George, 1996; Seidell, 1995]. Therefore, the workers in this group need to learn about eating habits, such as speed of eating, frequency of meals, content of diet, and techniques to control appetite. As for the workers in Group 3, they were all current smokers, and consumed more alcohol than the workers in the other terminal groups (Table 2). Since their obesity was derived from unfavorable eating or exercise habits, induced by smoking or heavy drinking, smoking cessation and alcohol control should be prioritized in intervention in this group. For the workers in Group 5, the rate of those who were married was lowest among the nine groups, and none ate nutritionally balanced meals. Thus, intervention efforts should aim at having this group eat balanced meals. The workers in Group 6 consumed relatively high levels of alcohol. Thus, alcohol control should be prioritized in this terminal group. The workers in Group 7 frequently drank and consumed relatively high levels of alcohol. Thus, alcohol control should also be prioritized in this group. Finally, although the workers in Group 8 did not consume large amounts of alcohol, all of them were frequent drinkers. In addition, although they were the youngest among the nine terminal groups, they did the least amount of physical exercise (Table 2). Thus, they should be educated about alcohol-control and the importance of physical exercise. We believe that the findings of the signal detection analysis are useful for developing effective tailored intervention on a population basis.

(3) Limitations of the study and conclusions

This study has several limitations. First, the external validity of the study is very limited. The findings are applicable only to other Japanese white-collar workers. However, the methodology used to facilitate matching the type of intervention and the targeted group is widely applicable to other situations. Second, questionnaire items concerning hereditary factors leading to obesity and work content were not included in our study. In order to obtain more complete findings on the interaction of factors relating to obesity, these factors should be included in a future study.

In conclusion, we evaluated the higher-order interaction of potential variables of obesity using signal detection analysis. The following results emerged from our study. (1) The subjects were categorized into nine subgroups. The obesity of three groups of workers, composed of workers who were at least 40 years old with a high degree of obesity, had different causes. Of these different causes, one was related to working conditions, one was related to smoking cessation, and one was related to excessive alcohol consumption. (2) Although the applicability of the findings is limited, the use of signal detection analysis might be widely applicable to other weight loss programs for facilitating the matching of the type of intervention to the targeted group.

REFERENCES

Anderson JV, Mavis BE, Robinson JI, Stoffelmayr BE. 1993. A work-site weight management program to reinforce behavior. *J Occup Med* **35**(8):800-804.

Avenell A, Brown TJ, McGee MA, Campbell MK, Grant AM, Broom J. 2004. What are the long-term benefits of weight reducing diets in adults? A systematic review of randomized controlled trials. *J Hum Nutr Dietet* **17**:317-335.

Basler HD. 1995. Patient education with reference to the process of behavioral change. *Patient Edu Counsel* **26**:93-98.

Battle EK, Brownell KD. 1996. Confronting a rising tide of eating disorders and obesity: treatment vs. prevention and policy. *Addict Behav* **21**(6):755-765.

Bild DE, Sholinsky P, Smith DE, Lewis CE, Hardin JM, Burke GL. 1996. Correlates and predictors of weight loss in young adults: the CARDIA study. *Int J Obes* **20**:47-55.

Bray GA. 1985. Complications of obesity. *Ann Intern Med* **103**(6 Pt 2):1052-1062.

Brownell KD. 1986. Public health approaches to obesity and its management. *Annu Rev Public Health* **7**:531-533.

Bull FC, Eyler AA, King AC, Brownson RC. 2001. Stage of readiness to exercise in ethnically diverse women: a US survey. *Med Sci Sports Exerc* **33**:1147-1156.

Cameron R, MacDonald MA, Schlegel RP, Young CI, Fisher SE, Killen JD, Rogers T, Horlick L, Shepel LF. 1990. Toward the development of self-help health behavior change program: weight loss by correspondence. *Can J Public Health* **81**:275-279.

Cook T, Flay B. 1978. The temporal persistence of experimentally induced attitude change: an evaluative review. In Berkowitz L (Ed.), *Advances in experimental social psychology* (pp. 1-57). New York, Academic Press.

Dale J, Williams S, Wellesley A, Glucksman E. 1999. Training and supervision needs and experience: a longitudinal, cross-sectional survey of accident and emergency department senior house officers. *Postgraduate Medical Journal* **75**(880):86-89.

DiClemente CC, Prochaska JO, Fairburst SK. 1991. The process of smoking cessation: an analysis of precontemplation, contemplation, and preparation stages of change. *J Consult Psycho* **59**:295-304.

Dishman RK, Oldenburg B, O'Neal H, Shephard RJ. 1998. Worksite physical activity interventions. *Am J Prev Med* **15**(4):344-361.

Eyler AA, Baker E, Cromer L, King AC, Brownson RC, Donatelle RJ. 1998. Physical activity and minority women: a qualitative study. *Health Educ Behav* **25**: 640-652.

Ferreira MF, Sobrinho LG, Pires JS, Silva ME, Santos MA, Sousa MF. 1995. Endocrine and psychological evaluation of women with recent weight gain. *Psychoneuroendocrinology* **20**(1):53-63.

Fielding JE. 1990. Worksite health promotion programs in the United States: progress, lessons and changes. In: Health Promotion International. Eynsham, Oxford, U.K. Oxford University Press **5**:75-84.

Flegal KM, Carroll MD, Kuczmarski RJ, Johnson CL. !998. Overweight and pbesity in the United Stetes: prevalence and trends, 1960-1994. *Int J Obes Relat Metab Disord* **22**: 39-47.

Foshee V, McLeroy KR, Sumner SK, Bibeau DL. 1986. Evaluation of worksite weight loss programs: a review of data and issues. *J Nutr Educ* **18**(1):s38-s43.

French SA, Jeffery RW, Forster JL, McGovern PG, Kelder SH, Baxter JE. 1994. Predictors of weight change over two years among a population of working adults: the health worker project. *Int J Obese* **18**:45-154.

Fukuda Y, Watanebe M, Kawazu S, Kumabe H, Koyama W. 1996a. Lifestyle and health. Health education based on the age of male adults (Part 1). *Jpn J Public Health Nurse* **52**(3):190-195. (In Japanese)

Fukuda Y, Watanabe M, Kawazu S, Kumabe H, Koyama W. 1996b. Lifestyle and health. Health education based on the age of male adults (Part 2). *Jpn J Public Health Nurse* **52**(4):315-319. (In Japanese)

Garfinkle L. 1985. Overweight and cancer. *Ann Intern Med* **103**(6 Pt 2):1052-1062.

Garrison RJ, Kannel WB, Stokes J, Castelli WP. 1987. Incidence and precursors of hypertension in young adults: the Framingham Offspring Study. *Prev Med* **16**:235-251.

Gerace TA, George VA. 1996. Predictors of weight increases over 7 years in fire fighters and paramedics. *Prev Med* **25**:593-600.

Hagihara A, Tarumi K, Nobutomo K. 2000. Work stressors, drinking with colleagues after work, and job satisfaction among white-collar workers in Japan. *Substance Use and Misuse* **35**(5):737-756.

Hennrikus DJ, Jeffery RW. 1996. Worksite intervention for weight control: a review of the literature. *Amer J Health Promotion* **10**(6):471-498.

Jeffery RW. 1993. Minnesota studies on community-based approaches to weight loss and control. *Ann Intern Med* **119**(7 Pt2):719-721.

Jeffery RW. 1995. Community programs for obesity prevention: the Minnesota Heart Health Program. *Obesity Research* **3 Suppl 2**:283s-288s.

Jeffery RW. 1995. Public health approaches to the management of obesity. In Brownell KD and Fairburn CG (Eds.), *Eating disorders and obesity: a comprehensive handbook* (pp. 558-563). New York, Gilford Press.

Jeffery RW, Forster JL, French SA, Kelder SH, Lando HA, McGovern PG, Jacobs DR Jr., Baxter JE. 1993. The Healthy Worker Project: a work-site intervention for weight control and smoking cessation. *AJPH* **83**(3):395-401.

Kahn HS, Tatham LM, Rodriguez C, Calle EE, Thun MJ, Health CW. 1997. Stable behaviors associated with adults' 10-year change in body mass index and likelihood of gain at the waist. *AJPH* **87**(5):747-754.

Kannel WB, Gordon T, Castelli WP. 1979. Obesity, lipids and glucose intolerance: the Framingham Study. *Amer J Clin Nutr* **32**:1238-1245.

Karasek RA, Theorell T. 1990. Healthy work. Stress, productivity, and the reconstruction of working life (pp. 31-82). New York, Basic Books.

Kataoka K. 1989. Himan to yase no kijun (Criteria for obese and skinny). *Naika* **64**:404-408. (In Japanese)

Kraemer HC. 1988. Assessment of 2 × 2 associations: generalization of signal detection methodology. *Amer Stat* **42**:37-49.

Kraemer HC. 1992. *Evaluating medical tests.* Newbury Park: Sage.

Klesges RC, Klesges LM, Haddock CK, Eck LH. 1992. A longitudinal analysis of the impact of dietary intake and physical activity on weight change in adults. *Am J Clin Nutr* **55**:818-822.

Kreuter MW, Farrell D, Olevitch L. Tailoring health messages: Customizing communication with computer technology. Mahwah, NJ, Lawrence Erlbaum Associate 1999; 1-270.

Kreuter MW, Wray RJ. 2003. Tailored and targeted health communication: Strategies for enhancing information relevance. *Am J Health Behav* **27**(Suppl 3): S227-S232.

Lasater TM, Sennett LL, Lefebvre RC, DeHart KL, Peterson G, Carleton RA. 1991. Community-based approach to weight loss: the Pawtucket "weigh-in". *Addict Behav* **16**:175-181.

Leighl N, Gattellari M, Butow P, Brown R, Tattersall MH. 2001. Discussing adjuvant cancer therapy. *J Clinical Oncology* **19**(6):1768-1778.

Masse LC, Ainsworth BE, Tortolero S. 1998. Mesuring physical activity in midlife, older, and minority women: issues from an expert panel. *J Womens Health* **7**:57-67.

Minkler M. 1999. Personal responsibility for health? 1999. A review of the arguments and the evidence at century's end. *Health Education and Behavior* **26**(1):121-140.

Morimoto K. 1991. *Raifusutairu to kenkou* (Lifestyle and health). Tokyo: Igaku Shoin, 2-45. (In Japanese)

Nubert HB, Feinleib M, McNamara PM, Castelli WP. 1983. Obesity as an independent risk factor for cardiovascular disease: a 26-year follow-up of patients in the Framingham Heart Study. *Circulation* **67**:968-977.

Owens JF, Matthews KA, Wing RR, Kuller LH. 1992. Can physical activity mitigate the effects of aging in the middle-aged women? *Circulation* **85**:1265-1270.

Perusse L, Bouchard C. 2000. Gene-diet interaction in obesity. *Am J Clin Nutr* **72**:1285s-1290s.

Petty R. 1977. The importance of cognitive responses in persuasion. *Advances in Consumer Research* **4**:357-362.

Petty R, Cacioppo J. 1981. *Attitudes and persuasion: Classic and contemporary approaches* (pp. 1-314). Dubuque, WC Brown.

Pirozzo S, Summerbell C, Cameron C, Glasziou P. 2003. Should we recommend low-fat diets for obesity? *Obes Review* **4**:83-90.

Prochaska JO, DiClemente CC. 1984. *The transtheoretical approach: Crossing traditional boundaries of change.* Homewood IL, Dorsey Press.

Prochaska JO, DiClemente CC, Velicer WF, Rossi JS. 1993. Standardized, individualized, interactive, and personalized self-help programs for smoking cessation. *Health Psychol* **12**:399-405.

Prochaska JO, Norcross JC, Diclemente CC. 1995. *Changing for good.* New York, Avon Books, 1-289.

Prochaska JO, Velicer WF, DiClemente CC, Fava J. 1988. Measuring processes of change: applications to the cessation of smoking. *J Consult Clin Psychol* **56**:520-528.

Ruggiero L, Redding CA, Rossi JS, Prochaska JO. 1997. A stage-matched smoking cessation programs for pregnant smokers. *Am J Health Promo* **12**:31-33.

Sapolsky HM, Altman D, Greene R, Moore JB. 1981. Corporate attitudes toward health care costs. *Millbank Memorial Fund Quarterly/Health and Society* **59**:561-581.

Saris WHM, Blair SN, van Baak MA, Eaton SB, Davies PSW, Pietro LDi, Fogelholm M, Rissanen A, Schoeller D, Swinburn B, Tremblay A, Westerterp KR, Wyatt H. How much physical activity is enough to prevent unhealthy weight gain? Outcome of the IASO 1st Stock Conference and consensus statement. *Obes Reviews* **4**:101-114.

Seidell JC. 1995. Obesity in Europe: scaling an epidemic. Int J Obes **19**(Suppl 3):s1-s4.

Shah M, French SA, Jeffery RW, McGovern PG, Forster JL, Lando HA. 1993. Correlates of high fat/calorie food intake in a worksite population: the healthy worker project. *Addict Behav* **18**:583-594.

Stamler R, Stamler J, Riedlinger WF, Algera G, Roberts RH. 1978. Weight and blood pressure: findings in hypertension screening of 1 million Americans. *JAMA* **240**: 1607-1610.

Steel Z, Jones J, Adcock S, Clancy R, Bridgford-West L, Austin J. 2000. Why the high rate of dropout from individualized cognitive-behavior therapy for bulimia nervosa? *Int J Eating Disorder* **28**(2):209-214.

Sternfeld B, Ainsworth BE, Tortolero S. 1999. Physical activity patterns in a diverse population of women. *Prev Med* **28**:313-323.

Sutton K, Logue E, Jarjoura D, Baughman K, Smucker W, Capers C. 2003. Assessing dietary and exercise stage of change to optimize weight loss interventions. *Obes Res* **11**: 641-652.

Tarumi k, Hagihara A, Morimoto K. 1993. An inquiry into the relationship between job strain and blood pressure in male white-collar workers. *Jpn J Ind Health* **35**:269-276.

U.S. National Commission on Diabetes. 1975. *Report of the National Commission on Diabetes to the Congress of the United States.* Bethesda (MD): U.S. Department of Health, Education and Welfare, Publication No. 76-11021.

Velicer WF, Prochaska JO. 1999. An expert system intervention for smoking cessation. *Patient Educ Couns* **36**:119-129.

Weinstein MS. 1983. *Health promotion and lifestyle change in the worksite.* Copenhagen, Denmark, WHO European Regional Office.

Winkleby MA, Flora JA, Kraemer HC. 1994. A community-based heart disease intervention: predictors of change. *AJPH* **84**:767-772.

Ziguras SJ, Stuart GW. 2000. A meta-analysis of the effectiveness of mental health case management over 20 years. *Psychiatric Services* **51**(11):1410-1421.

In: Weight Loss, Exercise and Health Research
Editor: Carrie P. Saylor, pp. 99-152

ISBN 1-60021-077-5
© 2006 Nova Science Publishers, Inc.

Chapter 6

THE DETERMINANTS OF PHYSICAL ACTIVITY: WHY ARE SOME PEOPLE ACTIVE AND OTHERS NOT?

Joan Wharf Higgins[1], Trina Rickert and Patti-Jean Naylor

Canada Research Chair, Health and Society
School of Physical Education,
University of Victoria PO Box 3015, STN CSC
Victoria BC Canada V8W 3P1 250-721-8377
Canadian Diabetes Association 360-1385 8th Avenue W
Vancouver BC Canada V6H 3V9 604-732-1331
School of Physical Education, University of Victoria
PO Box 3015, STN CSC Victoria BC
Canada V8W 3P1 250-721-7844

ABSTRACT

Physical inactivity has been identified as a health care burden (Katzmarzyk, Gledhill, and Shephard, 2000). It is a primary risk factor for both psychological and physical ill health, including many disease states that often originate during childhood years yet only become apparent in adulthood (Malina, 1996). Community-based initiatives promoting physical activity to prevent chronic disease have been found to be highly cost effective relative to traditional care (Baxter , Milner, Wilson, et al , 1997; Segal, Dalton, and Richardson, 1998; Tuomilehto, Lindstrom, Eriksson, et al., 2001). Despite the irrefutable evidence linking physical activity with physiological and psycho-social health benefits throughout the lifecourse (Bouchard, 2001; The Surgeon General's Call to Action, 2001), North Americans find little time in their daily life to be physically active. Approximately 54-57% of all North Americans are not active enough to reap such health benefits (Centers for Disease Control and Prevention,1999a). While traditional interventions have encouraged people to add physical activity to their daily activities or to change their daily routines, little attention has been paid to the contexts within which these changes must be made (Giles-Corti, and Donovan, 2002). These established approaches have much to recommend them, but the success rate of individualized exercise prescription

[1] jwharfhi@uvic.ca

interventions can be very low (Dishman, 1994). People can slip back into their normal, less-healthy behavior patterns in environments that do not support an active lifestyle. Research on the barriers to physical activity reveals that, in addition to overcoming personal, social, and psychological hurdles, policy and environmental factors also impede individuals' efforts to be active (Canadian Fitness and Lifestyle Research Institute, 2004; Centers for Disease Control and Prevention, 2001; King, Hawe, and Corne, 1999; Mitchell, and Olds, 1999; Salmon, Owen, Crawford, and Bauman, and Sallis, 2003; Wen, Thomas, Jones et al., 2002). Although the research literature is replete with studies of the individual determinants of physical activity, there is a collective gap in our understanding of the connections between individual determinants and those in the social, physical, economic and cultural environments. Advances in personal treatment approaches are important, but they seem to have limited impact on populations that continue to live in physical environments that have been called, with justification, "obesogenic" (Swinburn, Egger, and Raza, 1999). This chapter presents a socio-ecological framework for considering the multiple levels of influence on physical activity behavior, and provides some evidence that such comprehensive approaches are effective in promoting an active lifestyle.

INTRODUCTION

The purpose of this chapter is to present the evidence describing the determinants of physical activity, including best practices. In doing so, the chapter will draw on the current literature as well as the authors' own research detailing the results of a community-based diabetes prevention physical activity program. The chapter begins with an overview of the epidemiology of exercise, including a discussion of physical activity rates and the economics of exercise. This is followed by a presentation of the socio-ecological model which provides the framework for discussing the varying determinants of physical activity. The chapter closes with a section detailing best practices and interventions, and one that comments on advancing the field.

EPIDEMIOLOGY OF EXERCISE AND PHYSICAL ACTIVITY

The evidence is now quite clear on the benefits awarded through engaging in a physically active lifestyle, in terms of both preventing disease and promoting health and wellness (Corbin, 2001). There is considerable robust epidemiological evidence that physical inactivity is a health care burden (Pratt, Macera, and Wang, 2000), thought to be linked to at least 300,000 early deaths in the U.S. alone (Katzmarzyk et al., 2000; Manson, Skerrett, Greenland, and VanItallie, 2004). Inactivity represents a modifiable risk factor for, and predictor of, obesity and a host of chronic diseases, including heart disease, type 2 diabetes, cancer, osteoporosis, and several psychological disorders (Blair and Brodney, 1999; Blair and Church, 2004; Centers for Disease Control, 1999a; Hill, 2004; Molitch, Fujimoto, Hamman, and Knowler, 2003; Weinstein et al., 2004; Wessel et al., 2004).

The health benefits of physical activity can accrue at any point across the lifespan (Seefeldt, Malina, and Clark, 2002). For instance, there is consensus that physical activity not only promotes physical health among youth, but also positively impacts their social and mental health (Marshall, Biddle, Sallis, McKenzie, and Conway, 2002). The relationship between physical activity and physical fitness and reduced cardiovascular risk factors in youth aged 9 – 18 years has been demonstrated (Katzmarzyk, Malina, and Bouchard, 1999). McKelvie et al (2004) confirmed that a school-based, high impact exercise program can positively impact bone strength in prepubertal boys. For healthy, middle-aged men and women, physical activity has been demonstrated as critical to preserving high physical function over an eight year period, regardless of socioeconomic position, smoking and body weight (Hillsdon, Brunner, Guralnik, and Marmot, 2005). These authors suggest that activity levels delay the onset of sarcopenia, defined as the progressive loss of muscle mass and strength, which begins around 30 years of age.

Among postmenopausal women, walking reduced the risk of heart disease by 12-40% over 3.2 years (Manson et. al., 2002). Further, active individuals report better health, degree of independence and quality of life than inactive persons (Seefeldt et al., 2002).

Physical activity has been repeatedly shown to reduce the risk of functional limitations, prevents hip fractures or falls, contribute to healthy aging, and minimize risk of cardiovascular disease later in life (Bryant, Shetterly, Baxter, and Hamman, 2002).Older people may maintain independence in later life by increasing physical activity (Kaplan, 1992; LaCroix, Guralnik, Berkman, Wallace, and Satterfield, 1993; Peel, McClure, and Bartlett, 2005; Petrella, Lattanzio, Demeray, Varallo, and Blore, 2005; Seeman and Chen, 2002).

Furthermore, the benefits are also evident during recovery or rehabilitation from an illness: physical exercise is significantly associated with better physical, functional, and psychological well-being in breast and prostate cancer survivors during (Segal et al., 2002) and after treatment (Blanchard et al., 2002). For those managing a chronic illness, such as diabetes, an active lifestyle has been found to mitigate its negative effects on the body and extending longevity. The protective effect of physical activity is experienced regardless of body weight, blood pressure, cholesterol and smoking (Hu, Jousilahti, Barengo et al., 2005).

Because, as Blair and Church (2004) comment "the modern living environment in developed countries is characterized by low daily energy expenditure and an abundant and inexpensive food supply, making positive energy balance common" (p. 1232), physical inactivity is expected to soon become a leading cause of death in North America (Mokdad, Marks, Stroup, and Gerberding, 2004). The evidence supporting the salutary effects of physical activity is now unassailable (Blair and Church, 2004; Bouchard, 2001; Proper, Hildebrandt, Vander Beek, Twisk, and Van Mechelen, 2003; The Surgeon General's Call to Action, 2001), and should be pivotal to both clinical therapy and public health policy.

The new public health focus for chronic disease prevention emphasizes increasing population-wide energy expenditure through moderate-intensity physical activity in the context of everyday life (Owen, Leslie, Salmon, and Fotheringham, 2000). Health Canada (2004; 2003) recommends accumulating 30 to 60 minutes (which can be in ten minute bouts) of moderate intensity (around 50% of maximal aerobic capacity[2]) physical activity on most (preferably all) days of the week for sedentary people to realize significant health benefits. Flexibility activities four to seven days of the week, and strength activities two to four days of the week, are also included in the exercise prescription (2004). In the US, similar advisements recommending that moderate physical activity, such as thirty minutes of brisk walking five or

---

[2] Maximal capacity, also referred to as maximal oxygen uptake (VO$_2$ max), is defined as the maximum amount of oxygen the body can use to perform work (McArdle, Katch, & Katch, 2000).

more times a week, is sufficient to reap health benefits have appeared (The Surgeon General's Call to Action, 2001). Blair and Church (2004) suggest that 150 minutes each week of moderately intense activity protects against cardiovascular disease or all cause mortality even among obese individuals.

PHYSICAL ACTIVITY RATES

Despite the irrefutable evidence linking physical activity with physiological and psycho-social health benefits for people of all ages, North Americans find little time in their daily life to be physically active. Presently, the prevalence of physical inactivity is high and active lifestyles is low (Health Canada, 2004). More than 50% of American adults do not do enough physical activity to provide health benefits and 26% are not active at all in their leisure time. Activity decreases with age, and sufficient activity is less common among women than men and among those with lower incomes, less education and non-Caucasian groups (Centers for Disease Control, 1999a). Similarly in Canada, 57% of adults are insufficiently active for optimal health benefits (Canadian Fitness and Lifestyle Research Institute, 2003) and the majority (56%) are physically inactive (Craig and Cameron, 2004). The situation may actually be much worse: it has been suggested that the activity rate of Canadians is inflated due to small percentages of the adult population accounting for a large majority of total participation in the 10 most popular activities (Barber and Havitz, 2001). (The reader is advised to refer to Brownson, Boehmer and Luke (2005) for an excellent review of factors contributing to declining physical activity rates in the US). Such sedentary lifestyles are not exclusive to North Americans: developed countries, such as UK and Australia, report similar levels of inactivity among their citizens (Lewis and Ridge, 2005; WHO, 2003). Even in small children, physical activity rates have been found to be low, with only 20-25 minutes per day in moderate to vigorous physical activity; 35 minutes short of the daily recommended levels (Reilly et al., 2004).

Approximately one-fourth of young people in the US walk or bicycle nearly every day (Centers for Disease Control and Prevention, 1999a). In terms of active commuting, 41% of Canadian adults walk to or from work or school or to do errands, and 13% commute by bicycle (Cameron, Craig, Stephens, and Ready, 2002). In the US, walking is reported as the most common leisure-time physical activity, either in malls, parks or on treadmills (Eyler, Brownson, Bacak, and Housemann, 2003).

In a thorough review of the literature, Corbin (2001) documented the rates of physical activity throughout the lifespan. The data Corbin cites indicate that physical activity is highest during childhood, begins to decline in adolescence (roughly at about age 12), and continues to decline through adulthood to older adulthood. This pattern is referred to as "tracking." Investigations seeking to understand tracking patterns have been few and the results inconclusive. There is some evidence that sport participation in childhood and adolescence predicts physical activity in adulthood (Curtis, McTeer, and White,1999; Malina, 2001; Paffenbarger, Hyde, Wing and Steinmetz, 1984; Powell and Dysinger, 1987; Telama, Yang, Laakso and Viikari, 1997). Other studies have found that participation in endurance, fitness-type activities (Aarnio, Winter, Peltonen, Kujala, and Kaprio, 2002; Green, 2002), or intense and continuous participation throughout the school years, as well as use of local recreation centers, regardless of the type of activity (Nelson, Gordeon-Larsen, Adair, and Popkin, 2005; Telama, Yang, Viikari, Valimaki, Wanne, and Raitakari, 2005), predicts sustained exercise levels in adulthood.

THE ECONOMICS OF EXERCISE

In the US, coupled with pandemic rates of obesity, sedentary living is estimated to burden the health care system between $76 and $90 billion in direct health care costs annually (Manson et al., 2004; Pratt et al., 2000). The cost in human lives is estimated to range between 200,000 and 300,000 every year (Mokdad et al., 2000).

An economic analysis in 1999 revealed that $2.1 billion in Canadian direct health care costs were credited to physical inactivity. A 10% reduction in inactivity rates could reduce direct health care expenditures by $150 million a year (Katzmarzyk et al., 2000). A more recent economic analysis of the liability of physical inactivity in British Columbia (Colman and Walker, 2004) found that the significant proportions of the population who do not engage in vigorous (61%) or moderate (36%) physical activity, costs the province as much as $647 million per year; $185.7 million in direct health care costs alone. Moreover, physical inactivity accounts for 6.4% of premature deaths in BC. While this percentage may not sound troubling, it actually translates into a loss of 4,380 years of life – year in and year out – that are taken from our workforce, tax base and social and economic productivity. A mere 10% reduction in the rates of physical inactivity among British Columbians are anticipated to save $16.1 million annually by eluding hospital, drug, physician and other direct health care costs. As well, $19.9 million is forecast in terms of productivity gains, should the premature death rate decline due to increased physical activity levels. These savings amount to a total of $36 million each year (Colman and Walker, 2004).

Community-based initiatives promoting physical activity to prevent heart disease and diabetes have been found to be highly cost effective relative to traditional care (Baxter et al., 1997; Segal et al., 1998; Tuomilehto et al., 2001). There is also evidence from the exercise physiology and gerontology literatures that physical activity, in increasing seniors' levels of physical function, also functions to decrease dependence and the relative risk of admission to nursing homes (Guralnik, Simonsick, Ferrucci, et al., 1994; Schroeder, Nau, Osness, and Potteiger, 1998). For example, an evaluation of the Program for All-Inclusive Care for the Elderly (PACE) in New York found that seniors attending day health centers offering nutrition, exercise and social contact in addition the usual range of seniors' health services, reduced their overall health care costs by 5%, compared to seniors receiving only conventional care. Included in this figure was a 34% decrease in hospital costs and a 70% reduction in nursing home utilization (Rachlis, Evans, Lewis, and Barer, 2001).

THE SOCIO-ECOLOGICAL MODEL TO UNDERSTAND THE DETERMINANTS OF PHYSICAL ACTIVITY

Although it can be simple in its movements, the decision to engage in physical activity is complex. What at first glance seems an entirely personal choice is, upon deeper reflection, one that may not be a choice at all (Wright, MacDonald, and Groom, 2003). Rather it is a response to circumstances that enable or constrain an active lifestyle. As Singh-Manoux and Marmot (2005) comment, health-related behaviors, such as exercise, "are never truly 'voluntary'; they are a product of, and embedded in structures of society" (p. 2130). Indeed, a myriad of factors influence the intention, motivations, skills and ability of individuals to be active. Essentially, these variables can be classified as modifiable or non-modifiable determinants. Those that are nonmodifiable include age, gender, race, ethnicity, and to some extent health and socioeconomic status; modifiable factors include personal characteristics (knowledge, motivation, skills), community settings, living and environmental circumstances, educational levels, and support networks and cultural influences (Seefeldt et al., 2002). There are two types of targets for addressing modifiable factors: factors within and external to individual control (Cohen, Scribner, and Farley, 2000). Those within individual control include increasing knowledge, intent, motivation, and skills; those that target external factors address structural issues, such as income, social status, access to resources etc, outside the purview of individual control. In addition, individual-level focused interventions may target high risk persons or groups, or be community-wide in reach. Structural interventions, are by definition, population based.

As in the fields of epidemiology, public health and medicine, traditionally, much of the research in this area has over emphasized the individual determinants of physical activity failing to tend to other broader social and contextual factors (Cohen et al., 2000; Leung, Yen, and Minkler, 2004). And still, after two decades of investigating how to best motivate and enable individuals to be active, physical activity rates have declined. Explaining physical activity behavior is limited when only individual-level variables are considered (Henderson et al., 2001; Sallis, Kraft, and Linton, 2002). Gradually, the field has come to recognize that physical activity does not occur in a vacuum (Coogan and Coogan, 2004). For Fisher, Li, Michael, and Cleveland (2004), "individual-centered variables too often take center stage, with the result that environmental factors are either overlooked or ignored" (p. 46). It has often been difficult for researchers and practitioners alike to appreciate that physical activity behaviors are influenced by socio-ecological factors. As such, disease prevention and health promotion activity interventions have been plagued by the "paradox of self-responsibility: Even if we know the power of regular physical activity with respect to physical and mental health benefits, formidable barriers may reside in our work, family, neighborhood, and cultural circumstances." (McGinnis, 2001, p. 393). Note Leung, Yen, and Minkler (2004):

> A study on leisure physical activity might gather information about type and frequency of activity and may even monitor heart rate or pulse during activity, but is unlikely to take into consideration contextual or social factors (e.g. access to recreational facilities of safety of neighborhood environment) that influence whether and how a person engages in leisure physical activity (p. 500).

Or, as Henderson et al. (2001) note in much simpler words: "…regardless of how much interest or time an individual might have if no safe places to walk exist in his or her neighborhood, that person is not likely to be active in that way" (p. 27). Person-based approaches have much to recommend them, but the rate of recidivism from individualized prescription interventions can be very high (Dishman, 1994) as individuals slip back into their normal, less-active patterns in environments which have been termed "obesogenic" - where there are plentiful enticements to sit more and move less. Since it may be impossible to remove all the barriers for each and every individual, it may be more useful for organizations and communities to modify the larger environment to make it easier for everyone to be active. Coogan and Coogan (2004) suggest that the current sedentary epidemic is akin to the cholera epidemics of the 19th century:

> Throughout that century, cholera was blamed on individual characteristics, mostly "intemperance," poor character, and filthiness. In fact, cholera was a disease that could only be prevented by changing structural factors: the water supply and sanitation systems. In the same way, sedentariness is not solely an individual problem. It is a response to a society that has "designed out" options for physical activity. Thus, the most effective interventions to increase physical activity can be undertaken at the population (structural) level rather than at the individual level (p. 40).

Moreover, there are a dearth of methodological considerations and studies informing effective design and implementation interventions beyond an individual-level, 'one size fits all' approach (Fisher et al., 2004): "one would think that if we informed people of their risks they would rush home and, in the interests of good health, change behaviors that caused the risk. Some people do, but most do not" (Syme, 2002, p. 64). Corti, Donovan, and Holman (1996) found that the use of recreational physical activity facilities resulted from a complex relationship between personal and environmental factors, whereby preferences, perceived ability and age barriers, social circumstances and competing commitments also interacted with proximity to shops and accessibility of free facilities. There is much to be learned from the anti-tobacco efforts of recent years, in which policies and initiatives to alter the environment and norms of smoking have had far greater success in helping people kick the habit than the individualized smoking cessation campaigns (Hammond, McDonald, Fong, Brown, and Cameron, 2004). Community level approaches to promote physical activity that address places (i.e., the social structure and environment), in addition to people (i.e., health-related knowledge, skills, values, motivations), may produce similar payoffs (Sampson, 2003; Yoo et al., 2004).

Recently the physical activity field has moved beyond viewing physical activity as an individual practice to include the wider social and community contexts. The socio-ecological model is most helpful in this regard (Matson-Koffman, Brownstein, Neiner, and Greaney, 2005) as it acknowledges the multiple levels of influence on behavior that include: intrapersonal factors (i.e., characteristics, knowledge, skills), interpersonal factors (i.e., social support/influences, the quality and nature of human interactions, peers, family), and community factors (i.e., environmental/structural factors such as health policy, community's ability to create health promoting change) (Baker, Brennan, Brownson and Houseman, 2000). Socio-ecological models explain how "environments affect behavior and how environments and behavior affect each other" (Sallis and Owen, 1997, p. 404), and are important in increasing health promoting behaviors, including application in physical activity interventions (Baker et al., 2000) (Figure 1). An underlying theme is the importance and effectiveness of addressing problems on multiple levels. Therefore, interventions simultaneously influencing multiple levels and multiple settings may be expected to lead to greater and longer lasting changes and maintenance of existing health promoting habits. Overall, the goal of the socio-ecological model is to create a healthy community environments that provide health promoting information, access to resources and facilities, and social support to enable people to live healthier and more physically active lives (Stokols, Allen, and Bellingham, 1996).

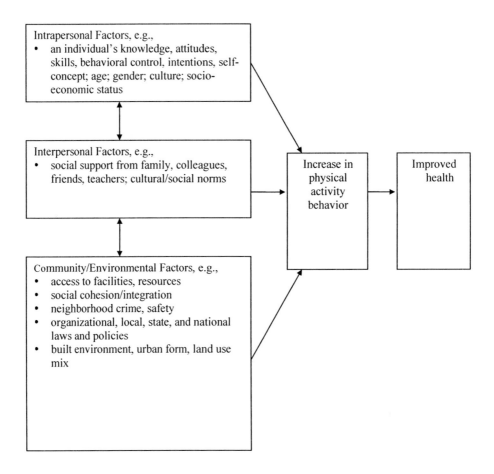

Figure 1. The Socio-ecological model applied to physical activity

LEVELS OF EVIDENCE FOR FACTORS INFLUENCING PHYSICAL ACTIVITY

The evidence accumulated to date for the three main factors within the socio-ecological model have been examined by Giles-Corti and Donovan (2002, 2003) who found that relative influences of these factors were found to be almost equally important on physical activity. More specifically, for intrapersonal variables they found that the odds of achieving recommended levels of walking were 48% higher among those with high levels of perceived behavioral control and the odds were nearly twice as high for those highly intent on being active within the next two weeks. Regarding intrapersonal factors, walking increased with the number of significant others who had exercised weekly with the participant during the previous three months (i.e. having others to exercise with, including a dog, was significantly influential). Examination of community and environmental factors influencing walking revealed that access to public spaces, particularly spatial access to recreational facilities (2002). More specifically, in examining the relative influence of individual, social environmental and physical environmental determinants of physical activity (adjusted for other determinants), these researchers (2003) found that exercising was more strongly associated with individual determinants. Logistical regression odds ratios for individual determinants showed the highest determinant scores of 8.14, social determinants scores of 3.72, and environmental determinants scores of 1.43. Overall, they report that their study findings suggest that exercise is enhanced for people with positive individual factors and positive social environments that are conducive to exercising. A supportive physical environment showed a significant, but a more moderate, influence on activity (2003).

DETERMINANTS OF PHYSICAL ACTIVITY

While we discuss the determinants according to the larger framework of the socio-ecological model independently below, please recognize that these determinants rarely occur in isolation from one another. As the reader will note, there are a plethora of intra-, interpersonal and community/environmental factors that can potentially mediate physical activity levels (Ball and Crawford, 2005). For example, low socioeconomic status as an intrapersonal factor is intimately tied to lower educational opportunities to learn about the benefits of an active lifestyle, and community or built environmental factors such as living in unsafe neighborhoods, or lack of access to facilities. Similarly, issues associated with gender or age (intrapersonal) and culture or social norms (interpersonal) may be inextricably linked with one another. This interconnectivity among factors is the reason that scholars call for comprehensive and coordinated interventions. In our concluding section we, too, contend that an appreciation of, and action across all dimensions is necessary to achieve physically active lifestyles for all.

Intrapersonal Factors

Individual determinants of physical activity relate to are factors such as knowledge, attitudes, intention, self-efficacy, behavioral control, and past experience experiences of being active; essentially those factors that are potentially within the grasp of an individual's control to change. Such variables have been the focus of much of the research in physical activity, particularly in the exercise psychology, motivation and adherence literatures (see for example, Calfas, Long, Sallis, Wooten, Pratt, and Patrick, 1996; Prochaska and Marcus, 1994). Each of these intrapersonal factors has been investigated and explored so that we have a sound *theoretical* grasp of the elements forming motivation, intention, self-efficacy, and attitudes. Behavior change theories such as the Theory of Planned Behavior, Social Learning Theory, Stages of Change, the Transtheoretical Model and Health Belief Model, among others (e.g., Azjen, 1985; Bandura, 1986; Duda, 2001; McAuley, Pena, and Jerome, 2001; Prochaska and Marcus, 1994), have been used to elucidate the components of intrapersonal factors. Integral to these concepts is how individuals perceive and evaluate: the importance of the benefits and costs of physical activity, the normative behavior and influences of others, their skills and abilities to perform the desired activity, and sense of control. Thus, oft cited personal barriers to doing physical activity include feeling too tired, lack of self-efficacy to engage in an exercise activity, cost, and no motivation or lack of enjoyment (Salmon et al., 2003). For two in five employed Canadians, constant tight timelines at work and lack of time due to work are barriers to activity. Other barriers to being active include long term illness or disability, feeling uncomfortable, lack of skill, obtaining enough physical activity at one's job and fear of injury (Craig and Cameron, 2004).

Self-presentation, how one monitors and controls how they are perceived by others, also appears to be emerging as an influential factor in the decision to be active. Although under-studied compared to other variables, self-presentation has been found as a motivator for some individuals who wish to improve their appearance (Leary, Chioidjian, and Kraxberger, 1994). Among older adults, there may be the additional perception that they are inept at physical activity due to age and health-related changes, and view the perception of exercise as an age-inappropriate activity (Bengoechea and Spence, 2003; Martin, Sinden, and Fleming, 2000). Health problems, or pain associated with health conditions, are likely to be the most common barrier cited by seniors, as well as a lack of ability to independently travel to, or access opportunities for exercise (Lim and Taylor, 2005). Thus, we are fairly confident that

> Individuals are more likely to begin and maintain activity programmes when they perceive that the activity is beneficial, enjoyable and leads to increased competence in a valued outcome. Individuals are more likely to sustain activities that enhance self-esteem and at the same time have minimal potential for negative consequences such as injuries, financial duress, and excessive peer pressure (Seefeldt et al., 2002, pg. 159).

Of all the health practices needing change in their lives, exercise is one of the most often cited (Canadian Institute for Health Information, 2005; Federal, Provincial and Territorial Advisory Committee on Population Health, 1999). In the US, 70% of adults acknowledge that they should exercise more often (Dishman and Buckworth, 1996). A study conducted in Alberta found that 90% of respondents agreed that physical activity is an important way to keep healthy and prevent serious health problems (Bengoechea and Spence, 2003). Despite these admissions, adherence rates to structured physical activity programs has hovered around 50% for the past three decades (Casperson and Merritt, 1995; Dishman, Washburn, and Schoeller, 2001; Morgan, 2001). For Morgan (2001), this failure to capture the attention and sustain interest in physical activity suggests that interventions have missed their mark. Morgan proposes a departure from prescriptive, structured and intensive exercise sessions and a move toward personalized approaches that emphasize moderate and purposeful activity. Providing information to increase knowledge and awareness is a necessary but insufficient strategy. For example, in a worksite intervention designed to test the efficacy of print materials and a website to promote physical activity, there was negligible change in employees' activity levels in response to information alone (Marshall, Leslie, Bauman,

Marcus, and Owen, 2003). Similarly, among university students who completed a health theory course or behaviorally-oriented physical activity intervention, no significant effects on physical activity outcomes were evident two years later (Calfas, Sallis, Nichols et al., 2000).

The following paragraphs describe the intrapersonal factors that are less modifiable, but no less influential. Evidence demonstrates that the least physically active North Americans are un- or under-employed, are smokers, experience more stress, and have poorer overall health, including physical disabilities. As well, race and gender also account for inactivity: African American and Hispanics, especially women, are among the least active Americans (Brownson et al., 2005), particularly those of low income (Seefeldt et al., 2002). As well, Asian Americans are much less likely to meet physical activity guidelines than US-born, non-Asians, although this is a population that does rely on active commuting (Kandula and Lauderdale, 2005). The twin influences of culture and gender on physical activity are less well understood, partly due to understudying women and non-Caucasian populations, and when doing so, relying on measures developed for white male populations (Eyler, Baker, Cromer et al., 1998). What we do know is that mothers with young children, faced with profound changes to the biological, social and employment aspects of their lives, have one of the lowest rates of activity (Armstrong, Bauman, and Davies, 2000), despite their acute understanding of the importance of regular activity (Lewis and Ridge, 2005). Moreover, the contextual circumstances in which women are physically active or not, are rarely captured or measured in research contributing to the gap of knowledge for such populations. In such instances, applying a gender lens to understanding the decision to be active would be required. Often, the 'ethic of care' and multiple-roles attributed to women's work eclipses their sense of entitlement to, and fundamentally underpins their decisions concerning, active living (Lewis and Ridge, 2005; Vertinsky, 1998). Examining the life transitions and patterns of physical activity among women aged 18-23 years, Brown and Trost (2003) found that when women get married, have children and start work, their physical activity levels decline. Enabling women to sustain their activity levels as they negotiate through this stage requires interpersonal and environmental solutions: the implementation of family-friendly policies in homes, workplaces and communities. In a qualitative inquiry examining how mothers frame physical activity, Lewis and Ridge (2005) suggest that

> Mothers of young children face considerable challenges, but they are far from being victims of a lack of knowledge and skills associated with physical activity. They have their own strategies for making physical activity both pleasurable and possible. The way forward in facilitating physical activity for women with young children is to better understand these strategies and then do whatever is practicable to support these (p. 2304).

Some of the strategies emerging from their study include creating more supportive social contexts, such as mother-baby friendly environments, promoting the broader health, social and pleasure benefits of activity and a legitimate part of motherhood, rather than as a means to losing baby weight or enhance their individual, post-partum mental and physical health. Seefeldt and colleagues (2001), in an excellent review of the literature, suggest that differences among cultural priorities (physical vs. academic competence), perceived confidence to perform certain activities and appropriateness of specific activities (e.g., swimming) may account for lower activity rates among ethnically diverse groups.

As with other health behaviors, socioeconomic status profoundly shapes an individual's capacity to engage in physical activity. Nearly half of the families with yearly incomes below $20,000 identify that high costs are a significant barrier to participation in physical activity (McCarger, 2000). Those who could benefit the most from including exercise in their lives, are the least active. Persons with college or university education, high incomes and 'professional' jobs are most likely to be active and least likely to be sedentary (Fisher et al., 2004; Eyler, Brownson, Bacak, and Housemann, 2003; Frankish, Milligan, and Reid, 1998). These are the individuals with the money, knowledge, organizational resources, support and motivation – the personal life skills - to engage in active living. Those with higher education and income levels are less likely to report barriers of cost, and lack of time, skill, motivation or enjoyment (Brownson, Baker, Housemann, Brennan, and Bacak, 2001; Craig and Cameron, 2004).

Drawing on demographic and psychographic survey data, Librett, Yorke, Buchner and Schmid (2005) found that Americans who volunteer their time in the community are more likely to be physically active than non-volunteers. The most active were those volunteering on environmental projects, such as maintaining trails, planting trees and cleaning up parks. Mindful of speculating on a causal relationship, the authors noted that "volunteer programs may offer opportunities to promote an active, healthy lifestyle" (p. 11).

Disseminating information on the benefits of exercise and tips for adding activity into one's daily routine is regarded as a cornerstone of health education strategies, despite its mixed success. In Canada, national guidelines encouraging sedentary adults to become more active were released in 1998. Unlike the positive response of Canadian seniors to the guidelines for older adults (Jiang, Gooper, Porter, and Ready, 2004), an evaluation of the utility of the guidelines for adults found that unprompted recall of the guidelines was low (7.4% in 1999, and 5.2% in 2002), particularly among the least educated, non-English speaking and inactive Canadians (Bauman, Craig and Cameron, 2005). Bauman and Finch (2000) also found a low recall and use of physical activity guidelines among professionals. Other community-wide media campaigns encouraging more people to be physical active have demonstrated success in increasing awareness, knowledge and recall of the issue, but less impact on changing actual behavior (Bauman, Bellew, Owen, and Vita, 2001; Finlay and Faulkner, 2005; Hillsdon, Cavill, Nanchahal, Diamond, and White, 2001; Marcus, Owen, Forsyth, Cavill, and Fridinger, 1998; Owen, Bauman, Booth, Oldenburg, and Magnus, 1995; Wimbush, MacGregor, and Fraser, 1998). Such minimal impact is not exclusive to physical activity campaigns: those addressing smoking, alcohol use reduction, oral health, mammography, seat belt use and other preventive health issues, have been found to initiate change in approximately 8% of the population (Snyder, Hamilton, Mitchell, Kiwanuka-Tondo, Fleming-Milici, and Proctor, 2004). Problems with translation have been identified as contributing to the ineffectiveness of information strategies. Because health communication is a two-way process, a person's ability to understand information is related to the clarity of the message itself, and the appropriateness of the channel, including cultural relevancy (Pirisi, 2000). Generic, one-way messages from experts about disease risks has been ineffective in engaging people to improve their health:

At the heart of the matter is a difficult question: What kind of communication promotes behavior change? Research suggests that it must be participatory, deeply meaningful, empathetic, empowering, interactive, personally relevant, contextually situated, credible and convenient (Neuhauser and Kreps, 2003, p. 18).

Indeed, in a primary-care based four month intervention characterized as 'interactive health communication,' Calfas et al. (2002) demonstrated improved physical activity behaviors among adult patients. After conducting a systematic review of this literature, Finlay and Faulkner (2005) note that without community-level partnerships and resources devoted to enabling more physical activity, a campaign's effectiveness at stimulating change is restricted. The disappointment of health communication interventions in helping people to change their health practices can arguably be blamed on both the inappropriateness of the communication effort, and their irrelevance to people's lives (*Choosing Health*, 2004; Neuhauser and Kreps, 2003).

Finally, the literature notes the role of technological change in ushering in an era of sedentary lifestyles. "Time that earlier generations spent performing more physical activities is now spent with computers, video games, television, and various labor-saving devices" (Matson-Koffman et al., 2005, p. 168). Higher levels of computer use are associated with increased likelihood of physical inactivity. One of the most common leisure-time behaviors, television viewing, is a sedentary behavior and there is a strong positive relationship between hours of television viewing and body mass index (Owen et al., 2000). Study findings revealed that television viewing may have detrimental effects on obesity independent of leisure time physical activity levels: participants who were highly active in their leisure time and reported watching more than four hours of television per day were twice as likely to be overweight as those who watched less than one hour of television per day (Salmon, Bauman, Crawford, Timperio, and Owen, 2000). This influence of modern society on physical activity levels was recently highlighted in a study of an Amish community (Bassett, Schneider, and Huntington, 2004). Pedometers and logsheets were provided to 98 Amish adults living in a North American farming community. Analyses of the data indicated an average of over 16,000 steps/day and 56 hours of activity for men and women, placing them in a very active category.

Interpersonal Factors

It seems that North Americans know they should be more physically active, but concerns of cost, safety, time, accessibility, as well as a lack of culturally, gender, age and skill appropriate opportunities, thwart even the best of intentions. Many Canadians (30-40%) expressed difficulty in finding someone to be active with, or to find a program where they can participate with their children (Canadian Fitness and Lifestyle Research Institute, 1999). Increasing outreach programs, creating social connections among people to be active, and provision of family-oriented services were recommended by Canadians as ways to increase their physical activity. Canadians view supportive services as very important in helping them be active, as well as convenient transportation, services to link up participants and specific instruction or coaching (Craig and Cameron, 2004).

The study of interpersonal level variables assumes that individuals are socially embedded, responding to and affecting their interpersonal environments (Lewis, 1997), thus relationships with family, friends, work colleagues and acquaintances are sources of influence on health related behaviors (McLeroy, Bibeau, Steckler, and Glanz, 1988). To a certain extent, individuals are defined in terms of their interpersonal relationships and this creates confidence and self-efficacy for exercise and health matters. Social support and social networks are important in creating health-enhancing interpersonal environments (Lewis, 1997), and the complexity of social environments must be recognized when approaching health issues (Lyons and Langille, 2000).

Numerous studies throughout the 1970's and 80's consistently revealed that a lack of social networks or ties predicted mortality for almost every cause of death and that "social network size or "connectedness" is inversely related to risk-related behaviors" (Berkman and Glass, 2000, p. 149), including physical inactivity. Social support for exercise is positively related with physical activity (Trieber, Baranowski, Braden, Strong, Levy, and Knox, 1991). Social networks also influence "cognitive and emotion states such as self-esteem, social competence and self efficacy, depression and affect" (Berkman and Glass, 2000, p. 149).

Thus, the most promising interpersonal factor influencing physical activity is social support for exercise from family, friends, neighbors, physicians or exercise program staff (Brownson, et al., 2001; Green, McAfee, Hindmarsh, Madsen, Caplow, and Buist, 2002), particularly for females (Wharf Higgins, Gaul, Gibbons, and Van Gyn, 2003). In their review of the literature, Seefeldt et al. (2002) suggest that there are mixed findings of the utility of social support due in part to methodological issues of investigating the affect of support on physical activity behavior. Yet, in a systematic review of the evidence for physical activity interventions conducted by the Centers for Disease Control Atlanta (Task Force on Community Preventive Services, 2002), non-family social support was strongly recommended based upon the evidence of efficacy. Social support that is direct and tangible (e.g., a ride to an exercise class) or informational (e.g., telephone counseling support to help overcome obstacles) is critical to sustaining an active lifestyle. Social environmental variables, such as exercise surroundings, having family who encourage exercise, and having at least one friend to exercise have been found to profoundly influence behavior. Girls whose parents provide logistical support (transportation, paying for enrollment in programs) or who modeled an active lifestyle, are more likely to be active than those with less involved parents (Davison, Cutting, and Birch, 2003). In fact, a positive association was found to exist: regardless of the type of parental involvement, the greater the involvement, the more likely that daughters were active.

Yet, support is generated by characteristics of people *and* places. The physical and social composition of the urban environment may promote isolation. Sedentary lifestyles associated with high rates of television viewing, computer use, crime concerns, little contact with neighbors and geographic isolation have created communities which are not active or interconnected (Srinivasan, O'Fallon, and Dearry, 2003). In examining neighborhood-level influences on physical activity among older adults, Fisher et al. (2004) found that seniors residing in more socially cohesive neighborhoods were more likely to report walking than those living in less cohesive surroundings, even after accounting for individual-level factors such as gender and health status.

Community and Environmental Factors

The socio-ecological model holds that different settings and environmental characteristics encourage or make it more difficult for people to be active (Owen et al., 2000; Sallis and Owen, 1997). A recent and highly promising tangent of inquiry regarding the obstacles to an active life explores the role of the built environment, urban form and land mix in affecting physical activity patterns. The concept of environmental influence refers not only to physical settings in direct contact with the individual, but the broader social, physical and policy milieu as well. For instance, just as individuals are affected by their socioeconomic status, so are communities. Richer neighborhoods enjoy more healthy amenities and facilities, while poorer areas have higher per capita outlets for alcohol, fast food and fewer retailers of fresh fruits and vegetables, recreation centers and parks (Cohen et al., 2000). Thus, the quality of the physical or built environments often reflect the amount of resources invested in that area and directly impact the healthful options of its residents. This phenomenon is referred to as spatial segregation (Diez Roux, 2003; Seguin and Divay, 2002). Below we discuss the influence of the built environment, with an in-depth discussion of how the urban design of our communities and cities affect physical activity. A look at the social and policy environments then follows.

Built Environment

The built environment is defined as human created or modified places (i.e., places in the physical environment built by people for people), such as schools, workplaces, homes, buildings, roads, parks, business and industrial areas (Northridge, Scla,r and Biswas, 2003; Srinivasan, et al. 2003). Approximately 80% of North Americans are urbanized, that is living in towns and cities, spending almost 90% of the time indoors (Hancock, 2002). Brownson et al. (2005), citing The National Household Transportation Survey, note that everyday – on average – adults drive a personal vehicle for 55 minutes traveling 29 miles. Not surprisingly, the built environment has been shaped by a paradigm that is centered on designing streets for the convenience of motorists (Frank, Engelke, and Schmid, 2003). In fact, two of the early studies in this regard emerged from psychology and urban planning when Handy (1992) and Cervero and Gorham (1995) examined the travel patterns of residents living in older communities and those living in suburban areas. In both studies, people who lived in older, more downtown areas were significantly more likely to either walk or cycle to work or commercial areas. Pikora, Giles Corti, Bull, Jamrozik and Donovan (2003) list four main physical environmental factors that may influence walking and bicycling: functional, safety, aesthetic and destination. Functional factors are attributes of the street or path that reflect the environment, such as type and width of the street, volume, speed and type of traffic, and direct routes to destinations. Safety incorporates the need to keep the environment safe for people, such as having adequate street lighting and pedestrian crossings, and perceived low levels of neighborhood safety (Frank et al., 2003; Jackson and Kochtitzky, 2003). Aesthetic attributes refer to an interesting and pleasing physical environment which includes the condition and size of trees, cleanliness, maintained parks and gardens, pollution level and architectural designs. Destination relates to the availability of community and commercial facilities in the neighborhood, for example post boxes, schools, parks, shops and transportation (bus stops, bike parking facilities and train stations). These are elements considered in urban design.

Urban design refers to the layout of a city, and the arrangement and appearance of the elements within it; it is concerned with the function and appeal of public spaces (Handy, Boarnet, Ewing, and Killingsworth., 2002). Design influences physical activity in that features of the built environment such as traffic safety, large distances between one's starting point and destination, limit travel choice and significantly influence people's decisions to walk or bike (Vandergrift and Yoked, 2004). These decisions shaped by the environment are also linked with individual factors, such as perceptions of lack of time and/or motivation and poor health.

Land use mix refers to the composition, organization or distribution of land uses within a geographical area or space, such as a building, neighborhood or entire city (Frank et al., 2003). It is the degree to which land uses are mixed or have a combination of uses within areas of a region (Ewing, Schmid, Killingsworth, Zlot, and Raudenbush, 2003). Single use areas are used only for one specific purpose, such as residential subdivisions, office/commercial centers, or industrial operations. Mixed-use development describes how far one needs to travel (proximity) between multiple destinations, whereby complementary land uses might include residential, commercial, entertainment and recreational destinations over a small area so there is minimum travel distance between activities (Frank et al., 2003). Distance is a barrier to non-motorized travel, thus mixed-use areas at the local level may have the greatest impact on physical activity and are thought to encourage travel behaviors involving activity, such as walking and biking. Investigating the relationship between pedestrian-friendly urban form and walking patterns among residents aged 70 years and older, Patterson and Chapman (2004) found that traditional urban design, characterized by mixed use services and pedestrian access, to be significantly associated with walking activities. This finding was echoed north of the border as well. Research conducted by the Heart and Stroke Foundation of Canada (2005) found that city-dwellers were twice as likely to walk or bike for both commuting and daily chore purposes. When asked if they found their community convenient to walk or bike in, 87% of city-dwellers responded positively, while only 60% of suburban and rural residents agreed.

Moreover, Canadians living in moderate to high density neighborhoods were 2.4 times more likely to achieve the recommended thirty minutes of activity each day then those in low density areas. Density is defined as a measure of urban design that provides information on how compactly built a place is (Frank et al., 2003) and the amount of activity in an area (Handy et al., 2002). Higher density areas reduce distances (or increase proximities) between destinations, thus higher density areas are thought to promote walking and biking because places are built more compactly and distances are shortened, thus destinations are closer in proximity to each other.

As a form of both transportation and exercise, walking tends to be particularly important for the elderly, disabled and lower income residents who may have fewer personal resources to access travel or physical activity opportunities. Physical activity and public health activities, and urban planners suggest that transportation systems that encourage active travel can serve to promote health and reduce traffic volume (Sallis, Frank, Saelens, and Kraft, 2004). Yet, walking and cycling patterns are more difficult to measure than motorized travel, and relatively inexpensive compared to vehicles, relegating walkers and cyclists invisible to, and undervalued by, transportation planners (Litman, 2004). Further, the higher status accorded motorized vehicles, combined with the automobile and oil industry lobbying efforts, has historically left pedestrians and cyclists without a strong voice at the planning table.

Aesthetic qualities of the built environment contribute to the attractiveness or appeal of a place (Handy et al., 2002). Examples include size and orientation of windows in buildings, landscaping including trees for shade along a street and public amenities such as benches and lighting. Thus, urban design features such as traffic, lighting, sidewalk maintenance, streetlights, and scenery also influence activity. Humpel, Owen, and Leslie (2002) found that accessibility of facilities, opportunities for activity, and aesthetic attributes had significant associations with physical activity and weather and safety showed less-strong relationships.

Street design is the layout and design of individual streets or networks, such as the length, size and connectivity of neighborhood streets/blocks (Frank et al., 2003). Connectivity is defined as "the directness and availability of alternative routes from one point to another within a street network" (Handy et al., 2002, p. 66). Street design can encourage walking or biking if it is attractive, perceived as safe (e.g., includes crosswalks, street lights), and connected to other streets. A common view held by urban planners, engineers and architects is that street design elements should be set by motorists' needs as a street's central purpose is to move motorized traffic efficiently and pedestrians hinder the flow of motorized traffic.

Utilitarian travel is for practical purpose or transportation to a destination, such as a trip to the store or work. Moderately intense activity, such as walking or bicycling, that can be purposive and incorporated into daily habits are more likely to be adopted and maintained because it is part of a daily routine, as well as because few financial resources are required (Frank et al, 2003). Walking, as a form of travel, has held very little interest for traditional transportation planners compared to motorized travel (Coogan and Coogan, 2004). This disinterest coincided with the historical public health research emphasis on vigorous activity. With a new appreciation of the health benefits of moderate activity, such as walking and cycling, as well as its role in serving utilitarian travel purposes, there is acknowledgement that activity can be built back into the lives of people by changing the ways communities are designed and structured (Frank et al., 2003).

Saelens, Sallis and Frank (2003) summarized research on the environmental correlates of walking and cycling and concluded that residents from communities with higher densities and greater connectivity and land use mix report higher rates of walking/cycling for utilitarian purposes than those from low-density, poorly connected and single land use neighborhoods. Recent work has confirmed these findings (Atkinson, Sallis, Saelens, Cain and Black, 2005; Sallis et al., 2004; Sharpe, Granner, Hutto andAinsworth, 2004): adults meeting recommendations for achieving moderate to vigorous physical activity levels were significantly more likely to live in higher density areas with well maintained and connected sidewalks, safe areas for walking or jogging, and have knowledge of walking or cycling routes. Zlot and Schmid (2005) used data from the Behavioral Risk Factor Surveillance System, the Nationwide Personal Transportation Survey, and the Trust for Public Land to investigate the association between community characteristics and walking/cycling behavior. San Francisco had the highest percentage of recreational walkers and cyclists, while more New Yorkers walked or cycled as a mode of transportation. Not surprisingly, a significant association between utilitarian walking/bicycling and parkland acreage was found.

One example of how to increase connectivity in an area would be to build pathways between residential subdivisions and retail developments for non-motorists (Frank et al., 2003). Choice of travel mode is influenced by the costs of different modes, such as length of time or how much money the trip will require. Frank et al. (2003) state that environmental changes can be focused on increasing the cost of one mode and decreasing the cost of another or making an area more welcoming to non-motorized travel. For example, traffic calming measures increase the cost of car travel through the use of speed bumps or narrow streets which slow cars down and decrease the incidence of potential accidents and encourage street use by non-motorists.

A groundbreaking national study by Ewing et al. (2003) in the US showed a direct association between community form and people's activity levels, weight and health. This was the first study to establish a link between the form of the community and people's health, revealing that sprawling counties were associated with people walking less during leisure time, weighing more (higher body mass index) and having a greater prevalence of hypertension than residents of compact counties. These findings were seen after controlling for age, education, gender, race and ethnicity. The degree of sprawl in a county was indicated with a sprawl index, whereby sprawling counties were spread-out and homes may be far from other destinations, such as services or businesses and the only route between destinations may be a high traffic road that is unpleasant or unsafe for bicycling or walking.

People in sprawling and compact areas were equally likely to report that they had exercised during leisure hours (e.g., golfing, gardening, walking, running), indicating that the degree of sprawl does not influence whether people exercise in leisure hours (Ewing et al., 2003). The study found that people in sprawling communities weighed more, suggesting that they may be missing out on health benefits that are available due to decreased levels of routine activity incorporated into daily life, such as climbing stairs, walking to a transit stop, biking to work or stores. The most likely way that community design influences weight is by encouraging or discouraging physical activity in daily life (Robert Wood Johnson, 2003b).

Social and Policy Environments

Intimately tied to the built environment are the social relationships, structures and policies that operate within the physical spaces. For example, issues of safety, traffic, crime, and access to resources impact residents' views about their neighborhood (Mullan, 2004), in addition to how its physical characteristics (i.e., the presence of sidewalks/paths, enjoyable scenery, hills) encourage or discourage physical activity (Ball, Bauman, Leslie, and Owen, 2001; Booth, Owen, Bauman, Clavisi, and Leslie, 2000). According to the 2002 Physical Activity Monitor, almost half of Canadians view supportive infrastructure as very important in helping them be active, such as safe streets and public spaces (48%), affordable facilities and programs (43%), access to paths, trails and green space (42%) (Craig and Cameron, 2004). Perceptions of safety and neighborhood instability also constrain walking among Americans (Balfour and Kaplan, 2002; Centers for Disease Control and Prevention, 1999b), and these subjective self-ratings have been found to match more objective measures of environmental attributes.

Socioeconomic status constrains the range of available choices for travel and activity within the built environment for people of low income (Frank et al., 2003). Physical activity levels were shown to be lower, and body weight higher, for people living in poverty areas, thus place of residence influences health behavior arguably due to few opportunities for, and access to affordable active living (parks, trails, indoor gyms) (Bengoechea and Spence, 2003;

Brownson et al., 2001; Ellaway Anderson, and Macintyre, 1997; Sallis, Bauman and Pratt,1998; Yen and Kaplan, 1998). In a review of the literature examining the epidemiology of walking, Eyler, et al. (2003) suggest that "providing places to walk (e.g., building walking trails, improving sidewalks and street lighting) may be the impetus for individuals who have never to begin this behavior" (p. 1535).

Deteriorated physical environments are linked to high crime rates (Srinivasan et al., 2003) and lack of neighborhood safety may discourage walking. Despite these social and environmental attributes, there is evidence that residents from low income areas walk more than residents of higher income neighborhoods, perhaps due to the expense of owning and operating automobiles (California Department of Health Services, 2004; Centers for Disease Control and Prevention, 2002; Niemeier and Rutherford, 1995).

The potent combination of socioeconomic and environmental affect on activity levels are exemplified in a recent study where the extent of neighborhood social (e.g., loitering, drinking alcohol, fighting, selling drugs, prostitution), and physical (e.g., grafitti, trash, needles, beer bottles) disorder and lack of safety were found to predict physical activity of children and youth living in 80 Chicago neighborhoods regardless of socioeconomic, demographic, and race/ethnic composition (Molnar, Gortmaker, Bull, and Buka, 2004). As the authors note, these are modifiable characteristics that will demand coordinated action from law enforcement, social services, community groups, waste management in addition to the traditional sectors responsible for youth and physical activity (i.e., education, recreation/parks, sporting organizations). Durkin, Laraque, Lubman and Barlow (1999) recommend changes to the built environment that involve injury prevention methods in low income neighborhoods, particularly to reduce car accidents with pedestrians, and the creation of safe and accessible play areas in preventing traffic injuries to children in urban communities.

For school children, proximity of their home to the school is the primary factor influencing walking patterns (Centers for Disease Control and Prevention, 2002). In addition to the factors previously identified as important for walking - extensive sidewalk coverage, short blocks, or a mixture of land uses - smaller schools that tend to be integrated in densely populated neighborhoods have more children who walk than larger centralized schools (Braza, Shoemaker, and Seeley, 2004). A blend of supportive built and social school environments further influence physical activity levels: those with physical activity facilities and amenities (e.g., basketball hoops, fields, goalposts, indoor gymnasium), and adult supervision were found to have four to five times higher rates of activity among students than in schools where the physical and social resources were deficient (Sallis, Conway, Prochaska, McKenzie, Marshall, and Brown, 2001, Sallis, Johnson, Calfas, Caparosa, and Nichols, 1997).

These data citing barriers that are beyond the control of the individual has spawned this exciting and new area of research – that of the community environment in influencing people's ability to be active. New research is identifying the modifiable environmental determinants and best evidence-based intervention strategies for whole populations, rather than individualized exercise prescriptions that target relatively proximate causes of inactivity (Owen et al., 2000; Vandergrift and Yoked, 2004). The field has recognized the high priority of investigating the role of environmental variables and develop models to predict conditions which promote and support physical activity (Handy et al., 2002) and incorporating environmental variables into health and physical activity research may inform advances in physical activity interventions (Saelens et al., 2003). The bulk of the research has been cross-section in nature. To establish causation, longitudinal and prospective designs will be required (Leslie, Saelens, Frank, Owen, Bauman, Coffee, and Hugo, 2005).

SUMMARY

This section has described the numerous variables influencing an individual's decision regarding, and capacity for, an active life. Yet, a lack of consistency in the design, analysis and reporting of physical activity interventions has produced ambiguous and equivocal results (Seefeldt et al., 2002). Because Eyler, Matson-Koffman and colleagues (2003) failed to identify one factor related to intrapersonal, interpersonal or community/environmental levels consistently associated with physical activity among various population groups, they contend "no single intervention fits all" (p. 103). As the next section details, implementation of a comprehensive strategy incorporating these multiple levels of influence are a requisite to the successful promotion of physical activity (Giles-Corti and Donovan, 2003; Seefeldt et al., 2002).

BEST PRACTICES AND INTERVENTIONS TO PROMOTE PHYSICAL ACTIVITY

Physical activity intervention research has only been conducted in the last 25 years (Dunn and Blair, 2002). More than 4000 studies have been published since 1991, undoubtedly due to the 1987 publication of Powell et al. who summarized the epidemiology of exercise on preventing death and disease. Over this quarter century, health surveys, studies, theories and interventions have influenced a change in focus from vigorous fitness oriented guidelines to moderate physical activity recommendations for health outcomes (Dubbert, 2002). Health strategies (interventions and research) are shifting from a focus on individual motivation for vigorous exercise to moderate intensity activities, such as walking in the context of everyday life (Pikora et al., 2003; Owen, et al., 2000). Concurrent with this shift, epidemiology and transportation research have reached as a consensus that the physical and social environments influence a person's propensity to walk or cycle (Coogan and Coogan, 2004). Because increased physical activity levels have been linked to behavioral, social and environmental correlates, community based interventions promoting activity are critical to increasing activity levels (Kahn, Ramsey, Brownson, Heath, Howze et al., 2002). Understanding how neighborhood attributes shape active living has practical and policy implications in that multi-sector and disciplinary action (e.g., transportation, urban planning, public health, environmental protection) is required (Leslie et al., 2005). As well, public health strategies for increasing physical activity that reach a broader range of people than commonly accessed through clinically oriented approaches or studies have proven to be successful in increasing physical activity levels (King, 1991). Support for intersectoral research alliances and collaboration for public health is seen in the literature (Craig, Brownson, Cragg, and Dunn, 2002; Srinivasan et al., 2003).

Interventions addressing components of the socio-ecological model (intrapersonal, interpersonal and environmental factors) suggest that it not only provides a useful means of understanding physical inactivity, but also tackling it. Indeed, the evidence argues that concurrent interventions at multiple levels offer the best hope for initiating and sustaining physical activity levels and should be encouraged (Pellman, Brandt and Macaran, 2002). In a comprehensive review of the evidence, five types of interventions were found to demonstrate strong or sufficient evidence for increasing physical activity levels (Task Force on Community Preventive Services, 2002): (1) Community-wide campaigns that included the use of mass media in concert with other strategies (support, counseling, education, community events, environmental/policy changes). Of the 10 studies reviewed, the median result was a five percent increase in physical activity rates among various sub-populations of rural, urban and ethnic and socioeconomic groups. (2) Point-of-decision prompts where signs encouraged people to use the stairs rather than elevators or escalators. Placed in a variety of settings (malls, bus stations, worksites), the median rise in stair use was 54% among obese and non-obese persons. (3) Creating or strengthening social support networks, such as a buddy system or walking clubs, has demonstrated a 44% increase in physical activity levels among adults of various ages and activity levels. (4) Individually-adapted and tailored behavior change programs that teach or enhance personal skills in goal setting and self-monitoring, reinforcement, problem-solving and prevention of relapse, as well as developing a social support network, promise a 35% increase in activity levels. (5) Creating or enhancing access to places for physical activity, for example exercise facilities in the workplace, or creation of cycling or walking trails. Typically, these programs also addressed individual and group factors, such as education, counseling, screening, support systems, resulting in a median increase in activity of 25%.

Cohen, Scribner and Farley (2000) have recently proposed a structural, ecological and pragmatic model of health behavior to guide interventions. They suggest four categories of structural and environmental influences to target in behavior change interventions: availability of protective or harmful products and services; physical structures or characteristics of products and services; social structures and policies, and media and cultural messages. The following are just but a few examples from the literature demonstrating that interventions in these four categories, as well as examples of those recommended by the Task Force, can enhance activity levels. A more in-depth discussion of school-based best practices closes this section.

- A home-based program used a contingent television devise to promote activity among obese 8-12 year olds. After 3 weeks, significant differences between intervention and control group participants in pedaling (64.4 vs. 8.3 minutes/week) and viewing time (1.6 vs. 21 hours per week) were achieved (Faith et al., 2001).
- A school lunch hour walking program organized for urban youth increased physical activity by 2400 steps/day (Bush, Leenders, Nicole, and O'Sullivan, 2004).
- Age, income and culturally appropriate physical recreational activities tailored for pre-adolescent African American, low-income girls in a community-based youth organization increased their enjoyment of, and sense of efficacy in, physical exercises (Klebanoff and Muramatsu, 2002).

- A national social marketing campaign funded by CDC to promote physical activity among 'tweens' (9-13 yrs) entitled "Verb. It's what you do" is seeking to establish 'brand loyalty' for physical activity similar to corporations' efforts to establish loyalty for products that encourage sedentary living. Marketing research has discovered that youth consider eating chips and watching TV to be fun. The VERB campaign will not lecture on the dangers of a couch-dwelling, high-fat life. Rather, it emphasizes that physical activity can be consistent with tween values: spending time with friends, having fun, gaining recognition, exploring the world around them. A longitudinal, dose-response study to evaluate the outcome of VERB is underway (6 communities have been sampled to receive high 'doses' of the VERB campaign) (Wong et al., 2004). FULL REF

- Taking an ecological and community-based approach to promoting walking through a media campaign coupled with support, Reger et al. (2002) demonstrated a 23% increase in walking among 50 to 65 year olds in West Virginia.

- "Concord A Great Place to be Active!" (Wen et al., 2002) was an Australian program designed to help women overcome personal, social and cultural barriers to physical activity. The community-wide campaign included social marketing, creation of activity opportunities and intersectoral commitment/involvement from local community, and was successful in motivating and sustaining walking behaviours for three years.

- A similar initiative occurred in Laval, Quebec (Nguyen, Gauvin, Martineau and Grignon, 2002) where the local public health region spearheaded the creation of walking clubs. Residents were trained as walking 'club' directors, and provided with resources to organize and implement walking groups. Over 800 residents joined the clubs and remained active members three years after its initiation.

- Construction of walking trails for rural, low income, African American populations enhanced their physical activity levels, particularly women and less educated residents were twice as likely to engage in more walking (Brownson, Houseman, Brown, Jackson-Homson, King, Malone and Sallis, 2000).

- The use of signs to promote stair use (Brownell, Stunkard and Albaum, 1980; Kahn et al., 2002), environmental prompts combined with incentives (Knadler and Rogers, 1987), and incentives to reward bicycle path use (Mayer and Geller, 1982) have been found effective in enhancing activity when compared to control groups' activity behaviors.

- Multiple strategies were found to be effective in increasing activity levels among naval base employees, including extending facility hours, acquiring more equipment, sponsorship of events and clubs, and mapping a one mile running route (Linenger, Chesson, and Nice, 1991).

- Worksite interventions that draw on a combination of tactics, such as installing locker rooms, providing onsite equipment, and delivering programs and counseling, as well as creating a supportive work culture for physical activity, have found physical activity levels to rise when compared to implementing just one component (Calfas et al., 1996; Erfurt, Foote and Heirich, 1991; Golaszewski, Barr, Blodgett, and Delprino, 1996; Hammond, Leonard, and Fridinger, 2000; Heirich, Foote, and Konopka, 1993; Proper et al., 2003; Veuori, Oja, and Paronen, 1994).

School-Based Interventions

Recent concerns regarding the sedentary lifestyles of adolescents (Wharf Higgins et al., 2003) has turned researchers' attention to the school setting and physical education (PE) classroom. The average child spends almost 50% of their waking hours in school (Fox, Cooper, and McKenna, 2004) explaining why most research addressing physical activity among children and youth have used schools as a site of intervention (Sallis et al., 2003). While there are calls for comprehensive school health promotion initiatives in the literature (Allensworth, Wyche, Lawson, and Nicholson, 1995; Story, 1999), in practice there are few examples, fewer evaluations providing evidence of their effectiveness, and less still that address environmental and policy components (Deschesnes, Martin, and Jomphe Hill, 2003; Lynagh, Schofield, and Sanson-Fisher, 1997). Most school programs adopt a curriculum and social skills approach. For example, "Active Winners," (Pate et al., 2003) a community-based physical activity intervention targeting African American 5th graders, offered in and after-school, summer programs, and community programs that were non-competitive, confidence building, enjoyable and socially oriented. The program was intended to influence the social and physical environments, and provide external cues to promote physical activity. However, its summative evaluation found no significant changes in activity levels after 18 months. Despite the intention to be ecological in nature, the process evaluations revealed that the programs failed to consider and address key social, cultural and environmental influences.

Several systematic reviews of the impact of school-based interventions on the physical activity levels of children and youth have been conducted (Dobbins, Lockett, Michel et al., 2001; Thomas, Ciliska, Wilson-Abra, Micucci, Dobbins and Dwyer, 2004; Stone, McKenzie, Welk and Booth, 1998). The most recent (Thomas et al., 2004) identified eight studies that specifically targeted physical activity and could be considered strong evidence. The majority of research involved the upper elementary years and interventions that lasted between 8 and 15 weeks, although SPARK (Sallis, McKenzie, Alcaraz, Kolody, Faucette, and Hovell, 1997) was eight months in duration. Thomas et al. (2004) concluded that all offered more opportunities to be active in the school day and all increased physical activity levels during the intervention period but these increases were not sustained. Effective programs were characterized by a multi-faceted approach seeking a balance between skill development and physical activity in PE, and increasing the amount of PE delivered (Thomas et al., 2004). There are many environments in which increases in dedicated physical education time have not been supported at the systems level (state or provincial government) and therefore a sole focus on physical education as the solution to physical inactivity has been debated (Fox, Cooper, and McKenna, 2004). In addition, many programs that focused on the curriculum and health education show no behavioral outcomes (Thomas et al., 2004).

There are however some notable examples from the research that do highlight the benefits of a more comprehensive and ecological approach rather than a sole focus on physical activity and curriculum. Most of these exemplar programs integrate healthy eating and incorporate a focus on changing the environment. Ground breaking work in this area is typified by the Child and Adolescent Trial for Cardiovascular Health (CATCH), a comprehensive intervention addressing environmental approaches. CATCH demonstrated significant changes in the fat content of school lunches, increased moderate to vigorous physical activity in PE and improved eating and physical activity behaviors of children (Luepker, Perry, McKinlay et al., 1996, McKenzie, Nader, Strikmiller, Yang Stone et al.,

1996). CATCH used a combination of policy change in the cafeteria and physical education, school curriculum, interactive education events, activities and communication tools to educate students and families.

The Middle-School Physical Activity and Nutrition (M-SPAN) (McKenzie et al., 2004; Sallis et al., 2003) also represents the shift to this more comprehensive school health-based model and provides evidence of the effectiveness of the approach. M-SPAN addressed policy and environmental aspects in a two-year school-based intervention to promote physical activity and healthy eating, focusing on the PE curriculum, providing before and after-school opportunities for activity, improving equipment and adult supervision, educating parents about the benefits of physical activity for their children and creating student and staff health committees. Sallis et al. (2003) found that in the schools assigned to the intervention, overall school activity levels increased. However, at the level of individual behavior, the transfer of the effect to outside of school behavior was statistically significant for boys only.

At the elementary school level, Action Schools! BC (McKay, Naylor, Rhodes et al., 2004) and the Annapolis Valley Health Promoting Schools Project (Veugelers and Fitzgerald, 2005) have adopted this approach and their findings provide preliminary support for the potential of comprehensive school health-based models for increasing physical activity levels in this younger age group. At the high school level the Healthy Youth Places initiative in England has also adopted this approach (Dzewaltowski, Estabrooks, and Johnston, 2002) but findings are not yet available. In addition to an environment / ecological approach and addressing multiple health issues the comprehensive school health model, it has been recognized that the engagement of multiple stakeholders in school-level coordination, context specific negotiated planning and linkages with community are critical. The emphasis on choice, involvement of those affected by the problem and local decision-making in these models represents best practice in health promotion and enhances the likelihood of sustainability (Syme, 2004).

Yet another critical shift evident in the literature is a move from a sport and movement skill-based approach toward a lifestyle physical activity approach. Sports-based curricula with its emphasis on competitive achievements and skill testing has been criticized for tending to the needs of only the most athletic of students (Gibbons, Van Gyn, Wharf Higgins, and Gaul, 2000; Gibbons, Wharf Higgins, Gaul, and Van Gyn, 1999). As PE becomes an elective in many high schools across Canada, enrollment has plummeted along with activity levels. US 2003 data reveal that about 55% of students in grades 9-12 enroll in PE, while less than 29% regularly attend (Centers for Disease Control and Prevention, 2004). This trend is mirrored at the elementary level as well, when children did not compensate for a lack of daily PE by adding to their out-of-school experiences (Dale, Corbin, and Dale, 2000). Research has also indicated that what is taught in school PE and the training of the teacher can influence student attitudes towards, and participation in, PE (Gibbons et al., 2000; 1999), as well as the quality and minutes of exposure to opportunities to be physically active (Sallis et al., 1997). Work in Canada has found that encouraging female high school students to enroll in PE, when it becomes an elective in grades 11 and 12, demands that teachers stray from the typical sports-based curriculum to emphasize lifelong physical activities where participation, rather than skill, is the basis for grading students' accomplishments (Gibbons et al., 1999).

In the US, school interventions that have followed national guidelines and standards seem to be effective in enhancing physical activity levels in school and after graduation. One such example is " Project Active Teen" (Dale and Corbin, 2000; Dale, Corbin, and Cuddihy, 1998) based on the HELP philosophy (Corbin and Lindsey, 1997). "H is for a **H**ealth focus, E is for a focus on **E**veryone regardless of ability level, L is for the focus on **L**ifelong activities, and P is for learning the skills to plan a **P**ersonal lifelong activity program" (Corbin, 2001, p. 352). The evidence from the school literature provides clear indication of the potential influence of settings on physical activity. The socio-ecological approach also suggests that a focus on more than one setting is necessary. This is illustrated by the work of Dale and colleagues (2000) who demonstrated that elementary school children did not compensate for a lack of daily PE by adding to their out-of-school experiences. In fact, Thomas et al. (2004) conducted a systematic review of school-based physical activity and healthy eating interventions and recommended that further research needs to focus on the community and family setting.

AN APPLICATION OF THE SOCIO-ECOLOGICAL MODEL: THE SAANICH PENINSULA DIABETES PREVENTION PROJECT

The Saanich Peninsula Diabetes Prevention Project, located on South Vancouver Island, British Columbia, was funded through Health Canada's Diabetes Prevention Strategy, 2001-2005. Comprised of three municipalities (population ~36,000), and four First Nations bands (population 4,600), the Saanich Peninsula hosts the Island's major international airport and ferry terminal. Top employers include farming and industrial parks, as well as tourism. Approximately half of the Peninsula's residents commute 12 miles to Greater Victoria for work (Capital Regional District, 2004). In a hybrid partnership of local community organizations and professionals working together, SPDPP delivered innovative recreation and health education programs designed to foster an active lifestyle among residents who may be at greater risk for type 2 diabetes, as well as other chronic health conditions. The project was initiated by the administrator of Panorama Recreation Center (a public recreation facility) and university faculty who assembled a team of eight intersectoral and multi-disciplinary partners, including representatives from community organizations serving persons with low incomes, and seniors; First Nations bands; Canadian Diabetes Association; the regional department of public health (nutrition, health promotion, Aboriginal Health, diabetes education); and, a citizen planning group. Since its inception, the SPDPP engaged an additional 26 organizations/agencies (e.g., Food Bank, schools, Native Friendship Centre, library) to be involved in various aspects of community-wide events, programs, and initiatives to strengthen local services supportive of diabetes-healthy living.

'A Taste of Healthy Living'

Scholars appeal for more research to identify "generic intervention strategies - enhanced social support, modifying access, and barriers" to prevent disease and promote health (Roussos and Fawcett, 2000, p. 392). The project's extensive two year community mobilization and needs assessment phase heeded this call, from which a program framework entitled "A Taste of Healthy Living" was developed. The program was designed to introduce participants to a "menu" of physical activities, and foster social inclusion while addressing the identified transportation, economic and resource barriers. The eight week program was offered to distinct groups of people living with low incomes, seniors and individuals clinically at risk for type 2 diabetes. The First Nations bands decided to integrate culturally appropriate walking programs into their schools and communities rather than participate in "A Taste of Healthy Living." The walking programs are detailed elsewhere (Wharf Higgins, Rickert, and Rutherford, 2004). With the assistance of SPDPP staff and a program facilitator each group of participants tailored the program content to their collective interests and incorporated individualized participant goals. In a "support group" format, the program offered a variety of low or no cost recreational activities, transportation to and from venues, and access to experts (e.g., fitness leaders, nurses and community resources). Participants also received, at no cost, t-shirts, water bottles, pedometers, and print materials related to their interests (e.g., community contacts, health education resources). Participants met at the recreation center to begin each session with a discussion of the previous week's goals, and would then engage in a variety of activities, for example, testing their blood sugar levels and attending educational sessions with a community health nurse; touring the recreation facility weight room, pool, walking trail and other amenities; participating in trail hikes, chair exercises, yoga, tai chi and Swiss ball classes; and participating in discussions about, being introduced to, and visiting community resources (e.g., Food Bank, Good Food Box program, computer services at library, free lunches at local churches). This section presents findings from a total of twelve programs delivered over a two year period; five for low income residents (n=35), and four each for seniors (n=30), and two each for clinically at risk (n=15) individuals.

Procedure

The SPDPP utilized a community-based research (CBR) design, working *with* project partners and citizens at risk of developing type 2 diabetes in all aspects of the project from needs assessment to evaluation. The CBR process is characterized by collaborative investigation, education and action to support those with less power in community settings (Hall, 2001). According to Leung and colleagues (2004), the application of CBR principles is important to help make epidemiological findings locally relevant and context specific in the development of meaningful policy and practice (Leung et al., 2004). They also acknowledge the labor and time intensive nature of CBR as well as the challenge and importance of developing relationships with people in different disciplines and sectors. However, working outside disciplinary silos, utilizing a multidisciplinary approach, and forming partnerships built on trust and equity in a collaborative process are important so that communities determine their priorities, and participate in identifying suitable intervention methods and solutions for enabling change.

Data Collection

The following methods of data collection were implemented: participant questionnaires (pre-and post program); participant focus group interviews (post-program); program facilitator exit interviews; participant logbooks/journals (post program transcription and analysis). All questions asked of participants and program facilitators followed the theoretical framework Precede/Proceed (Green and Kreuter, 1999) that oriented the overall project research design. Precede/Proceed is a health promotion planning and evaluation framework that is best described as socio-ecological: it asks planners to consider the intrapersonal, interpersonal and community and environmental determinants relevant to the targeted health issue. In the post-program interviews, participants and facilitators were asked to contemplate and reflect on what factors predisposed (or motivated), enabled and reinforced or supported participation in the program and its activities. In addition, during interviews, participants were asked to reflect on program aspects they would maintain and change, the influence of the program on their eating and physical activity knowledge and behaviors, and access to and familiarity with community resources to support healthy living. The response rate for the pre- and post-program questionnaire was 61% (n=49); 83% of participants attended the post-program focus group discussion (n=66), and 33% submitted completed logbooks (n=26). The majority of those who completed pre-program questionnaires were female (n=50) and Caucasian (n=63); between the ages of 40-64 (n=34) or 65 + (n=27). Forty percent (n=32) reported earning less than $20,000 (CAN)/year, the majority of these being women aged 40-45 (n=35).

DATA ANALYSIS

Data were transcribed/imported by SPDPP staff and analyzed/interpreted by the first two authors. EXCEL software facilitated questionnaire data analysis and NVivo was used to manage and organize the focus group, interview, and journal data and integrate coding with qualitative linking, shaping, and modeling. Various techniques were used to analyze data (i.e., text searches for co-occurrence of theme words and key concepts and using proximity function, and Boolean searches). The Precede/Proceed framework provided the initial conceptual orientation for data analysis (Patton, 1990). First, using an editing analysis approach (Crabtree and Miller, 1992), open coding of predisposing, reinforcing, and enabling factors were identified. As patterns and themes began to emerge across focus group and interview transcripts, and journals, and relationships between categories became apparent, each one was revisited to link connections between them as axial coding, memoing, clustering and factoring, and other inductive analytic strategies were employed (Miles and Huberman, 1994). Thus, interpretation of data occurred through a method of constant comparison (Henderson, 1991) whereby relevant literature was revisited and located in order to make sense of the patterns and themes captured in the categories.

Limitations

The limitations of the study include: participant self-selection and self-report of personal goals for change, which is inherent in a CBR approach, particularly because of the purposeful emphasis on participant ownership and control of program activities. Thus, we were reluctant to impose evaluation directives/outcomes and standardized tests/procedures for all and additional data were not collected to confirm participants' self-reports about improved health behaviors or outcomes (e.g., fitness tests, food recall diaries). Participants declined the opportunity to endure such measurements, and we abided their decisions, nurturing trust and respect. This measurement failure (Weiss, 1998) is common to academic-community partnerships and the realities of community-based grant funding limitations (Zapka, Valentine Goins, Pbert, and Ockene, 2004). The decision to be participatory and sample purposively (Patton, 1990) resulted in compromising the overall sample size; a weakness in the ability to conduct and calculate statistics beyond descriptive percentages and generate interpretive statistical relationships. While more of a key learning outcome, than a limitation, the participants' own comfort level with and trust of the research process, particularly the citizens living with low income, influenced results since the use of logbooks as a data collection method did not work well with all participant groups. For low income participants, entries proved to be too personal or bothersome to complete, however logbooks were well received and utilized by the seniors and clinically-at-risk participants. A final limitation is the short timeline in which programs were implemented and evaluated. Visible and/or measurable changes in population health outcomes may not be detectable for 3-10 years (Roussos and Fawcett, 2000), particularly when the emphasis was on social, rather than bio-medical determinants of health.

However, the participatory, ecological and multi-method design lends credibility to and support for our findings (Vogel, 2002). The conventional reliance on quantitative methods to gather data from primarily individually, behaviorally and educationally oriented interventions has provided some insight into why some people engage in healthy living and others do not, but we lack a full understanding of how and why such choices are made (Syme, 2002). We were not seeking to predict behaviors but understand the complexity of them. The time we spent in the field established the trustworthiness and transferability of our data (Guba and Lincoln, 1989) and "obtaining a sample was not simply a matter of recruiting people into the research but, rather, a complex social process of gaining access into the community itself" (Sixsmith, Boneham, and Goldring, 2003, p. 579).We were able to triangulate through various data collection sources/methods (both quantitative and qualitative), researchers and theory and in doing so, captured multiple perspectives, and a more substantive description and confirmation of, participants' and facilitators' experiences in the program (Berg, 1998).

Results: Findings Related to Participants' Lives

Three major themes were identified in the data analysis of "Taste of Healthy Living" programs confirming the intrapersonal, interpersonal and environmental influences on active living. The first focuses on the advantages of monitoring tools (intrapersonal), the second on supportive environments (interpersonal), and the third on participants' acquired knowledge to support behavior changes and self-reported and perceived improvements in health (community/environmental).

Intrapersonal: The Power of The Pedometer

The pedometer, a simple tool, was found to motivate, enable and reinforce participants' physical activity levels. It provided a benchmark of how participants' daily routines translated into healthy living and encouraged doing a little more each day. One participant explained in a post-program focus group "the pedometer was motivating [me] to use it everyday. I looked forward to reading the number of steps every night; I really loved wearing it." Fellow participants similarly remarked

> When I first got it [pedometer] I think I might have done 500 steps in a week, and then it started to double each week, and it showed me that I was progressing and that I was doing something. It built my self-esteem, and with self-esteem going up I got more active. The little self-esteem that I was given by comin' to this program was worth a million dollars...it's priceless.
>
> The pedometer was great, I wore it for the first two weeks and did daily stuff and now I bike 30 minutes or walk for an hour to get 10,000 steps and I've changed my eating a little.

With very few exceptions, the majority of participants and program facilitators remarked that this monitoring tool acted as key mediators influencing their lives. They cited the motivating influence on their intention to continue being physically active as a resource that enabled them to monitor their progress, experience success, and begin to integrate healthy behaviors as part of their daily routine. Perhaps because it can take months before the effects of lifestyle changes are noticed by individuals, receiving immediate feedback about an activity (e.g., number of steps recorded on a pedometer) seemed to have motivated those who had not previously experienced longer-term success. These findings mirror the exercise psychology literature where strategies for reinforcement control and self-monitoring have been found effective in motivating and sustaining behavior change (Buckworth and Dishman, 2002).

Participants reported increased knowledge related to making simple yet important changes to their lifestyle. Those who completed a post-program questionnaire reported learning more about healthy living. For example:

- 78% (n=62) of participants somewhat or strongly agreed with the statement "a person can get type 2 diabetes from not exercising or being physically active on a regular basis;"
- 81% (n=65) somewhat or strongly agreed with the statement "a person can get type 2 diabetes from not having a healthy body weight;"
- 95% (n= 76) somewhat or strongly agreed with the statement "a person can reduce their risk of getting type 2 diabetes."

Qualitative data from post-program focus group interviews confirmed these findings:

> Very useful and goal-oriented to really make us change our lifestyle to one of active and healthful living [seniors' group, participant, focus group].
>
> Information received was all very helpful I have passed the information I have gained to my son and other young adults because the info is so pertinent [seniors' group, participant, focus group].

Acquiring knowledge about behavior change and community resources, motivated, reinforced, and enabled participants to increase their levels of physical activity These changes, according to participants, reportedly helped to them lower blood glucose and cholesterol levels, contributed to weight loss, and enhanced coping with stress and depression. For example, one low income participant noted the influence activity had on her health, "It makes me feel better. I've always known this, that if I can put one foot in front of the other that eventually it'll help my depression."

Interpersonal: A supportive environment

The support group format also functioned as a motivating factor for individuals and in nurturing connections among participants. The goal-setting activity was personal and individualized in which participants determined their own aspirations (e.g., become more active, feel better about themselves, connect to the community). This goal-setting provided a sense of control or input and created a relevant and meaningful purpose for each that they also perceived to be shared as well. This role of leisure has been described as problem-focused coping (Folkman et al., 1991). Group discussions of participants' progress and challenges led off each session, which generated group problem-solving and strategizing that helped individuals attain their goals, and fostered bonding between group members. Further, the notion that participants could modify or adapt their goals as the program ensued fostered "new ways to do things," as well as "experiencing success at every session, and hearing about everyone's successes including my own" [seniors' group, participant, focus group]. With low income participants, the connections made and problem-solving strategies learned motivated them to continue meeting as a group and to continue to be physically active after the program's completion.

Trusting, confidential, and reciprocal relationships were formed and as one low income participant mentioned, the group "holds together and supports each other" and the program was an opportunity "meet people of other social and financial levels and not feel....isolated" and "to meet people who can understand and were helpful and they like me to help them which...gives me something for my self worth." Thus, interacting with others (i.e., social support and inclusion) encouraged, motivated and supported physical activity and individual change. One low income participant commented, "it gave me the shot I that needed to do something about the way things were going". Another stated,

> We got to meet and know people but we maintained confidentiality so we were able to talk. It felt good - like I trust them and they trust me. I think that's good. I think you need an element of trust in any relationship. [low income group, participant, focus group].

Echoing earlier work arguing that leisure satisfies the need for affiliation (Tinsely and Eldredge, 1995), and provides a sense of purpose, belonging and acceptance (Hutchinson, Loy, Kleiber, and Dattilo, 2003), the socialization aspect of the programs also served to enable participants' involvement. Participants of the low income groups explained, "I'm not as shy or not wanting to meet people. I used to stay home all the time and watch t.v., and now I'm coming out every Monday" and "just the fact that everybody was there and those that normally wouldn't normally participate in things felt that they could." A senior participant mentioned that "Going to Panorama [has] been positive to help me meet people in the community and it's just opening up a different world to all these connections in all these different ways."

In addition to creating new relationships within the group, the programs inspired participants' sense of belonging to and knowledge of the community and its resources to support healthy living. Of the participants responding to the post-program questionnaire, 95% (n=76) reported that the consequences of the program included being somewhat or strongly informed about what was available in the community to help improve health, knowledgeable about who to contact in the community regarding health questions or issues, and, supported by the community to live a healthy lifestyle. In the words of one of the low income participants, "this program made us aware that there are organizations and people out there."

Community/Environmental: Increasing Awareness of and Access to Community Resources

Finally, participants' enhanced knowledge and use of community resources, in addition to the variety of new opportunities for healthy living they experienced, created a supportive environment at the community level for them to integrate physical activity into their daily life. For example, as one low income group participant noted in the post-program focus group "If you don't have money and you don't know of any places to get inexpensive stuff, you're stuck. So, it was really good to tell people the things in the community." Access to amenities and services, shaping individual participation in physical activity, was influenced by increased awareness and the availability of programs and services. Others low income participants commented that "there's all kinds of support out there" and "when you're aware you can see that our community has all these different...programs...it trickles down to you on an individual level."

Providing physical activity instructors for specific sessions "...made participants feel part of the Panorama experience, where they learned that physical activity is not an elitist exercise, but part of everyday life for many people" [low income group, program facilitator, exit interview]. Hence, facilitators noted that low income participants felt sufficiently comfortable to inquire about Panorama facilities and programs. In fact, eleven low income participants reported their use of the recreation subsidy following the program's completion. One participant explained, "as part of the group subsequently I got the subsidy pass...[and] alerted my neighbor that there's such a thing as the subsidy program." Additionally, participants recommended that future programs should be located at the recreation center, rather than at one of the project partner's organization. Toward the end of the program group members viewed Panorama as a place where they can come "to help themselves, as opposed to Peninsula Community Services [the social service agency where the program was initially held] where they come to be helped" [low income group, program facilitator, exit interview].

DISCUSSION

While limited by the number of program participants completing the evaluation, and the self-reporting nature of the data, the results point to the success of the SPDPP in having a positive effect on participants' lives. Adopting a socioecological view to fostering physical activity in populations at risk of type 2 diabetes, and addressing some of the intrapersonal, interpersonal and environmental factors prohibiting their involvement in an active lifestyle, the SPDPP was able to help participants emerge from the programs feeling more knowledgeable, experienced and supported to engage in active living. The programs provided information, as well as opportunities for information sharing, social support and resources (e.g., water bottle, pedometer, goal setting) which not only encouraged individual behavior change (e.g., drinking more water, doing activity) but influenced others' behaviors as well, further reinforcing the behavior change. Together these factors built self-esteem and trusting relationships, and social connections were formed, which further motivating physical activity. As Berkman and Kawachi (2000) explain, "Individuals are embedded in societies and populations...environments place constraints on individual choice" (p. 7-8) and this includes the choice to be physically active, which is influenced by one's place in society. Furthermore, "psychological states, behaviors and aspects of the physical or built environment are influenced by social environments and vice versa" (p. 6). "A Taste of Healthy Living" programs provided opportunities to try new activities, learn about community resources supporting healthy living, and break down the walls of "suburbanization...where people keep to themselves and one's social life is private with lives centered inside the house rather than the neighborhood or community" (Putnam, 2000, p. 208).

Moreover, the project's activities – by engaging local community organizations as partners in the delivery of programs – promises to be sustained once external funding ceased. Data collected from SPDPP partners (n=11) at the project's termination found that their involvement enhanced connections in the Saanich Peninsula community. Partners reported becoming more acquainted with their target populations, which subsequently informed the design of appropriate community recreation programs and services. An important, but often unanticipated, benefit has been the enhanced understanding by project partners of the work that each does in the community. Frequently isolated in their disciplinary 'silos,' many were unaware of the duplication or gaps in service or knowledge. Collaborative efforts helped the SPDPP to avoid creating redundant and uncoordinated programs or resources (Mattessich and Monsey, 1992). Specifically, partners reported that their involvement in the SPDPP:

- enhanced "face-to-face" contact or networking and relationships with different agencies, particularly when partner meetings were held at different organizations;
- meant they were more "apt to initiate a phone call or connect based on the fact that now there are personal relationships;"
- strengthened relationships with community representatives due to regular meetings/communications, resulting in greater access to information and participating in joint initiatives "because there is some familiarity" with each other;
- more awareness of community agencies and services, including discovering that organizations "who were duplicating services within the community didn't even know that the other people existed";better 'internal' communication, discussions and relationships within organizations;
- 72.5% of partners indicated that the increased cooperation with other organizations was "very much of a benefit" as a result of their involvement with the SPDPP; 100%

of partners noted that their organization had benefited "a lot" or "quite a lot" from the collaborative relationships.

As in the literature, these findings offer some evidence that community-based partnerships, such as SPDPP, have helped to influence individual behavior, but the strongest evidence demonstrates that collaborative relationships contribute to changes in programs, services, and practices addressing community or environmental factors of influence (Butterfoss and Francisco, 2004). As Provan, Veazie, Teufel-Shone, and Huddleston (2004) note, "the capacity of a community to attend to the health needs of its citizens is enhanced substantially when the many organizations that have a stake in promoting health and delivering health and human services work together" (p. 175).

THE WAY FORWARD

The physical activity field has a sound grasp on how to address the intrapersonal factors influencing physical activity; nurturing an individual's values, attitude, motivation, skills and efficacy toward an active lifestyle. The science needs to progress from the laboratory to real-life settings where we are asking people to take up and sustain activity (O'Neal and Blair, 2001). Qualitative, community-based and case study research can help elucidate the best means of integrating physical activity into peoples' lives, particularly in the design of interventions, whether they be health communication materials, school or worksite policies, mother-baby friendly programs, or strategies for making neighborhoods safer and more conducive to play (Fisher et al., 2004). Mindful of the need to balance health promotion interventions informed by epidemiological evidence with citizens' experiential knowledge of health in choosing what and how to address issues (Roussos and Fawcet, 2000), collecting data directly from populations for whom health promotion initiatives are designed may produce more appropriate and effective programs and policies (Thomas et al., 2004). In the literature (Smedley and Syme, 2000; Neuhauser, Schwab, Syme and Bieber, 1998) there is acknowledgement that "… programs typically do not invite people to design and implement the programs intended to help them. People need to be directly involved in helping to shape these programs to fit their lives. We need to help them do that" (Syme, 2002, pg. 66).

Equally critical is research that gathers insights into collaboration among practitioners, professionals and researchers because it "is essential to integrate knowledge across sectors" (Craig et al. 2002, p. 36). Socio-ecological models will play a significant role in enhancing our understanding of all levels of influence, their interactions, and by definition, the collaborative relationships required to work across levels. For instance, how do affective (e.g., enjoyment), social support (e.g., walking groups) and urban design (e.g., presence of sidewalks etc.) aspects connect and influence physical activity behavior (Bengoechea and Spence, 2003; Eyler, et al., 2003)? This will demand a trans-disciplinary research agenda.

Community-based research (CBR) that facilitates collaborative, equitable partnerships throughout the research process (Israel et al., 2002), may further such a trans-disciplinary agenda. This type of research might focus on increasing physical activity levels by bringing together professionals from various disciplines, as well as community citizens to work together, sharing and building skills, knowledge and resources with goals to produce social change and improve health, and in ways that benefit all parties (Fisher et al., 2004), such as in the SPDPP experience. The experience of Faith and his colleagues (2001), and others (Sallis, Patrick, Frank et al., 2002; Simons-Morton, Calfas, Oldenburg, and Burton, 1998) suggest that pediatricians and primary care providers might play a unique and influential role both in and outside of clinical care. For example, helping parents reconstruct their home environments to simultaneously reduce TV viewing and increase physical activity, or providing patients with a combination of counseling information, supervised exercise sessions and access to exercise equipment . The literature on school interventions is clear that enhancing physical activity levels among students must move beyond the school zone. Community residents and stakeholders have unique knowledge of the specific context of their neighborhoods and schools, thus engaging community partners' participation in designing opportunities for children are key to implementing authentic and sustainable strategies. Because of this "insider" knowledge, community partners can craft solutions appropriate to, and tailored for, their locality. The built environment literature appears to be dominated by engineers, city planners, academics and other professionals and there is a need for power sharing and the formation of collaborative, equitable partnerships with multiple disciplines and community members.

In fact, scholars maintain that collaborative research is essential to furthering progress (Katz, 2004; Handy et al., 2002; Syme, 2002). Professionals from disciplines such as sport and exercise sciences, behavioral epidemiology, health psychology and health care, transportation, urban design and planning, and architects (Owen et al., 2000) as well as schools, government and local citizens need to contribute to research, apply findings and work together to address intrapersonal, interpersonal and environmental factors influencing physical activity. For example, partnerships could be formed to implement traffic calming and pedestrian-oriented measures and policy changes to support activity. Community initiatives involving partnerships, such as the walking school bus programs (Pedestrian Bicycle Information Center, 2004), are being developed to encourage activity, change perceptions of neighborhood environments, and bring about social change so that youth feel safe to walk to school, go for a bike ride or play outside.

CBR may also be effective in making lasting change to design activity back into people's daily home and work lives because it involves the community throughout all stages of the research process. As such, it hold promise in addressing local needs or health problems (within the realm of the built environment and physical activity) that are relevant to the community. Mixed-use development has its greatest relevance at smaller scales in terms of influencing physical activity (Frank et al., 2003), therefore community level changes to incorporate land use mixing rather than single use could encourage walking or biking in the community. For example, changing areas around transit stations to contain mixed-uses could encourage walking because a variety of destinations are provided within a short distance. According to Handy et al. (2002) 25% of trips are <1 mile in length. CBR can create relevant initiatives and programs to promote the health benefits of walking and encourage walking.

Incorporating activity into people's lives requires ensuring that it is "practical, safe, and enjoyable to expend extra energy traveling to and from work, going to school, shopping, running errands, socializing, and having fun" (Bredenberg, 2003, p. 1). CBR emphasizes a focus on multiple determinants of health, the individual, as well as larger contexts within which individuals live, such as families, community, and social and economic circumstances (Israel et al., 2002;). This is complementary to research within the built environment since the field is complex, for example determinants of travel behavior are embedded in cultural and attitudinal approaches to travel (Krizek, 2000). Advocacy, citizen and professional groups have contributed to changing concepts, guidelines and thoughts around street design so that the automobile does not dominate (Frank et al., 2003) and CBR may complement future development in the area of street design and environmental changes which reflect the acceptance of and respect for non-motorized transportation.

RESEARCH ON CAUSAL RELATIONSHIPS

In an exhaustive review of the literature regarding policy and environmental interventions for promoting physical activity, Matson-Koffman et al. (2005) note that this type of work is lacking. Moreover, there was a dearth of experimental or quasi-experimental research designs that included control groups, relying predominantly on self-reported measures, and even fewer addressed minority populations. We simply do not know enough about the associations of policy, social and physical environmental attributes with physical activity and cause-effect relationships (Bauman, Sallis, Dzewaltowski, and Owen, 2002; Craig et al., 2002; Humpel et al., 2002). Regarding community design and health, Dr. Ewing (Robert Wood Johnson, 2003a) states that the sprawl/health connection can be viewed as a causal chain with urban form affecting people's daily lives and activities, which affects transportation mode choice, which affects physical activity levels, affecting weight and health. However, the associations between overweight and sprawl are not causal, therefore further studies designed to support cause and effect are needed to bolster evidence. Further research could examine whether or not there is a dose response (or grading) of these environmental variables, whether or not there is a directional relationship, how strong or weak relationships are between environmental variables/attributes, weight and physical activity, and how changes in environmental variables effect physical activity behaviors. For example, non-motorized trips have shown high sensitivity to variations in the local physical environment (Rodríguez and Joo, 2003).

CONCLUSION

Physical inactivity is a health problem and contributes to premature death, chronic disease and obesity (Frank et al., 2003). The literature has, as Seefeldt et al. (2002) note, "identified an impressive list of determinants that influence lifestyle choice" (p. 160). The vast majority of this list has been generated through studies addressing individually, behaviorally- oriented psychological and social variables (Craig, et al., 2002), thus equal attention must be paid to investigating the policy and physical environment factors discussed in this chapter (Sallis et al., 2002; Salmon et al., 2003). In fact, Cohen et al. (2000) suggest that when the prevalence of a high-risk behavior is high (such as physical inactivity), and the hope is to reach and facilitate change in as many people as possible, then a structural/policy/environmental approach is warranted. Strong support exists for the development of policies that will improve the health of today's adults, as well as that of children, the next generation of adults (Marmot, 2000). Public policy can support the adoption of healthier behaviors and creation of supportive environments, or safe, attractive and convenient places for physical activity. Policies and strategies that emphasize population-wide physical activity have been shown to be related to better opportunities and infrastructure (e.g., existing facilities) for physical activity. More specifically, policy orientation influences the environment and individual behavior, and has shown an association with high participation rates, perceived opportunities for being physically active (e.g., awareness of programs), and high numbers of recreation/sports facilities (Ståhl, Rütten, Nutbeam, and Kannas, 2002).

When physical activity determinants are viewed from a socio-ecological perspective, there are many gaps in our collective knowledge for addressing the litany of factors that conspire against an active lifestyle. For instance, what is the role of specific determinants across the lifespan and for the sedentary, moderately active and highly active populations? To what extent do social, cultural and economic factors predispose or reinforce the decision to be active? The role and influence of technology has been relatively understudied, although holds great promise for engineering activity back into out lives (e.g., through online prompting, monitoring, support mechanisms, activity contingent video and TV monitors).

It is critical to operate collaboratively across disciplines to promote healthier and more active environments (Killingsworth, 2003), and to disseminate and translate the knowledge generated (Dunn and Blair, 2002). This will demand the collaborative efforts of public health, sociology, urban planning, marketing and communications, transportation, political science, public health and social policy, to name just a few. Given current rates of obesity and chronic diseases and evidence of the health benefits of physical activity and activity as a modifiable risk factor, Jackson and Kochtitzky (2003) state that it is dishonest to tell citizens to be active when there are no safe or supportive places to do so. Research is needed to examine and further untangle the web of causal relationships between intrapersonal, interpersonal and environmental determinants of physical activity. Currently, the theoretical and applied sciences of physical activity are enjoying unprecedented attention from the public, professionals, politicians, and funding agencies. The field has 'come a long way' since 1980, particularly in the last five years which has witnessed prolific and intense interest in the community/built environment domain. While there is general consensus that further advances will require a socio-ecological approach (Altman, 1995; Emmons, 2000; Rootman and Edwards, 2004; Salmon et al., 2003) as Dunn and Blair (2002) so eloquently sum, "there is much for us to do" (p. 9).

REFERENCES

Aarnio, M., Winter, T., Peltonen, J., Kujala, U., and Kaprio, J. (2002). Stability of leisure-time physical activity during adolescence – a longitudinal study among 16-, 17- and 18-year old Finnish youth. *Scandanavian Journal of Medicine and Science in Sports, 12*, 179-185.

Allensworth, D.D., Wyche, J., Lawson, E., and Nicholson, L. (1995). *Defining a comprehensive school health program: an interim statement*. Division of Health Sciences Policy, National Academy Press, Washington DC.

Altman, D.G. (1995). Strategies for community health intervention: Promises paradoxes, pitfalls. *Psychosomatic Medicine, 57*(3), 226-233.

Armstrong, T., Bauman, A., and Davies, J. (2000). *Physical activity patterns of Australian adults. Results of the 1999 National Physical Activity Survey.* Canberra; Australian Institute of Health and Welfare.

Atkinson, J., Sallis, J., Saelens, B., Cain, K., and Black, J. (2005). The association of neighborhood design and recreational environments with physical activity. *American Journal of Health Promotion, 20*, 304-309.

Azjen, I. (1985). From intentions to actions: a theory of planned behavior. In J. Kuhl and J. Beckman (Eds.), *Action-control: from cognition to behavior* (pp.11-39). NY: Springer.

Baker, E.A., Brennan, L.K., Brownson, R., and Houseman, R.A. (2000). Measuring the determinants of physical activity: current and future directions. *Research Quarterly for Exercise and Sport, 71*(2), 146-158.

Balfour, J., and Kaplan, G. (2002). Neighborhood environment and loss of physical function in older adults: evidence from the Alameda County Study. *American Journal of Epidemiology, 155*, 507-515.

Ball, K., Bauman, A., Leslie, E., and Owen, N. (2001). Perceived environmental aesthetics and convenience and company are associated with walking for exercise among Australian adults. *Preventive Medicine, 33*, 434-440.

Ball, K., and Crawford, D. (2005). Socioeconomic status and weight change in adults: a review. *Social Science and Medicine, 60*, 1987-2010.

Bandura, A. (1986). *Social foundations of thought and action: a social-cognitive theory.* Englewood Cliffs: Prentice-Hall.

Barber, N., and Havitz, M. (2001). Canadian participation rates in ten sport and fitness activities. *Journal of Sport Management, 15*, 51-76.

Bassett, D., Schneider, P., and Huntington, G. (2004). Physical activity in an old order Amish community. *Medicine and Science in Sports and Exercise, 36*(1), 79-85.

Bauman, A., Bellew, B., Owen, N., and Vita, P. (2001). Impact of an Australian mass media campaign targeting physical activity in 1998. *American Journal of Preventive Medicine, 21*(1), 41-47.

Bauman, A., Craig, C., and Cameron, C. (2005). Low levels of recall among adult Canadians of the CSEP/Health Canada physical activity guidelines. *Canadian Journal of Applied Physiology, 30*(2), 246-252.

Bauman, A., and Finch, C. (2000). Awareness of and attitudes to the new physical activity recommendations - perceptions of attenders of the 5th IOC World Congress on Sport Sciences. *Journal of Science and Medicine in Sport, 3*, 493-501.

Bauman, A., Sallis, J., Dzewaltowski, D., and Owen, N. (2002). Toward a better understanding of the influences on physical activity: The role of determinants, correlates, causal variables, mediators, moderators, and confounders. *American Journal of Preventative Medicine, 23*, 5-14.

Baxter, T., Milner, P., Wilson, K., Leaf, M., Nicholl, J., Freeman, J., et al. (1997). A cost effective, community based heart health promotion project in England: Prospective comparative study. *British Medical Journal, 315*(7108), 582-585.

Bengoechea, E., and Spence, J. (2003). *2002 Alberta survey on physical activity: A concise report.* Edmonton: Alberta Centre for Active Living.

Berg, B. (1998). *Qualitative research methods for the social sciences.* MA: Allyn and Bacon.

Berkman, L., and Glass, T. (2000). Social integration, social networks, social support, and health. In L. Berkman and I. Kawachi (Eds.), *Social epidemiology* (pp. 137-173). New York: Oxford University Press.

Berkman, L.F., and Kawachi , I. (2000). A historical framework for social epidemiology. In L. Berkman and I. Kawachi (Eds.), *Social epidemiology* (pp. 3-12). New York: Oxford University Press.

Blair, S., and Brodney, S. (1999). Effects of physical inactivity and obesity on morbidity and mortality: Current evidence and research issues. *Medicine and Science in Sports and Exercise, 31*(S6), 46-662.

Blair, S., and Church, T. (2004). The fitness, obesity, and health equation. *Journal of the American Medical Association, 292*(10), 1232-1234.

Blanchard, C., Courneya, K., Rodgers, W., and Murnaghan, D. (2002). Determinants of exercise intention and behavior in breast and prostate cancer survivors: An application of the theory of planned behavior. *Cancer Nursing, 25(2),* 88-95.

Booth, M., Owen, N., Bauman, A., Clavisi, O., and Leslie, E. (2000). Social-cognitive and perceived environmental influences associated with physical activity in older Australians. *Preventive Medicine, 31*, 15-22.

Bouchard, C. (2001). Physical activity and health: Introduction to the dose-response symposium. *Medicine and Science in Sports and Exercise, 33*(6), 347-350.

Braza, M., Shoemaker, W., and Seeley, A.(2004). Neighborhood design and rates of walking and biking to elementary school in 34 California communities. *American Journal of Health Promotion, 19*(2), 128-136.

Bredenberg, J. (2003). *Designing activity into our daily lives*. Robert Wood Johnson Foundation. Retrieved on February 20, 2004, from *http://www.rwjf.org/news/special/design.jhtml?liquidandpf*

Brown, W., and Trost, S. (2003). Life transitions and changing physical activity patterns in young women. *American Journal of Preventive Medicine, 25*(2), 140-143.

Brownell, K., Stunkard, A., and Albaum, J. (1980). Evaluation and modification of exercise patterns in the natural environment. *American Journal of Psychiatry, 137*, 1540-1545.

Brownson, R.., Baker, E.., Housemann, R.., Brennan, L.., and Bacak, S.. (2001). Environmental and policy determinants of physical activity in the United States. *American Journal of Public Health, 91*(12), 1995-2003.

Brownson, R., Boehmer, T., and Luke, D. (2005). Declining rates of physical activity in the United States: what are the contributors. *Annual Review of Public Health, 26*, 421-443.

Brownson, R., Housemann, R., Brown, D., Jackson-Homson, J., King, A., Malone, B., and Sallis, J. (2000). Promoting physical activity in rural communities - walking trail access, use and effects. *American Journal of Preventive Medicine, 18*(3), 235-240.

Bryant, L., Shetterly, S., Baxter, J., and Hamman, R. (2002). Modifiable risks of incident functional dependence in Hispanic and non-Hispanic white elders: the San Luis Valley Health and Ageing Study. *Gerontologist, 42*, 690-697.

Buckworth, J., and Dishman, R. (2002). *Exercise psychology*. Champaign, IL: Human Kinetics.

Bush, K., Leenders, A., Nicole, Y., and O'Sullivan, M. (2004). Implementation of a walking program for urban youth during school hours. *Physical Educator, 61*,(1), 2-14.

Butterfoss, F., and Francisco, V. (2004). Evaluating community partnerships and coalitions with practitioners in mind. *Health Promotion Practice, 5*(2), 108-114.

Calfas, K., Long, B., Sallis, J., Wooten, W., Pratt, M., and Patrick, K. (1996). A controlled trial of physician counseling to promote the adoption of physical activity. *Preventive Medicine, 25*, 225-233.

Calfas, K., Sallis, J., Nichols, J., Sarkin, J., Johnson, M., Caparosa, S., Thompson, S., Gehrman, C., and Alcaraz, J. (2000). Project GRAD: two-year outcomes of a randomized controlled physical activity intervention among young adults. *American Journal of Preventive Medicine, 18*(1), 28-37.

Calfas, K., Sallis, J. Zabinski M., Wilfley, D., Rupp, J., Prochaska, J., Thompson, S., Pratt M., and Patrick, K. (2002). Preliminary evaluation of a multicomponent program for nutrition and physical activity change in primary care: PACE+ for adults. *Preventive Medicine, 34,* (2), 153-161.

California Department of Health Services. (1999). *California Children's Healthy Eating and Exercise Practices Survey.* Retrieved March 2005 from *http://www.dhs.ca.gov/ps/cdic /cpns/research/calcheeps.htm*

Cameron, C., Craig, C., Stephens, T., and Ready, T. (2002). Translating evidence-based physical activity interventions into practice, the 2010 challenge. *American Journal of Preventive Medicine, 22* (4S), 8-9.

Canadian Fitness and Lifestyle Research Institute (2003). *2001 Physical activity monitor.* Retrieved March 28, 2003, from *http://www.cflri.ca/cflri/pa/surveys/2001survey /2001survey.html*

Canadian Fitness and Lifestyle Research Institute (2004). *Twenty year trends of physical activity among Canadian adults.* Retrieved July 15, 2004, from *http://www.cflri.ca/cflri /news/2004/0401b_1.html*

Canadian Institute for Health Information. (2005). *Select highlights on public views of the determinants of health.* Ottawa: Canadian Institute for Health Information.

Capital Regional District, Regional Planning Services. (2004). *Population, dwelling unit, and employment projections for the capital region's growth strategy alternatives, 1996-2026, vol. 1 – results June, 2000.* Retrieved August 6, 2004, from *http://www.crd.bc.ca/ regplan/rgs/reports/vol1.htm*

Casperson, C., and Merritt, R. (1995). Physical activity trends among 26 states, 1986-1990. *Medicine and Science in Sports and Exercise, 27*, 713-720.

Cavill, N. (1998). National campaigns to promote physical activity: can they make a difference? *International Journal of Obesity, 22*(Suppl. 2), S48-S51.

Centers for Disease Control and Prevention: National Centre for Chronic Disease Prevention and Health Promotion (1999a*). Physical activity and health: A report of the surgeon general.* Retrieved July 15, 2004, from *http.//www.cdc.gov/nccdphp/sgr/ chapcon.htm*

Centers for Disease Control and Prevention. (1999b). Neighborhood safety and the prevalence of inactivity – selected states, 1996. *Morbidity and Mortality Weekly Report, 47*, 143-146.

Centers for Disease Control and Prevention. (2001). Increasing physical activity: A report on recommendations of the Task Force on Community Preventive Services. *Morbidity and Mortality Weekly Report, 50*, 1–14.

Centers for Disease Control and Prevention. (2002) School transportation modes – Georgia 2000. *Morbidity and Mortality Weekly Reports*, 51(32), 704-705.

Centers for Disease Control and Prevention. (2004b). Participation in high school physical education --- United States, 1991—2003. *Morbidity and Mortality Weekly, 53*(36);844-847.

Cervero, R., and Gorham, R. (1995). Commuting in transit versus automobile neighborhoods. *Journal of the American Planning Association, 61*, 210-225.

Choosing Health. (2004). White Paper . UK Government. Retrieved November 17, 2004 from *http://www.dh.gov.uk/PublicationsAndStatistics/Publications/PublicationsPolicyAndGu idance/PublicationsPolicyAndGuidanceArticle/fs/en?CONTENT_ID=4094550andchk= aN5Cor*

Cohen, D., Scribner, R., and Farley, T. (2000). A structural model of health behavior: a pragmatic approach to explain and influence health behaviors at the population level. *Preventive Medicine, 30*, 146-154.

Colman, R., and Walker, S. (2004). *The Cost of Physical Inactivity to British Columbians.* Victoria: BC Ministry of Health Services.

Coogan, P., and Coogan, M. (2004). When worlds collide: observations on the integration of epidemiology and transportation behavioral analysis in the study of walking. American *Journal of Health Promotion, 19*(1), 39-44.

Corbin, C. (2001). The "untracking" of sedentary living: A call for action. *Pediatric Exercise Science, 13*, 347-356.

Corbin, C., and Lindsey, R. (1997). *Teacher's Edition: Fitness for Life.* (4th edition). Glenview, IL: Scott, Foresman and Co.

Corti, B., Donovan, R.., and Holman, C. (1996). Factors influencing use of physical activity facilities: Results from qualitative research. *Health Promotion Journal of Australia, 6*(1), 16-21.

Crabtree, B., and Miller, W. (1992). *Doing qualitative research.* Newbury Park, CA: Sage.

Craig, C., Brownson, R., Cragg, S., and Dunn, A (2002). Exploring the effect of the environment on physical activity: A study examining walking to work. *American Journal of Preventative Medicine, 23*, 338-358.

Craig, C., and Cameron, C. (2004). Increasing physical activity: Assessing trends from 1998-2003. Ottawa, ON: Canadian Fitness and Lifestyle Research Institute. Retrieved July 15, 2004, from *http://www.cflri.ca/pdf/e/2002pam.pdf*

Curtis, J., McTeer, W., and White, P. (1999). Exploring effects of school sport experiences on sport participation in later life. *Sociology of Sport Journal, 16*, 348-365.

Dale, D., and Corbin, C. (2000). Physical activity participation of high school graduates following exposure to conceptual or traditional physical education. *Researcher Quarterly in Exercise and Sport, 71*, 61-68.

Dale, D., Corbin, C., and Dale, K. (2000). Restricting opportunities to be active during school time: do children compensate by increasing physical activity levels after school? *Research Quarterly in Exercise and Sport, 71*, 240-248.

Dale, D., Corbin, C., and Cuddihy, T. (1998). Can conceptual physical education promote physically active lifestyles? *Pediatric Exercise Science, 10*, 97-109.

Davison, K., Cutting, T., and Birch, L. (2003). Parents' activity-related parenting practices predict girls' physical activity. *Medicine and Science in Sports and Exercise, 35*(9), 1589-1595.

Deschesnes, M., Martin, C., Jomphe Hill, A. (2003). Comprehensive approaches to school health promotion: how to achieve broader implementation? *Health Promotion International, 18*(4), 387-396.

Diez Roux, A. (2003). The examination of neighborhood effects on health: Conceptual and methodological issues related to the presence of multiple levels of organization. In I. Kawachi and L. Berkman (Eds.), *Neighborhoods and health* (pp. 45-64). NY: Oxford University Press.

Dishman, R. (1994). Introduction: Consensus, problems and prospects. In R. Dishman (Ed.), *Advances in exercise adherence* (pp. 1–27). Champaign, IL: Human Kinetics.

Dishman, R., and Buckworth, J. (1996). Increasing physical activity: a quantitative synthesis. *Medicine and Science in Sports and Exercise, 28*, 706-719.

Dishman, R., Washburn, R., Schoeller, D. Measurement of physical activity. (2001). *Quest, 53*, 295-309.

Dobbins, M., Lockett, D., Michel, I., Beyers, J., Feldman, L., Vohra, J., and Micucci, S. (2001). *The effectiveness of school-based interventions in promoting physical activity and fitness among children and youth: a systematic review.* Effective Public Health Practice Project, Ministry of Health and Long Term Care, Ontario, Canada. September.

Dubbert, P. (2002). Physical activity and exercise: Recent advances and current challenges. *Journal of Consulting and Clinical Psychology, 70*(3), 526-536.

Duda, J. (2001). Achievement goal research in sport: pushing the boundaries and clarifying some misunderstandings. In G. Roberts (ed.), *Advances in motivation in sport and exercise* (pp. 129-182). Champaign, IL: Human Kinetics.

Dunn, A., and Blair, S. (2002). Translating evidence-based physical activity interventions into practice, the 2010 challenge. *American Journal of Preventive Medicine, 22* (4S), 8-9.

Durkin, M., Davidson, L., Kuhn, L., O'Connor, P., and Barlow, B. (1994). Low-income neighborhoods and the risk of severe pediatric injury: A small-area analysis. *American Journal of Public Health, 84*(4), 587-592.

Durkin, M., Laraque, D., Lubman, I. and Barlow, B. (1999). Epidemiology and prevention of traffic injuries to urban children and adolescents. *Pediatrics, 103*(6), Retrieved on March 2, 2004, from *http://pediatrics.aappublications.org/cgi/reprint/103/6/e74.pdf*

Dzewaltowski, D., Estabrooks, P., and Johnston, J. (2002). Healthy youth places: promoting nutrition and physical activity. *Health Education Research, 17*(5), 541-551.

Ellaway, A., Anderson, A., and Macintrye, S. (1997). Does area of residence affect body size and shape? *International Journal of Obesity, 21*, 304-308.

Erfurt, J., Foote, A., and Heirich, M. (1991). Worksite-wellness programs: incremental comparisons of screening and referral alone, health education follow-up counseling, and plant organization. *American Journal of Health Promotion, 5*, 438-448.

Ewing, R., Schmid, T., Killingsworth, R., Zlot, A., and Raudenbush, S. (2003). Relationship between urban sprawl and physical activity, obesity, and morbidity. *American Journal of Health Promotion, 18*(1), 47-57.

Eyler, A., Baker, E., Cromer, L., King, A., Brownson, R., and Donatell, R. (1998). Physical activity and minority women: a qualitative study. *Health Education and Behavior, 25*, 640-652.

Eyler, A., Brownson, R., Bacak, S., and Housemann, R. (2003). The epidemiology of walking for physical activity in the United States. *Medicine and Science in Sports and Exercise, 35*, 1529-1536.

Eyler, A., Matson-Koffman, D., Rohm-Young, D., Wilcox, S., Wilbur, J., Thompson, J., et al. (2003). Quantitative study of correlates of physical activity in women from diverse ration/ethnic groups. *American Journal of Preventive Medicine, 25*(3Si), 93-103.

Faith, M., Berman, N., Heo, M., Pietrobelli, A., Gallagher, D., Epstein, L., Eiden, M., and Allison, D. (2001). Effects of contingent television on physical activity and television viewing in obese children. *Pediatrics, 107*, 1043-1048.

Federal, Provincial and Territorial Advisory Committee on Population Health. (1999). *Toward a healthy future: Second report on the health of Canadians.* Ottawa: Minister of Public Works and Government Services Canada.

Finlay, S-J and Faulkner, G. (2005). Physical activity promotion through the mass media: inception, production, transmission and consumption. *Preventive Medicine, 40*, 121-130.

Fisher, J., Li, F., Michael, Y., and Cleveland, M. (2004). Neighborhood-level influences on physical activity among older adults: a multilevel analysis. *Journal of Aging and Physical Activity, 11*, 45-63.

Fox, K., Cooper, A., and McKenna, J. (2004). The school and promotion of children's health enhancing physical activity: perspectives from the United Kingdom. *Journal of Teaching in Physical Education, 21*, 128-144.

Folkman, S., Chesney, S., McKusick, L., Ironson, G., Johnson, D., and Coates, T. (1991). Translating coping theory into an intervention. In J. Eckenrode (Ed.), *The social context of coping* (pp. 239-260). NY: Plenum Press.

Frank, L., and Engelke, P., Schmid, T., and Killingsworth, R. (2000). How land use and transportation systems impact public health: A literature review of the relationship between physical activity and urban form. *ACES: Active Community Environments Initiative, Working Paper #1, Georgia Institute of Technology, and Center for Disease Control, Atlanta.* Retrieved on February 24, 2004, from *http://www.cdc.gov/nccdphp/dnpa/pdf/aces-workingpaper1.pdf*

Frankish, C., Milligan, C., and Reid, C. (1998). A review of relationships between active living and determinants of health. *Social Science and Medicine, 47*(3), 287-301.

Gibbons, S.L., Van Gyn, G., Wharf Higgins, J., and Gaul, C. (2000). Reversing the trend: Girls' participation in physical education. *Journal of the Canadian Association for Health,* Physical Education, Recreation and Dance, 66(1), 26-32.

Gibbons, S., Wharf Higgins, J., Gaul, C., and Van Gyn, G. (1999). Listening to female students in high school physical education. *AVANTE , 5(*2), 1-20.

Giles-Corti, B., and Donovan, R. (2002). The relative influence of individual, social and physical environment determinants of physical activity. *Social Science and Medicine, 54*, 1793–1812

Giles-Corti, B., and Donovan, R. (2003). Relative influences of individual, social environmental, and physical environmental correlates of walking. *American Journal of Public Health, 93*(9), 1583-1589.

Golaszewski, T., Barr, D., Blodgett, C., and Delprino, R. (1996). Continued development of an organizational heart-health assessment. *AWHP Worksite Health, Spring*, 32-35.

Green, K. (2002). Physical education and the "coach potato society" – part one. European *Journal of Physical Education, 7*, 95-97.

Green, L., and Kreuter, M. (1999). *Health promotion planning, an educational and ecological approach.* Mountain View, CA: Mayfield.

Green, B., McAfee, T., Hindmarsh, M., Madsen, L., Caplow, M., and Buist, D. (2002). Effectiveness of telephone support in increasing physical activity levels in primary care patients. *American Journal of Preventive Medicine, 22*(3), 177-183.

Guba, E., and Lincoln, Y. (1989). *Fourth generation evaluation.* CA: Sage.

Guralnik, J., Simonsick, E., Ferrucci, L. et al. (1994). A short physical performance battery assessing lower extremity function: Association with self-reported disability and prediction of mortality and nursing home admission. *Journal of Gerontology in Medicine and Science, 49*, M85-M94.

Hall, B. (2001). I wish this were a poem of practices of participatory research. In P., Reason and H. Bradbury (Eds.), *Handbook of action research* (pp. 171-178). London: Sage Publications.

Hammond, D., McDonald, P., Fong, G., Brown, K., and Cameron, R. (2004). The impact of cigarette warning labels and smoke-free bylaws on smoking cessation. *Canadian Journal of Public Health, 95*(3), 201-204.

Hammond, S., Leonard, B., and Fridinger, F. (2000). The Centers for Disease Control and Prevention director's physical activity challenge: an evaluation of a worksite health promotion intervention. *American Journal of Health Promotion, 15*, 17-20.

Hancock, T. (2002). Indicators of environmental health in the urban setting. *Canadian Journal of Public Health, 93*(S1), S45-S51.

Handy, S. (1992). Regional versus local accessibility. *Built Environment, 18*, 253-267.

Handy, S., Boarnet, M., Ewing, R., and Killingsworth, R. (2002). How the built environment affects physical activity: Views from urban planning. *American Journal of Preventative Medicine, 23*(2S), 64-73.

Health Canada (2003a). *Stairway to health.* Retrieved February 16, 2004, from *http://www.hc-sc.gc.ca/pphb-dgspsp/sth-evs/english*

Health Canada, Center for Chronic Disease Prevention and Control (CDC). Population and Public Health Branch. (2002). *Diabetes in Canada* (2nd ed.). Retrieved February 24, 2003, from *http://www.hc-sc.gc.ca/pphb-dgspsp/publicat/dicdac2/english/03foreword _e .html*

Health Canada, Physical Activity Unit (2003). *Canada's physical activity guide to healthy active living.* Retrieved October 29, 2003, and April 3, 2004, from *http://www.hc-sc.gc.ca/hppb/paguide*

Health Canada, Population Health, Gauvin, L. (2004). *Social disparities and involvement in physical activity: Shaping the policy agenda in healthy living to successfully influence population health.* Retrieved April 3, 2004, from *http://www.hcsc.gc.ca/hppb/phdd/ overview_implications/01_overview.html*

Heart and Stroke Foundation of Canada. (2005). *Heart and Stroke Foundation 2005 Report Card on Canadians' Health - has the suburban dream gone sour?* Heart and Stroke Foundation of Canada. Retrieved from www.heartandstroke.ca on February 10, 2005.

Heirich, M., Foote, A., and Konopka, B. (1993). Work-site physical fitness programs: comparing the impact of different program designs on cardiovascular risks. *Journal of Occupational Medicine, 35*, 510-517.

Henderson, K. (1991). *Dimensions of choice: A qualitative approach to recreation, parks, and leisure research.* State College, PA: Venture Publishing.

Henderson, K., Neff, L., Shapre, P., Greaney, M., Royce, S., and Ainsworth, B. (2001). "It takes a village" to promote physical activity: the potential for public park and recreation departments. *Journal of Park and Recreation Administration, 19*(1), 23-41.

Hill, J. (2004). Physical activity and obesity. *The Lancet, 363*, 182.

Hillsdon, M., Brunner, E., Guralnik, J., and Marmot, M. (2005). Prospective study of physical activity and physical function in early old age. *American Journal of Preventive Medicine, 28*(3), 245-250.

Hillsdon, M., Cavill, N., Nanchahal, K., Diamond, A., and White, I. (2001). National level promotion of physical activity: results from England's ACTIVE FOR LIFE campaign. *Journal of Epidemiology and Community Health, 55*(10), 755-761.

Hu, G., Jousilahti, P., Barengo, N., Qiao, Q., Lakka,T., and Tuomilehto, J. (2005). Physical activity, cardiovascular risk factors, and mortality among Finnish adults with diabetes. *Diabetes Care, 28*, 799-805.

Humpel, N., Owen, N., and Leslie, E. (2002). Environmental factors associated with adults' participation in physical activity: A review. *American Journal of Preventative Medicine, 22*(3), 188-199.

Hutchinson, S., Loy, D., Kleiber, D., and Dattilo, J. (2003). Leisure as a coping resource: Variations in coping with traumatic injury and illness. *Leisure Sciences, 25*, 143-161.

Israel, B., Shulz, A., Parker, E., Becker, A., Allen III, A., and Guzman, J. (2002). Critical issues in developing and following community based participatory research principles. In M. Minkler and N. Wallerstein (Eds.), *Community Based Participatory Research for Health*, (pp. 53-76). San Francisco: Jossey-Bass.

Jackson, R., and Kochtitzky, C. (2003). *Creating a healthy environment: The impact of the built environment on public health.* Retrieved March 4, 2004, from *http://www.cdc.gov/healthyplaces/articles/Creating%20A%20Healthy%20Environment .pdf*

Jiang, X., Cooper, J., Porter, M., and Ready, A. (2004). Adoption of Canada's physical activity guide and handbook for older adults: impact on functional fitness and energy expenditure. *Canadian Journal of Applied Physiology, 29*, 395-410.

Kahn, E., Ramsey, L., Brownson, R., Heath, G., Howze, E.,. Powell, E., Stone, E., Rajab, M., and Corso, P. (2002). The effectiveness of interventions to increase physical activity. *American Journal of Preventative Medicine, 22*(4S), 73-107.

Kandula, N., and Lauderdale, D. (2005). Leisure time, Non-leisure time, and occupational physical activity in Asian Americans. *Annals of Epidemiology, 15*(4), 257-265.

Kaplan, G. (1992). Maintenance of function in the elderly. *Annals of Epidemiology, 2*, 823-834,

Katz, D. (2004). Representing your community in community-based participatory research: Differences made and measured. *Preventing Chronic Disease, Public Health Research, Practice and Policy, [On-line serial],1*(1),1-4. *http://www.cdc.gov.pcd/issues/ 2004/jan/katz.htm*

Katzmarzyk, P., Gledhill, N., and Shephard, R. (2000). The economic burden of physical inactivity in Canada. *Canadian Medical Association Journal. 163*(11), 1435-1440.

Katzmarzyk, P., Malina, R.M., and Bouchard, C. (1999). Physical activity, physical fitness and coronary heart disease risk factors in youth: the Quebec family study. Preventive Medicine, 29, 555-552.

Killingsworth, R.E. (2003). Health promoting community design: A new paradigm to promotehealthy and active communities. *American Journal of Health Promotion, 17*(3), 169-170.

King, A.C. (1991). Clinical and community interventions to promote and support physical activity participation. In L. Green and M. Kreuter (Eds.), *Health Promotion Planning: An Educational and Environmental Approach*, (pp. 183-212). Mountain View, CA: Mayfield.

King, L., Hawe, P., and Corne, S. (1999). What is local government's capacity for partnership in promoting physical activity? A case study. *Health Promotion Journal of Australia, 9,* 39-43.

Klebanoff, R., and Muramatsu, N. (2002). A community-based physical education and activity intervention for African-American Preadolescent Girls: A strategy to reduce racial disparities in health. *Health Promotion Practice, 3*(2), 276-285.

Knadler, G., and Rogers, T. (1987). Mountain climb month program: a low-cost exercise intervention program at a high-rise work-site. *Fitness Business, October*, 64-76.

Krizek, K. (2000). Pretest-posttest strategy for researching neighborhood-scale urban form and travel behavior. *Transportation Research Record, 1722*, 48-55.

LaCroix, A., Guralnik, J., Berkman, L., Wallarce, R., and Satterfield, S. (1993). Maintaining mobility late in life. II. Smoking, alcohol consumption, physical activity and body mass index. *American Journal of Epidemiology, 137*, 858-869.

Leary, M., Chioidjian, L., and Kraxberger, B. (1994). Self-presentation can be hazardous to your health: impressions management and health risk. *Healthy Psychology, 13*, 461-470.

Leslie, E., Saelens, B., Frank, L., Owen, N., Bauman, A., Coffee, N., and Hugo, G. (2005). Residents' perceptions of walkability attributes in objectively different neighbourhoods: a pilot study. *Health and Place, 11*, 277-236.

Leung, M., Yen, I., and Minkler, M. (2004). Community based participatory research: a promising approach for increasing epidemiology's relevance in the 21st century. *International Journal of Epidemiology, 33*(3), 499-506.

Lewis, F. (1997). Perspectives on models of interpersonal health behavior. In K. Glanz and F. Lewis (Eds.), *Health behavior and health education: Theory, research and practice* (2nd ed., pp. 227-235). San Francisco: Jossey-Bass Publishers.

Lewis, B., and Ridge, D. (2005). Mothers reframing physical activity: Family oriented politicism, transgression and contested expertise in Australia. *Social Science and Medicine, 60*, 2295-2306.

Librett, J., Yore, M., Buchner, D., and Schmid, T. (2005). Take pride in America's health: volunteering as a gateway to physical activity. *American Journal of Health Education, 36*(1), 8-13.

Lim, K., and Taylor, L. (2005). Factors associated with physical activity among older people – a population-based study. *Preventive Medicine, 40*, 33-40.

Linenger, J., Chesson, C., and Nice, D. (1991). Physical fitness gains following simple environmental changes. *American Journal of Preventive Medicine, 7*, 298-310.

Litman, T. (2004). *Economic value of walkability*. Victoria Transport Policy Institute. Retrieved November 12, 2004 from www.vtpi.org.

Luepker, V., Perry, C., McKinlay, M., Nader, P., Parcel, G., Stone, E. et al (1996). Outcomes of a field trial to improve children's dietary patterns and physical activity. The Child and Adolescent Trial for Cardiovascular Health. CATCH collaborative group. *Journal of the American Medical Association*, 275(10), 768-776.

Lynagh, M., Schofield, M., and Sanson-Fisher, R.. (1997). School health promotion programs over the past decade: a review of the smoking, alcohol and solar protection literature. *Health Promotion International, 12*(1), 43-60.

Lyons, R., and Langille, L. (2000). *Healthy lifestyle: Strengthening the effectiveness of lifestyle approaches to improve health.* For Health Canada, Population and Public Health Branch, Atlantic Health Promotion Research Centre: Dalhousie University and Canadian Consortium of Health Promotion Research Centres.

Malina, R. (1996). Tracking of physical activity and physical fitness across the lifespan. Research Quarterly for Exercise and Sport, 167, 48-57.

Malina, R. (2001). Adherence to physical activity from childhood to adulthood: a perspective from tracking studies. *Quest, 53,* 346-355.

Manson, J., Skerrett, P., Greenland, P., and VanItallie, T. (2004). The escalating pandemics of obesity and sedentary lifestyle. *Archives of Internal Medicine, 164*(3), 249-258.

Marcus, B., Owen, N., Forsyth, L., Cavill, N., and Fridinger, F. (1998). Physical activity interventions using mass media, print media, and information technology. *American Journal of Preventive Medicine, 15*, 362-378.

Marmot, M. (2000). Multilevel approaches to understanding social determinants. In L. Berkman and I. Kawachi (Eds.), *Social epidemiology* (pp. 349-367). New York: Oxford University Press.

Marshall, A., Leslie,E., Bauman,A., Marchus, B., and Owen, N. (2003). Print versus website physical activity programs, a randomized trial. *American Journal of Preventive Medicine, 25*(2), 88-94.

Marshall, S., Biddle, S., Sallis, J., McKenzie, T., and Conway, T. (2002). Clustering of sedentary behaviors and physical activity among youth: a cross-national study. *Pediatric Exercise Science, 14*, 401-417.

Martin, K., Sinden, A., and Fleming, J. (2000). Inactivity may be hazardous to your image: the effects of exercise participation on impression formation. *Journal of Sport Exercise Psychology, 22*, 283-291.

Matson-Koffman, D., Brownstein, J., Neiner, J., and Greaney, M. (2005). A site-specific literature review of policy and environmental interventions that promote physical activity and nutrition for cardiovascular health: what works? *American Journal of Health Promotion, 19*(3), 167-193.

Mattessich,P., and Monsey, b. (1992). *Collaboration: What makes it work - a review of research literature on factors influencing successful collaboration.* St. Paul, Minn: Amherst H. Wilder Foundation.

Mayer, J., and Geller, E. (1982). Motivating energy efficiency travel: a community-based intervention for encouraging biking. *Journal of Epidemiology and Community Health, 12*, 99-112.

McArdle, W., Katch, F., and Katch, V. (2000). *Essentials of exercise physiology* (2nd ed.). Baltimore, MD: Lippincott Williams and Wilkins.

McCarger, L. (2000). *Should the 1988 Canadian guidelines for healthy weights be updated?* Edmonton: University of Alberta.

McCauley, E., Pena, M., Jerome, G. (2001). Self-efficacy as a determinant and outcome of exercise. In G. Roberts (Ed.), *Advances in motivation in sport and exercise*, (pp. 235-261). Champaign, IL: Human Kinetics.

McGinnis, J.M. (2001). Does proof matter? Why strong evidence sometimes yields weak action. *American Journal of Health Promotion, 15*(5), 391-396.

McKay, H.A., Naylor, P.J. Rhodes, R., Warburton, Reed K., MacDonald, H., et al. (2004). Action Schools! BC Phase I Pilot Evaluation Report. Retrieved March 1, 2005 from *http://www.healthservices.gov.bc.ca/cpa/publications/actionschoolsreport.pdf.*

McKelvie, K., Petit, M., Khan, K., Beck, T., and McKay, H.A. (2004). Bone mass and structure are enhanced following a 2-year randomized controlled trial of exercise in prepubertal boys. *Bone*, 34, 755-764.

McKenzie, T., Nader, P., Strikmiller, P., Yang Stone, E., Perry, C.L. et al (1996). School physical education: effect of the Child and Adolescent Trial for Cardiovascular Health. *Preventive Medicine, 25*(4), 423-431.

McKenzie, T., Sallis, J., Prochaska, J., Conway, T., Marshall, S., and Rosengard, P. (2004). Evaluation of a two-year middle-school physical education intervention: M-SPAN. *Medicine and Science in Sports and Exercise, 36*(8), 1382-1388

McLeroy, K., Bibeau, D., Steckler, A., and Glanz, K. (1988). An ecological perspective on health promotion programs. *Health Education Quarterly, 15*(4), 351-377.

Miles, M., and Huberman, A. (1994). *Qualitative data analysis*. Newbury Park, CA: Sage.

Mitchell, S., and Olds, R. (1999). Psychological and perceived situational predictors of physical activity: A cross-sectional analysis. *Health Education Research, 14*, 305-313.

Mokdad, A., Marks, J., Stroup, D., and Gerberding, J. (2004). Actual causes of death in the United States, 2000. *Journal of the American Medical Association, 291*(10), 1238-1245.

Molitch, M., Fujimoto, W., Hamman, R., and Knowler, W. (2003). The diabetes prevention program and its global implications. *Journal of the American Society of Nephrology, 14*, S103-107.

Molnar, B., Gortmaker, S., Bull, F., and Buka, S. (2004). Unsafe to play? Neighborhood disorder and lack of safety predict reduced physical activity among urban children and adolescents. *American Journal of Health Promotion, 18*(5), 378-386.

Morgan, W. (2001). Prescription of physical activity: a paradigm shift. *Quest, 53*, 366-382.

Mullan, E. (2003). Do you think that your local area is a good place for young people to grow up? The effects of traffic and car parking on young people's views. *Health and Place, 9*(4), 351-360.

Nelson, M., Gordon-Larsen, P., Adair, L., and Popkin, B, (2005). Adolescent physical activity and sedentary behavior, patterning and long-term maintenance. *American Journal of Preventive Medicine, 28*(3), 259-266.

Neuhauser, L., and Kreps, G. (2003). Rethinking communication in the e-health era. *Journal of Health Psychology, 8*(1), 7-23.

Neuhasuer, L., Schwab, M., Syme, S., and Bieber, M. (1998). Community participation in health promotion: Evaluation of the California Wellness Guide. *Health Promotion International, 12*, 211-222.

Niemeier, D., and Rutherford, G. (1995). *Non-motorized transportation*. Washington, DC : Federal Highways Administration, US Dept. of Transportation. Publication FHWA-PL-94-019.

Nguyen, M.N., Gauvin, L., Martineau, I., and Grignon, R. (2002). Promoting physical activity at the community level: Insights into health promotion practice from the Laval walking clubs experience. *Health Promotion Practice, 3*(4), 485-496.

Northridge, M., Sclar, E., and Biswas, P. (2003). Sorting out the connections between the built environment and health: A conceptual framework for navigating pathways and planning healthy cities. *Journal of Urban Health, 80*(4), 556-558.

O'Neal, H., and Blair, S. (2001). Enhancing adherence in clinical exercise trials. *Quest, 53*, 310-317.

Owen, N., Bauman, A., Booth, M., Oldenburg, B., and Magnus, P. (1995). Serial mass-media campaigns to promote physical activity: reinforcement or redundant? *American Journal of Health Promotion, 84*, 244-248.

Owen, N., Leslie E., Salmon J., and Fotheringham, M. (2000). Environmental determinants of physical activity and sedentary behavior. *Exercise and Sport Sciences Reviews, 28*, 153-158.

Paffenbarger, R., Hyde, T., Wing, A., and Steinmetz, C. (1984). A natural history of athleticism and cardiovascular health. *Journal of the American Medical Association, 252*, 491-495.

Parks, S., Housemann, R., and Brownson, R. (2003). Differential correlates of physical activity in urban and rural adults of various socioeconomic backgrounds in the United States. *Journal of Epidemiology and Community Health, 57*(1), 29-35.

Pate, R., Saunders, R., Ward, D., Felton, G., Trost, S., and Dowda, M. (2003). Evaluation of a community-based intervention to promote physical activity in youth: Lessons from active winners. *American Journal of Health Promotion, 17*(3), 171-182.

Patterson, P., and Chapman, N. (2004). Urban from and older residents' service use, walking, driving, quality of life, and neighborhood satisfaction. *American Journal of Health Promotion, 19*(1), 45-52.

Patton, M.Q. (1990). *Qualitative evaluation and research methods.* CA: Sage. Pedestrian Bicycle Information Center. (2004). *The walking school bus information website.* Retrieved on March 11, 2004, from www.walkingschoolbus.org/

Peel, N., McClure, R., and Bartlett, H. (2005). Behavioral determinants of healthy aging. *American Journal of Preventive Medicine, 28*(3), 298-304.

Pellman, T., Brandt, E., and Macaran, A. (2002). Health and behavior: the interplay of biological, behavioral, and social influences: summary of an institute of medicine report. *American Journal of Health Promotion, 16*, 206-219.

Petrella, R., Lattanzio, C., Demeray, A., Varallo, V., and Blore, R. (2005). Can adoption of regular exercise later in life prevent metabolic risk for cardiovascular disease? *Diabetes Care, 28*, 694-701.

Perdue, W.C., Gostin, L.O., and Stone, L.A. (2003). Public health and the built environment: Historical, empirical, and theoretical foundations for an expanded role. *Journal of Law, Medicine and Ethics, 31*(4), 557-566.

Pikora, T., Giles-Corti, B., Bull, F., Jamrozik, K., and Donovan, R. (2003). Developing a framework for assessment of the environmental determinants of walking and cycling. *Social Science and Medicine, 56*, 1693-1703.

Pirisi, A. (2000). Low health literacy prevents equal access to care. *The Lancet, 356*, 1828.

Powell, K., and Dysinger, W. (1987). Childhood participation in organized school sports and physical education as precursors of adult physical activity. *American Journal of Preventive Medicine, 3*, 276-281.

Powell, K., Thompson, P., Caspersen, C., Kendrick, J. (1987). Physical activity and the incidence of coronary heart disease. *Annual Review of Public Health, 8*, 253-187.

Pratt, M., Macera, C., and Wang, G. (2000). Higher direct medical costs associated with physical inactivity. *Physician in Sports Medicine, 28*, 63-70.

Prochaska, J., and Marcus, B. (1994). The transtheoretical model – the applications to exercise. In R. Dishman (Ed.), *Advances in exercise adherence* (pp. 161-180). Champaign, IL: Human Kinetics.

Proper, K., Hildebrandt, V., Vander Beek, A., Twisk, J., and Van Mechelen, W. (2003). Effect of individual counseling on physical activity fitness and health, a randomized controlled trial in a workplace setting. *American Journal of Preventive Medicine, 24*(3), 218-226.

Provan, K., Veazie, M., Teufel-Shone, N., and Huddleston, C. (2004). Network analysis as a tool for assessing and building community capacity for provision of chronic disease services. *Health Promotion Practice, 5*(2), 174-181.

Putnam, R. (2000). *Bowling alone: The collapse and revival of American community*. New York: Simon and Schuster.

Rachlis, M., Evans, R., Lewis, P., and Barer, M.L. (2001). *Revitalizing Medicare: Shared Problems, Public Solutions*. A study prepared for the Tommy Douglas Research Institute. Vancouver, B.C. Retrieved November, 2001 from *http://www.tommydouglas.ca*.

Reger, B., Cooper, L., Booth-Butterfield, S., Smith, H., Bauman, A., Wootan, M., Middlestadt, S., Marcus, B., and Greer, F. (2002). Wheeling walks: a community campaign using paid media to encourage walking among sedentary older adults. *Preventive Medicine, 35*, 285-292.

Reilly, J., Jackson, D., Montgomery, C., Kelly, L., Slater, C., Grant, S., and Paton, J. (2004). Total energy expenditure and physical activity in young Scottish children: mixed longitudinal study. *The Lancet, 363*, 211-212.

Robert Wood Johnson Foundation (2003a). *The health effects of sprawl: Interview with Reid Ewing*. Retrieved February 20, 2004, from *http://www.rwjf.org/news/special/ sprawlqa.jhtml?liquidandpdf*

Robert Wood Johnson Foundation (2003b). *The health effects of sprawl: Overview of report findings*. Retrieved February 20, 2004, from *http://www.rwjf.org/news/special /sprawlFindings.jhtml*

Rodríguez, D., and Joo, J. (2003). The relationship between non-motorized mode choice and the local physical environment. *Transportation Research, D9*, 151-173.

Rootman, I., and Edwards, P. (2004). The best laid schemes of mice and men… ParticipACTION's legacy and the future of physical activity promotion in Canada. *Canadian Journal of Public Health, 95*(S2), S37-44.

Roussos, S., and Fawcett, S. (2000). A review of collaborative partnerships as a strategy for improving community health. *Annual Review of Public Health, 21*, 369-402.

Saelens, B., Sallis, J., and Frank, L. (2003). Environmental correlates of walking and cycling: Findings from the transportation, urban design, and planning literature. *Annals of Behavioral Medicine, 25*(2), 80-91.

Sallis, J., Bauman, A., and Pratt, M. (1998). Environmental and policy interventions to promote physical activity. *American Journal of Preventive Medicine, 15*(4), 379-397.

Sallis, J., Conway, T., Prochaska, J., McKenzie, T., Marshall, S., and Brown, M. (2001). The association of school environments with youth physical activity. *American Journal of Public Health, 91*(4), 618-620.

Sallis, J., Frank, L., Saelens, B., and Kraft, K. (2004). Active transportation and physical activity: opportunities for collaboration on transportation and pubic health research. *Transportation Research Part A, 38,* 249-268.

Sallis, J., Johnson, M., Calfas, K., Caparosa, S., and Nichols, J. (1997). Assessing perceived physical environmental variables that may influence physical activity. *Research Quarterly for Exercise and Sport, 68*(4), 345-351.

Sallis, J., Kraft, K., and Linton, L. (2002). How the environment shapes physical activity, a transdisciplinary research agenda. *American Journal of Preventive Medicine, 22*(3), 208.

Sallis, J., McKenzie, T., Alcaraz, J., Kolody, B., Faucette, N., and Hovell, M. (1997). The effects of a 2-year physical education program on physical activity and fitness in elementary school children. *American Journal of Public Health*, 87(8), 1328-1334.

Sallis, J., McKenzie, T., Conway, T., Elder, J., Prochaska, J., Brown, M., Zive, M., Marshall, S., and Alcarez, J. (2003). Environmental interventions for eating and physical activity: A randomized controlled trial in middle schools. *American Journal of Preventive Medicine, 24*(3), 209-217.

Sallis J., and Owen N. (1997). Ecological models. In K. Glanz, F.M. Lewis, and B.K. Rimer (Eds.), *Health Behavior and Health Education: Theory, Research and Practice*, (2nd ed., pp. 403-424). San Francisco: Jossey-Bass.

Sallis, J., Patrick K., Frank, E., Pratt M., Wechsler, H., and Galuska, D. (2002). Interventions in health care settings to promote healthful eating and physical activity in children and adolescents. *Preventive Medicine, 31*, S112-S120.

Salmon, J., Bauman, A., Crawford, D., Timperio, A, and Owen, N. (2000). The associations between television viewing and overweight among Australian adults participating in varying levels of leisure-time physical activity. *International Journal of Obesity, 24*, 600-606.

Salmon, J., Owen, N., Crawford, D., Bauman, A., and Sallis, J. (2003). Physical activity and sedentary behavior: A population-based study of barriers, enjoyment, and preference. *Health Psychology, 22*(2), 178-188.

Sampson, R. (2003). Neighborhood level context and health: Lessons from sociology. In I. Kawachi and L. Berkman (Eds)., *Neighborhoods and Health*, (pp. 132-146). NY: Oxford University Press.

Satariano, W., and McAuley, E. (2003). Promoting physical activity among older adults: From ecology to the individual. *American Journal of Preventative Medicine, 25*(3S), 184-192.

Schroeder, J., Nau, K., Osness, W., and Potteiger, J. (1998). A comparison of life satisfaction, functional ability, physical characteristics, and activity level among older adults in various living settings. *Journal of Aging and Physical Activity*, 6, 340-349.

Seefeldt, V., Malina, R., and Clark, M. (2002). Factors affecting levels of physical activity in adults. *Sports Medicine, 32*(3), 143-168.

Seeman, T., and Chen, X. (2002). Risk and protective factors for physical function in older adults with and without chronic conditions: MacArthur studies of successful ageing. *Journal of Gerontology, 57B*, S135-144.

Segal, L., Dalton, A. and Richardson, J. (1998). Cost-effectiveness of the primary prevention of non-insulin dependent diabetes mellitus. *Health Promotion International, 13*(3), 197-209.

Segal, R., Reid, B., Johnson, D., Laplante, J., Jette, M., Evans, W., and Smith, J. (1997). Progressive resistance exercise training in men with advanced prostate cancer. *Clinical Investigative Medicine, 20,* S58.

Seguin, A., and Divay, G. (2002). *Urban Poverty: Fostering Sustainable and Supportive Communities.* Discussion Paper F/27, Family Network. Toronto: Canadian Policy Research Networks.

Sharpe, P., Granner, M., Hutto, B., and Ainsworth, B. (2004). Association of environmental factors to meeting physical activity recommendations in two South Carolina counties. *American Journal of Health Promotion, 18*(3), 251-257.

Simons-Morton, D., Calfas, K., Oldenburg, B., and Burton, N. (1998). Effects of interventions in health care settings on physical activity or cardiorespiratory fitness. *American Journal of Preventive Medicine, 15*(4), 413-430.

Singh-Manoux, A., and Marmot, M. (2005). Role of socialization in explaining social inequalities in health. *Social Science and Medicine, 60*, 2129-2133.

Sixsmith, J., Boneham, M., and Goldring, J. (2003). Accessing the community: Gaining insider perspectives from the outside. *Qualitative Health Research, 13*(4), 578-589.

Smedley, B.D., and Syme, L. (2000). *Promoting health: Intervention strategies from social and behavioral research.* Washington, DC: Institute of Medicine, National Academy Press.

Snyder, L., Hamilton, M., Mitchell, E., Kiwanuka-Tondo, J., Fleming-Milici, F., and Proctor, D. (2004). A meta-analysis of the effect of mediated health communication campaigns on behavior change in the United States. *Journal of Health Communication, 9*, 71-96.

Srinivasan, S., O'Fallon, L.R., and Dearry, A. (2003). Creating healthy communities, healthy homes, healthy people: Initiating a research agenda on the built environment and public health. *American Journal of Public Health, 93*(9), 1446-1450.

Ståhl, T., Rütten, A., Nutbeam, D., and Kannas, L. (2002). The importance of policy orientation and environment on physical activity participation, a comparative analysis between Eastern Germany, Western Germany and Finland. *Health Promotion International, 17*(3), 235-246.

Stokols, D., Allen, J., and Bellingham, R. (1996). The social ecology of health promotion: Implications for research and practice. *American Journal of Health Promotion, 10*(4), 247-251.

Stone, E., McKenzie., Welk, G., and Booth, M. (1998). Effects of physical activity interventions in youth: review and synthesis. *American Journal of Preventive Medicine*, 15(4), 298-315.

Story, M. (1999). School-based approaches for preventing and treating obesity. *International Journal of Obesity and Related Metabolic Disorders*, 23 (S2), S43-S51.

Swinburn, B., Egger, G., and Raza, F. (1999). Dissecting obesogenic environments: The development and application of a framework for identifying and prioritizing environmental interventions for obesity. *Preventive Medicine, 29,* 563-570.

Syme, L. (2002). Promoting health and preventing disease. *Social Marketing Quarterly, VIII*(4), 64-66.

Syme, L. (2004). Social determinants of health: The community as an empowered partner. *Preventing Chronic Disease, Public Health Research, Practice and Policy, [serial online] 1*(1),1-5. *http://www.cdc.gov.pcd/issues/2004/jan/syme.htm*

Task Force on Community Preventive Services. (2002). Recommendations to increase physical activity in communities. *American Journal of Preventive Medicine, 22(4S),* 67-72.

Telama, R., Yang, X., Laakso, L., and Viikari, J. (1997). Physical activity in childhood and adolescence as predictor of physical activity in young adulthood. *American Journal of Preventive Medicine, 13,* 317-323.

Telama, R., Yang, X., Viikari, J., Valimaki, I., Wanne, O., and Raitakari, O. (2005). Physical activity from childhood to adulthood, a 21-year tracking study. *American Journal of Preventive Medicine, 28*(3), 267-273.

The Surgeon General's Call to Action to Prevent and Decrease Overweight and Obesity. (2001). Rockville, MD: U.S. Department of Health and Human Services.

Thomas, H., Ciliska, D., Wilson-Abra, J., Micucci, S., Dobbins, M., and Dwyer, J. (2004). *Effectiveness of physical activity enhancement and obesity prevention programs in children and youth.* Report to Health Canada 6795-15-2002/5440007.

Thomas, J., Harden, A., Oakley, A., Oliver, S., Sutcliffe, K., Rees, R., et al. (2004). Integrating qualitative research with trials in systematic reviews. *British Medical Journal, 318,* 1010-1012.

Thomas, J., and Nelson, J. (2001). *Research methods in physical activity* (4th ed.). Champaign, IL: Human Kinetics.

Tinsley, H., and Eldgred, B. (1995). Psychological benefits of leisure participation: A taxonomy of leisure activities based on their need-gratifying properties. *Journal of Counseling Psychology, 42*(2), 123-132.

Trieber, F., Baranowski, T., Braden, D., Strong, W., Levy, M., and Knox, W. (1991). Social support for exercise: Relationship to physical activity in young adults. *Preventive Medicine, 20*(6), 737-750.

Tuomilehto, J., Lindstrom, J., Eriksson, J., Valle, T., Hamalainen, H., Ilanne-Parikka, P., Keinanen-Kiukaanniemi, S., Laakso, M., Louheranta, A., Rastas, M., Salminen, V., Aunola, S., Cepaitis, Z., Moltchanov, V., Hakumaki, M., Mannelin, M., Martikkala, V., Sundvall, J., Uusitupa, M., and the Finnish Diabetes Prevention Study Group. (2001). Prevention of type 2 diabetes mellitus by changes in lifestyle among subjects with impaired glucose tolerance. *The New England Journal of Medicine, 344*(18), 1343-1350

Vandergrift, D., and Yoked, T. (2004). Obesity rates, income, and suburban sprawl: an analysis of US states. *Health and Place, 10,* 221-229.

Vertinsky, P. (1998). "Run, Jane, Run": central tensions in the debate about enhancing women's health through exercise. *Women and Health, 27*(4), 81-111.

Veugelers, P., and Fitzgerald, A.L. (2005). Effectiveness of school programs in prevention childhood obesity: a multi-level comparison. *American Journal of Public Health,* 95, 432-435.

Vogel, E. (2002). *An initial overview of the capacities of diabetes educators.* Ottawa Canada: Centre for Chronic Disease Prevention and Control, Health Canada.

Vuori, I., Oja, P., and Paronen, O. (1994). Physically active commuting to work – testing its potential for exercise promotion. *Medicine and Science in Sports and Exercise, 26,* 844-850.

Weinstein, A., Sesso, H., Min Lee, I., Cook, N., Manson, J., Buring, J., and Gaziano, J. (2004). Relationship of physical activity vs. body mass index with type 2 diabetes in women. *Journal of the American Medical Association, 292*(10), 1188-1194.

Weiss, C. (1998). *Evaluation* (2nd ed.). Upper Saddle River, NJ: Prentice Hall.

Wen, L., Thomas, M., Jones, H., Orr, N., Moreton, R., King, L., Hawe, P., Bindon, J., Humphries, J., Schicth, K., Corne, S., and Bauman, A. (2002). Promoting physical activity in women: Evaluation of a 2-year community-based intervention in Sydney, Australia. *Health Promotion International, 17*(2), 127–137.

Wessel, T., Arant, C, Olson, M., Johnson, D., Reis, S., Sharaf, B., et al. (2004). Relationship of physical fitness vs. body mass index with coronary artery disease and cardiovascular events in women. *Journal of the American Medical Association, 292* (10), 1179-1187.

Wharf Higgins, J., Gaul, C., Gibbons, S., and Van Gyn, G. (2003). Factors Influencing Physical Activity Levels Among Canadian Youth. *Canadian Journal of Public Health, 94*(1), 45-51.

Wharf Higgins, J., Rickert, T., and Rutherford, M. (2004). The Vancouver island race: A collaboration between the Saanich Peninsula diabetes prevention project and Saanich adult education centre. *Canadian Association for Health, Physical Education, Recreation and Dance Journal, 70*(2), 23-26.

Wilcox, S., Castro, C., King, A., Housemann, R., and Brownson, R. (2000). Determinants of leisure time physical activity in rural compared with urban older and ethnically diverse women in the United States. *Journal of Epidemiology and Community Health, 54,*667-672.

Wimbush, E., MacGregor, A., and Fraser, E. (1998). Impacts of a national mass media campaign on walking in Scotland. *Health Promotion International, 13*(1), 45-53.

Wong, F., Huhman, M., Heitzler, C., Asbury, L., Bretthauer-Mueller, R., McCarthy, S. et al., (2004). VERB A social marketing campaign to increase physical activity among youth. *Preventing Chronic Disease [On-line serial], 1*(3), 1-7. *http://www.cdc.gov/pcd/issues/2004/jul/toc.htm*

World Health Organization (WHO). (2003). *Consultation document to guide the development of a WHO global strategy on diet, physical activity and health.* Retrieved January, 2005 from *http://www.who.int/hpr/gs.consultation.document.shtml.*

Wright, J., MacDonald, D., and Groom, L. (2003). Physical activity and young people: beyond participation. *Sport, Education and Society, 8*(1), 17-33.

Yen, I., and Kaplan, G. (1998). Poverty area residence and changes in physical activity level: Evidence from the alameda county study. *American Journal of Public Health, 88*(11), 1709-1712.

Yoo, S., Weed, N., Lempa, M., Mbondo, M., Shada, E., and Goodman, R. (2004). Collaborative community empowerment: an illustration of a six-step process. *Health Promotion Practice, 5*(3), 256-265.

Zapka, J., Valentine Goins, K., Pbert, L., and Ockene, J. (2004). Translating efficacy research to effectiveness studies in practice: Lessons from research to promote smoking cessation in community health centers. *Health Promotion Practice*, 5(3), 245-255.

Zlot, A., and Schmid, T. (2005). Relationships among community characteristics and walking and bicycling for transportation or recreation. *American Journal of Health Promotion, 20*, 314-317.

In: Weight Loss, Exercise and Health Research
Editor: Carrie P. Saylor, pp. 153-178

Chapter 7

CROSS-CULTURAL COMPARISON OF COLLEGE STUDENTS' PHYSICAL ACTIVITY BEHAVIOR IN THE REPUBLIC OF CHINA AND UNITED STATES OF AMERICA ON THE BASIS OF THE TRANSTHEORETICAL MODEL

Sharon Chai Flath[1] and Bradley J. Cardinal
Department of Publis Health
Oregon State University, Orgeon
Department of Exercise and Sport Science
Oregon State University, Oregon

ABSTRACT

This was a cross-cultural comparative study that examined college students' physical activity behavior in both the Republic of China (ROC) and United States of America (USA) on the basis of the full Transtheoretical Model (TTM) of behavior change. Although current investigations do support TTM as a powerful model of physical activity behavior change, there remains a need for examining other variables and constructs relative to those proposed in TTM. From a health promotion planning or intervention perspective, the integration of some of the PRECEDE/PROCEED (PRE) constructs might provide unique insight into physical activity behavior. A total of 1,132 participants were recruited into this study, with 531 coming from the ROC and 601 coming from the USA. In spite of similar recruitment techniques, the participants from the ROC were older and had lower BMIs than those in the USA. They also spent more time sitting in comparison to their American counterparts. The scales and subscales used in this study were completed in the participants' native language (i.e., Chinese or English). Prior to their use in this study, all of the questionnaires were translated into Chinese using a multiple-step methodology, including back translation, and they were found to have

[1] *Correspondence:* Sharon Chai Flath, Department of Public Health, 256 Waldo Hall, Oregon State University, Corvallis, OR 97331. Phone: (541) 737-3825; FAX: (541) 737-4001; E-Mail: flaths@onid.orst.edu

reasonable internal consistency. Results showed that the best predictive model for the stages of physical activity behavior change was based on concomitants coming from both TTM and PRE together. Specifically, the variables that contributed the most to the participants' stage of change for physical activity classification in a stepwise analysis, in order of entry, were the behavioral processes of change, nationality, predisposing, cognitive processes of change, and gender. The overall classification accuracy was 49%. Other than the maintenance stage (66%-68% classification accuracy), this study found that the preparation stage (65.5%-70.4% classification accuracy) was especially reliably predicted, which suggests that the preparation stage might be less transitory than previous thought. Furthermore, the concurrent validity of the stage of change measure used in this study was significantly related to the International Physical Activity Questionnaire (IPAQ). This is the first application of IPAQ in the ROC (Taiwan) and the results of the present study support its continued use as a physical activity measure within a new country. As nationality was a key concomitant of stage of change classification, the present study suggests there may be a need for more non-Eurocentric research with TTM before concluding that behavior change strategies and techniques hypothesized in the model (e.g., behavioral and cognitive processes of change, decisional balance, and self-efficacy) are fully generalizable in physical activity behavior change interventions using mixed culture samples. Likewise, there may be some unique contributions to such interventions by incorporating constructs from a broader health promotion planning or intervention model.

INTRODUCTION

Our population suffers from obesity, heart disease, stroke, cancer, sleep apnea, depression, and chronic pain. Though there are many other ills, these ones have specifically been linked to a sedentary lifestyle. Indeed, an aptly named condition has gained popularity: Sedentary Death Syndrome (SeDS). It is estimated that 70% of the U.S. population is affected by SeDS (Chakravarthy and Booth, 2002). Alarmingly, these conditions have not been exclusively limited to middle and older aged citizens. College students are experiencing some of these conditions at an increasing rate. So much so that the U.S. Department of Health and Human Services (2000) has identified the need for increased physical activity behavior among college students as a national health priority. It appears that a significant decrease (62.5%) in physical activity occurs between high school and college (Cullen et al., 1999). Correspondingly college students' health declines when activity declines. The challenge, then, is to understand why and how this trend can be reversed.

To date, research addressing sedentary lifestyle habits in both the US and the Republic of China (ROC) has largely been targeted at school children, middle-aged adults, and elderly adults (Robert Wood Johnson Foundation 2002; Lee 1998; Lu et al. 2000; Lin, 2000; Stone et al., 1998; Wu, and Jwo, 2005). However, the university student population has received little research attention. Also, the physical education requirement has been reduced or eliminated in many colleges and universities in the US (Hensley, 2000). A similar or perhaps worse situation exists in the ROC's 150 colleges and universities according to the National Council on Physical Fitness and Sports in Taiwan (1999). Also, in 1997 the Ministry of Education in Taiwan eliminated the physical education requirement and as a result most universities chose to eliminate their physical education classes. The result of this elimination has not been studied. It is urgent to understand how to help college students adopt patterns of active living in order to prevent the consequences of sedentary lifestyle-mediated disorders.

There is strong international interest in this topic (Killoran, Fentem, and Caspersen, 1994). However, at present, there is very little scientifically based knowledge about physical activity and health promotion within the context of ethnicity and culture, let alone international cross-cultural diversity. This void has resulted in several recent pleas for researchers in exercise and sports science to engage in more cross-cultural research aimed at fostering international understanding and appreciation (Duda and Hayashi, 1998, Zeigler, 2000).

One promising approach for studying physical activity behavior is that proposed in the Transtheoretical Model (TTM) of behavior change. The TTM attempts to identify and isolate key variables associated with successful behavior change. These variables are the behavioral and cognitive processes of change, decision-making, self-efficacy, and the stages of change.

THE INTERNATIONAL PROBLEM OF PHYSICAL INACTIVITY

Commonly known health beliefs and practices, or different medicine practices, may be important determinants of health behaviors that are culturally specific (Hufford, 1997; Jack, Harrison, and Airhihenbuwas, 1994; Kramer, 1992; Huff and Kline, 1999). Also, the norms, values, and beliefs of western culture may not meet the needs of other cultural settings. That is, an acceptable and effective intervention in one population may not be acceptable or effective for another. Therefore, it is a challenge to study cross-cultural exercise behavior change and, at the same time, to keep the development of interventions as generic as possible to meet the needs of a culturally diverse population. This need has largely been ignored by scholars in the sub-discipline of sport and exercise psychology (Duda and Allison, 1990; Duda and Hayashi, 1998).

THE BENEFITS OF PHYSICAL ACTIVITY

The benefits of exercise and physical activity are well established in the literature (U.S. Department of Health and Human Services [USDHHS], 2000; American College of Sports Medicine [ACSM], 1995). Also, sedentary living is a major public health problem (Sparling et al., 2002). According to the Centers for Disease Control and Prevention (CDC, 1995; 1997; 2000), approximately 60% of Americans are not sufficiently active on a regular basis, and 25 % are not active at all. It is a dire situation for the future health of the US (Sparling, 2003). In Taiwan it is estimated that only 25 % of people are doing regular routine exercise (Wu and Jwo, 2005). Furthermore, greater than 50% of people 40 years old or older and greater than 75% of people 20 years old or younger, lack adequate levels of physical activity (Huang et al., 1991; Liu, 1995). Rates of taking part in physical activity also decline throughout high school, college, and then even more sharply after college graduation (Casperson et al., 2000; Hensley, 2000; Sparling and Snow, 2002).

STATUS OF RESEARCH IN THE COLLEGE STUDENT POPULATION

The college student population has received surprisingly little research attention in physical inactivity. Most of the research in this area has been devoted to adult or elderly participants (Marcus, Rakowski, and Rossi, 1992; Armstrong et al., 1993; Wyse, Mercer, and Ashford, 1994; Buxton et al., 1995; Cardinal, 1995; Robert Wood Johnson Foundation, 2002). Sedentary living habits usually are established at a young age (e.g., preadolescents and adolescents; Cardinal, Engels and Zhu, 1998; Nigg and Courneya, 1998; Walton et al., 1999; Robert Wood Johnson Foundation, 2002). The sedentary habits of children and youth, at least in part, have been shown to track into adulthood (Reynolds, 1990).

A recent health survey indicated that a person's physical activity pattern as a college senior persevered in the years after graduation (Sparling and Snow, 2002). That is, six years after graduation, 85% of those who were active remained active. Similarly, 81% of those who were inactive remained inactive. The college years are probably the last opportunity for a major social institution to shape young adults' physical activity habits (Leslie et al., 2001; Sparling and Snow, 2002).

More than 12 million students currently are enrolled in the colleges and universities of the US. Approximately 20% of the students are overweight and few engage in physical activity on a regular basis. The *Healthy People 2010* document (US Department of Health and Human Services [USDHHS], 2000) discusses the need for studies in the college age group and listed one of the six major health-risk behaviors as inadequate physical activity. It is also a goal of the USDHHS to target college students and create course work for them so that young people will be able to find, understand, and use information and services to enhance their health. There are very few studies that have focused on college students' physical activity behavior in either America or the Republic of China (Lu et al., 2000; Lin, 2000; Wu et al., 2003; Sparling, 2003).

Before 1995 in Taiwan, physical education was required in the college curriculum. With required physical education programs from elementary school throughout high school and college in Taiwan, young people historically had at least three to five full hours of moderate to vigorous physical activity every week. Since physical education classes were changed to elective, many universities rely on students themselves to decide whether to be active or not. Unfortunately, many are choosing not to be active (Huang, Chiang, Lan, Fang, and Kwei, 1991; Liu, 1995; Wu and Jwo, 2005). A similar situation has been found in the US, with a large drop off in physical activity from high school to college (Cullen et al., 1999).

Exercise-promotion efforts need to reach everybody. Despite the lack of research attention, studying college students will be an ideal starting point because the school setting is an important avenue to reach a large segment of the population, which, as previously noted, is the last window of opportunity for a major social institution to influence physical activity behavior (Leslie, Sparling, and Owen, 2001; Sparling and Snow, 2002).

Many research studies indicate that physical activity interventions using theoretical frameworks can increase the physical activity behavior of sedentary adults (Dunn et al., 1999; Marcus et al., 1998). One promising approach in the field of physical activity behavior change is the Transtheoretical Model (TTM), which has been extensively studied in the US in an attempt to identify promising exercise and physical activity behavior change strategies.

However, few health and physical activity promotion and intervention curricula have been developed using such models (Buckworth, 2001).

THE TRANSTHEORETICAL MODEL OF BEHAVIOR CHANGE

On the basis of the TTM, behavior change is viewed as a complex process that unfolds over time through a series of stages. These stages account for the temporal, motivational and constancy characteristics of human behavior. The model has four overarching dimensions (Burbank and Riebe, 2002; Kosma, Cardinal, and Rintala, 2002). They are: (1) stages of change (2) processes of change (3) self-efficacy, and (4) decision balance. Marshall and Biddle's (2001) meta-analysis indicated that there were 80 published studies involving at least one of the four dimensions. Only a few studies have examined all four main dimensions simultaneously (Gorely and Gordon, 1995; Hellman, 1997; Nigg and Courneya, 1998; Cardinal, Tuominen and Rintala, 2003). For example, Gorely and Gordon indicated 8 of the 13 core constructs from TTM accounted for 57% of the variance in a sample of older (M age= 56 year) Australian adult's stage of change classification. Hellman reported that 50% of the variance in a sample of cardiac rehabilitation patients' (M age = 73.5 year) stage of change for exercise adherence was accounted for by their perceived self-efficacy, benefits (surrogate measure of pros), interpersonal support (not a core construct in the TTM), and barriers (surrogate measure of cons). The hypothesized processes of change contributed no unique variance in this study. Among a sample of adolescents (M age = 15 year), Nigg and Courneya found all of the hypothesized constructs from TTM to be significantly related to the participants' stage of change for exercise behavior. Cardinal, Tuominen and Rintala found that self-efficacy accounted for the most variance between stages ($\eta^2 = 0.32$), followed by the behavioral processes of change ($\eta^2 = 0.07$). The largest variance being accounted for in their series of univariate comparisons of the individual processes of change came from counter-conditioning ($\omega^2 = 0.26$), self-efficacy ($\omega^2 = 0.32$), and self-liberation ($\omega^2 = 0.14$). Both counter-conditioning and self-liberation are behavioral processes of change.

THE PRECEDE/PROCEED HEALTH PROMOTION MODEL

While TTM has proven to be a valuable and powerful tool for the study of intrapersonal behaviors, other levels of study that merit analysis include interpersonal, institutional, community, and policy levels. These require the examination of additional variables in conjunction with those hypothesized in TTM. In health promotion, Green and Kreuter's (1991) PRECEDE/PROCEED model is popular. "PRECEDE" refers to the predisposing, reinforcing, and enabling constructs in educational or environmental diagnosis and evaluation, whereas "PROCEED" refers to policy, regulatory, and organizational constructs in educational and environmental development. Corbin and Lindsey (1994) have extracted three dimensions from the model and applied and developed a research tool that can be used within the context of exercise adherence. Their tool examines the predisposing, reinforcing, and enabling factors that might influence physical activity behavior.

COMPARATIVE STUDIES OF PHYSICAL ACTIVITY ON THE BASIS OF THE TRANSTHEORETICAL MODEL

Although studies of the TTM have been conducted in countries other than the United States (U.S.) (e.g., Australia, Canada, and throughout the European Union), there has only been one true comparative study published at present (Cardinal, Tuominen, and Rintala 2003). This study focused on translating the TTM measures into the Finnish language, and assessing the translated instruments' psychometric properties relative to English versions of the measures among an American sample. Their study provides a model for successfully translating psychological inventories from one language to another.

Though other international studies of inactivity/activity have been performed using TTM (Marcus and Owen 1992), the groups being studied were never directly compared. That is, nationality was not used as an independent variable. Also, most of the TTM studies have relied mainly on the Caucasian mainstream. There is evidence of cultural variation in style, and the meaning of activity, even when ethnic groups seem to adopt the sport forms of the mainstream (Duda and Allison, 1990). For example, Kearney, Graal, Damkjaer, and Engstrom (1999) found that substantial inter-country variation existed based on descriptive statistical analysis among 15 member states of the European Union with regard to their stage of change for regular physical activity, motivational factors, and perceived barriers to their involved physical activity. The authors also noted gender differences within their sample, with the percentage of females being higher in the precontemplation stage, and the percentage of males being higher in the maintenance stage. However, no direct statistical comparisons were made between the countries involved in this study, nor were such comparisons made for gender. Furthermore, at present, there are no cross-cultural comparative studies that have been conducted between western and eastern countries.

COMPARISON OF LIFE IN THE U.S. AND ROC

Both the ROC and the U.S. represent advanced economies, but in spite of this, there remain a number of socio-cultural and geo-political differences between the two countries (Wright, 2001). For example, the government in the ROC operates as a Republic, with a nearly ten-decade long democracy (a conservative regime). The government in the U.S. operates as a Federal Republic, with a strong democratic tradition (an advanced liberal regime). This may impact people's psychosocial concomitants for physical activity behavior because of different funding arrangements and different emphases on physical education in the school system, different degrees of access to higher education between the two countries, and semi-mandatory military service for males in the ROC. Also, in the year 2000, the gross national product per capita in the ROC was $13,954 with a GDP growth rate of 5.9% vs. $35,083 with a GDP growth rate 4.1% in the U.S. This may impact people's psycho-social concomitants for physical activity behavior because those in the U.S. have different purchasing power and discretionary income that can potentially be applied to leisure-time pursuits.

Relative to physical activity involvement, recent evidence suggests that those in the ROC may be experiencing similar trends in participation as those in the U.S. (Wu et al., 2002; Lu,

2000; Lin, 2000; Huang et al., 1991). That is, a large proportion of adults in the ROC appear to be remaining sedentary, or having only moderate levels of physical activity in their leisure. And, occupational and commuting forms of physical activity have declined over the past 15 years. These trends seem similar to the situation in the U.S. (U.S. Department of Health and Human Services, 2000). In terms of other related consumer health behaviors, the average daily caloric supply for a male in the ROC is 2,203 kcal, and 1,591 kcal for a female (First Nutrition and Health Survey in Taiwan [NHSIT] 1993-96). In the U.S., it is 2,821 kcal for a male and 1,841 kcal for a female (The Continuing Survey of Food Intakes by Individuals in the United States, by race [CSFII] 1994-96). Finally, the prevalence rate of heart disease is high in both the ROC and the U.S. (Killoran, Fentem, and Caspersen, 1994, National Vital Statistic Report [NVSR] 2002). This is true for both men and women between ages 20-29.

SUMMARY AND PURPOSE

It is well established that physical activity is an important health behavior for the prevention of morbidity and mortality, as well as the promotion of health and wellness. In spite of its benefits, too few people throughout the industrialized world engage in physical activity on a regular basis. To improve this situation, theory based research has been recommended. A particularly promising theory is TTM. TTM is comprised of four main dimensions. To date, few researchers have employed the entire TTM in their studies, let alone additional variables in conjunction with those in TTM. Moreover, researchers have only begun to take up the challenge of performing true cross-cultural, comparative studies with TTM, or other potential constructs related to physical activity and exercise behavior (e.g., predisposing, reinforcing, and enabling factors). The current study seeks to improve upon this situation by addressing whether the stages of change, processes of change (behavioral and cognitive), self-efficacy, and decisional balance are moderated by nationality or gender. The general research question of interest relates to the external and internal validation of the TTM, as well as improving its predictive utility by examining other theoretical variables from a health promotion planning model.

METHOD

Participants

College students were invited to take part in this study from Oregon State University (OSU) and National Taiwan Normal University (NTNU). The authors contacted class representatives or available instructors to invite classes' students for the survey. The first author, who is fully conversant in English and Chinese, employed similar procedures at each respective university. Study participation was voluntary. Similar weather conditions were chosen between the two countries throughout the data collection period, with normal daily high temperatures around 23 degrees Centigrade, and monthly precipitation between 6.35-9.14 cm. In accordance with the selected university's Institutional Review Boards, informed consent by the participants was obtained prior to their participation in the study.

A minimum of 1,100 participants were required for this study. The sample size was determined using power analysis (Kraemer and Thiemann, 1987). This sample size allowed an 80% chance of finding a moderate ($d = 0.45$) effect size difference with alpha set at $p < 0.01$ and a two-tail (bi-directional) test.

MEASURES

Conceptually, the stages of change seek to capture the temporal, motivational, and constancy dimensions of health behavior change. Participants' stage of change for physical activity behavior was assessed using a previously validated measure (Reed et al., 1997). Specifically, participants were informed that:

> "Physical activity includes activities such as brisk walking, jogging, swimming, and aerobic dancing, biking, rowing, etc. Primarily sedentary activities, such as bowling, or playing golf with a cart, would not be considered an appropriate level of physical activity. REGULAR PHYSICAL ACTIVITY = 3 TIMES OR MORE PER WEEK. Please mark the box that best describes your present level of physical activity behavior."

Participants who endorsed the statement: "Yes, I have been participating for more than 6 months," were classified as being in the maintenance stage. Those who endorsed the statement, "Yes, I have been participating for less than 6 months," were classified as being in the action stage. Those who endorsed the statement, "No, but I am planning to start in the next 30 days," were classified as being in the preparation stage. Those who endorsed the statement, "No, but I am planning to start in the next 6 months," were classified as being in the contemplation stage. Those who endorsed the statement, "No, and I don't plan to start in the next 6 months," were classified as being in the precontemplation stage.

To provide construct related validity evidence of the participants' stage of change for physical activity placement, participants also completed the "International Physical Activity Questionnaire" (IPAQ). On this measure, participants reported their frequency of vigorous sessions of physical activity during the previous week (e.g., heaving, lifting, digging, aerobics, or fast bicycling), moderate (e.g., carrying light loads, bicycling at a regular pace, or double tennis), walking (walking at work/school and at home, travel from place to place, and any other solely for recreation, sport, exercise or leisure), and sitting (weekdays while at work/in classroom, while doing course work and during leisure time). This measure was used for the first time in conjunction with the TTM and the people of Taiwan (Craig et al., 2003).

Conceptually, the processes of change are the activities, events and strategies that help people successfully change their behavior. The processes of change were assessed using a 30-item measure (Nigg and Riebe, 2002). Half of the items assessed the behavioral processes of change (i.e., counter-conditioning, helping relationships, reinforcement management, self-liberation, and stimulus control); and the remaining half assessed the cognitive processes of change (i.e., consciousness raising, dramatic relief, environmental reevaluation, self-reevaluation, and social liberation). A sample behavioral item is, "Instead of taking a nap after work/school, I do physical activity," and a sample cognitive item is, "I feel more confident when I do physical activity regularly." Participants responded to each item using a five-point Likert scale (1 = "never," 5 = "repeatedly").

A person's situation specific self-confidence in the face of barriers constitutes barrier self-efficacy. To assess the participants' barrier self-efficacy for exercise, an 18-item measure was used (Rossi et al., 2000). A sample item is, "I am confident I can participate in regular physical activity when it is raining or snowing." Participants responded to each item using a five-point Likert scale (1 = "not at all confident," 5 = "very confident").

On the basis of decision theory (Janis and Mann, 1977), it was anticipated that a person would not adopt or maintain a regular physical activity program unless her/his pros exceed her/his cons. This was referred to as decisional balance. To assess the decisional balance construct, a 10-item measure of potential positive (i.e., pros) and potential negative (i.e., cons) consequences of physical activity involvement were used (Plotnikoff, 2001). A sample pro item is, "I would feel more confident about health by getting physical activity." A sample con item is, "Physical activity would take too much of my time." Participants responded to each statement using a five-point Likert scale (1 = "not at all important," 5 = "extremely important").

Corbin and Lindsey's (1994) 15-item "Physical Activity Adherence Questionnaire" was used to assess the predisposing, reinforcing, and enabling factors associated with physical activity behavior. There were seven predisposing factors on the scale. A sample item is, "I have been a regular exerciser most of my life." There are four enabling factors. A sample item is, "I have a place to exercise and equipment that I can use in or near my home." There are also four reinforcing factors. A sample item is, "I have a doctor and/or employer who encourage me to exercise." Participants responded to each statement on a three-point Likert scale (1 = "very true," 3 = "not true.").

PROCEDURES

All measures were completed in the participants' native language. In translating the measures from English to Chinese, the methodology outlined by Banville, Desrosiers, and Genet-Volet (2000) was used. First, the authors translated all measures into Chinese. Second, three native speaking Chinese (one with a Ph.D. in Education, one a Ph.D. candidate in Public Health, and one a Ph.D. candidate in Human Development and Family Studies) without access to the original version, helped back-translate all the measures into English. Third, these three versions in Chinese were compared, discussed, and modified to reconcile any differences among them. Lastly, the revised instrument was given to a small group of Chinese students at NTNU for pilot testing. The authors continued to collaborate on refining the measures on the basis of any difficulties expressed or observed. Cronbach alpha was used to assess the psychometric properties of the Chinese versions of the measures.

ANALYSIS

The Statistical Package for the Social Sciences (SPSS version 11.5) was used to manage and analyze all data in this study. Scales and subscales employed in this study were examined by Cronbach alpha (α) for internal consistency. A number of demographic variables were compared using either chi-square (χ^2) or t-test. Concurrent validity of stage of change was assessed by comparing it to the IPAQ using both χ^2 or F-test. Finally, univariate analyses and direct and stepwise discriminant function analysis were used to identify important concomitants as well as to generate a classification matrix. As appropriate and to assist in the interpretation of significant and non-significant findings derived from probability (p) testing, measures of magnitude including the contingency coefficient (c), effect size (d), or eta-squared (η^2) were used.

RESULTS

Preliminary Analysis

As shown in Table 1, 16 of scales and sub-scales employed in this study had acceptable levels of internal consistency (i.e., Cronbach $\alpha > .70$) and 9 did not (i.e., Cronbach $\alpha < .70$). Because measurement reliability is important in the detection of statistical significance (Traub, 1994), only certain scales and sub-scales were retained for use in this study. The scales/sub-scales used for analyses in this study were: Predisposing (Cronbach $\alpha = .77$), Reinforcing (Cronbach $\alpha = .60$), Enabling (Cronbach $\alpha = .73$), Behavioral Processes in their entirety (Cronbach $\alpha = .92$), Cognitive Processes in their entirety (Cronbach $\alpha = .87$), the long form of Self-efficacy (Cronbach $\alpha = .87$), Pros (Cronbach $\alpha = .57$) and Cons (Cronbach $\alpha = .61$). The three measures with less than desirable reliability that were retained for use in this study each have theoretical importance, which, for the purposes of this study, trumped their less than ideal reliability.

Table 1. Reliability Coefficients

Variables	Alpha value ($N = 1{,}133$)	Number of Items
Predisposing	$= .77$	7
Reinforcing	$= .61$	4
Enabling	$= .74$	4
Behavior processes	$= .92$	15
Counter conditioning	$= .75$	3
Helping relationship	$= .88$	3
Reinforcement management	$= .81$	3
Self-liberation	$= .79$	3
Stimulus control	$= .70$	3
Cognitive processes	$= .87$	15
Consciousness raising	$= .79$	3
Dramatic relief	$= .64$	3
Self-evaluation	$= .67$	3

Table 1. Reliability Coefficients (Continued)

Variables	Alpha value N= 1,133)	Number of Items
Environmental re-evaluation	= .83	3
Self-liberation	= .59	3
Self-Efficacy		
Negative affect	= .79	3
Excuse making	= .63	3
Must exercise alone	= .90	3
Inconvenient to exercise	= .62	3
Resistance from others	= .85	3
Bad weather	= .84	3
Self-efficacy short form	= .67	6
Self-efficacy long form	= .87	18
Decisional Balance		
Pros	= .57	5
Cons	= .61	5

Participant Characteristics

A total of 1,132 participants were recruited into this study. In terms of national origin, 531 (46.9%) were from Taiwan and 601 (53.1%) were from the US. The majority of participants were male ($n = 596$, 52.6%) and held freshman class standing ($n = 564$, 49.8%). On average, participants were 20.0 years of age ($SD = 1.6$) and had BMIs of 22.6 ($SD = 3.6$).

The 2 (national origin) by 2 (gender) analysis is shown in Table 2. While there was a statistically significant relationship between these two variables (χ^2 (1, $N = 1,132$) = 3.91, $p <$ .05), the magnitude of the relationship was small (i.e., $c = .06$).

Table 2. Nationality by Gender

Nationality	Gender Female	Male	Total
US	268	333	601
TW	268	263	531
Total	536	596	1,132

χ^2 (1, N =1,132) = 3.91, p <. 05, c = .06

The 2 (national origin) by 5 (grade level) analysis is shown in Table 3.

This relationship was statistically significant (χ^2 (4, N = 1,132) = 115.30, p < .001) and of large magnitude (i.e., c = .32). The main difference was that the Taiwan sample was more evenly distributed across grade levels than the US sample, which tended to include mostly underclassmen. Still, though, the majority of participants in both samples held either freshman or sophomore class standing (i.e., 64.8% Taiwan and 85.3% US).

Table 3. Nationality by Grade Level

Nationality			Grade			
	Freshman	Sophomore	Junior	Senior	Graduate	Total
US	386	127	54	32	2	601
TW	178	166	98	84	5	531
Total	564	293	152	116	7	1,132

χ^2 (4, N =1,132) = 115.3, p < .001, c = .32

On average the American students were younger than the Chinese students (M age = 19.5 years, SD = 1.4 vs. M = 20.5 years, SD = 1.7; t (1,130) = -10.27, p < .001, d = .62), and had significantly higher BMIs (M = 23.8, SD = 3.8, vs. M = 21.2, SD = 2.9; t (1,130) = 12.57, p < .001, d =. 74).

DEMOGRAPHIC VARIABLES AND THE STAGES OF CHANGE

As shown in Table 4, the 2 (national origin) by 5 (stage of change) analysis revealed a statistically significant relationship between these two variables (χ^2 (4, N = 1,132) = 120.79, p < .001) and the relationship was large (i.e., c = .31). More than twice as many of the US participants were in the Maintenance stage as compared to those from Taiwan. Also, about three times more of the Taiwan participants were in the Contemplation stage and nearly seven times more were in the Precontemplation stage.

Table 4. Nationality by Stage of Change

Nationality			Stage of Change			
	MA	AC	PR	CO	PC	Total
US	257	98	206	32	8	531
TW	116	77	186	97	55	601
Total	373	175	392	129	63	1,132

Note: MA = maintenance; AC = action; PR = Preparation; CO = contemplation; PC = precontemplation. χ^2 (4, N =1,132) = 120.8, p < .001, c = .31

As shown in Table 5, the 2 (gender) by 5 (stage of change) association was also statistically significant (χ^2 (4, N = 1,132) = 24.58, p < .001), but the magnitude of this association was small (i.e., c = .15). Likewise, as shown in Table 6, the 5 (grade level) by 5 (stage of change) analysis was statistically significant (χ^2 (16, N = 1,132) = 59.6, p < .001), but the magnitude of the relationship was small (i.e., c = .22).

Table 5. Stage of Change by Gender

Stage	Gender		
	Female	Male	Total
Maintenance	143	230	373
Action	83	92	175
Preparation	196	196	392
Contemplation	78	51	129
Precontemplation	36	27	63
Total	536	596	1,132

χ^2 (4, N =1,132) = 24.6, p <. 001, c = .15

Table 6. Grade Level by Stage of Change

Grade Level			Stage of Change			
	MA	AC	PR	CO	PC	Total
Grade						
Freshman	203	96	205	44	16	564
Sophomore	108	42	81	40	22	293
Junior	37	23	59	22	11	152
Senior	23	14	45	20	14	116
Graduate	2	0	2	3	0	7
Total	373	175	392	129	63	1,132

Note. MA = maintenance; AC = action; PR = Preparation; CO = contemplation; PC = precontemplation. χ^2 (4, N =1,132) = 24.6, p <. 001, c = .22

On average and over the course of one week, IPAQ data indicated that the American students reported more physical activity than the Chinese students (Table 7). The American students' sitting time (M sitting time per day = 5.3 hours) was 2.5 hours less per day than the Chinese students (M sitting time per day = 7.8 hours). The Chinese female students' sitting time was the highest, followed by the Chinese male students, then the American male students, with the least sitting time being reported by the American female students. IPAQ data also indicated that US students spent 9.5% more vigorous physical active time, 15 % more moderate physical active time, and 22% less physically inactive time than Chinese students.

CONCURRENT VALIDITY OF THE STAGE OF CHANGE MEASURE

With stage of change as a categorical independent variable and IPAQ scores (IPAQ Short Form, 2003) as a continuous dependent variable, a statistically significant relationship was observed, F (4, 1,130) = 43.67, p < .001, η^2 = .13. Overall, 13% of the participants' physical activity behavior was accounted for in this analysis. Moreover, the 5 (stage of change) by 3 IPAQ category (i.e., insufficiently active, sufficiently active and highly active) (See Table 8) revealed a statistically significant and large association between the two measures, χ^2 (8, N =

1,131) = 193.5, $p < .001$, $c = .38$; thus supporting the concurrent validity of the stage of change measure within this mixed culture sample.

Table 7. IPAQ Physically Active Time and Sitting Time Comparisons by Nationality

Category (per day)	Nationality	Mean	SD	df	t	p	d
Sitting Time	US	5.3	2.9	1129	-12.3	< .001	.56
	TW	7.8	3.8				
Vigorous time	US	68.2	58.9	1130	.5	< .60	.03
	TW	66.2	71.4				
Moderate time	US	59.8	58.6	1130	-2.54	< .011	.16
	TW	70.1	78.8				
Insufficient time	US	73.5	70.8	1130	-3.75	< .001	.13
	TW	94.1	112.5				

Table 8. Stage of Change by IPAQ Category

IPAQ Category	Stage of Change					
	MA	AC	PR	CO	PC	Total
Insufficiently Active	9	8	49	49	15	130
Sufficiently Active	23	25	74	30	10	162
Highly Active	341	142	269	50	37	839
Total	373	175	392	129	62	1,132

Note. MA = maintenance; AC = action; PR = Preparation; CO = contemplation; PC = precontemplation. χ^2 (4, $N = 1132$) = 193.5, $p < .001$, $c = .38$

UNIVARIATE COMPARISON BY STAGE OF CHANGE

Means scores for the behavioral processes, cognitive processes, cons, enabling, predisposing, pros, reinforcing, and self-efficacy constructs showed a general linear trend from precontemplation (low) through maintenance (high). Table 9 summarizes these results and provides post-hoc contrasts across the hypothesized concomitants.

There were also significant age and BMI differences across the stages of change. Those data are shown in Table 10.

Prior to running the multivariate statistics, bivariate correlations among the hypothesized concomitants were examined for multicollinearity. Three of the 28 bivariate relationships did exceed .70. Specifically, the relationship between enabling and predisposing was .71, enabling and reinforcing was .70, and the cons and pros (decisional balance) was .71; however, multicollinearity was not considered a major issue for the multivariate analysis.

Table 9. Univariate Summary of Stage of Change Theoretical Concomitants

Variable	MA	AC	PR	CO	PC	$F_{4,1127}$	p	η^2	Tukey Post Hoc Contrast
Transtheoretical Model									
Behavior processes									
M	50.7	47.8	41.7	35.8	31.3	108.5	<.001	.28	MA,AC>PR>CO>PC
SD	10.4	9.7	9.3	7.7	10.3				
Cognitive processes									
M	37.5	37.3	30.6	30.2	27.2	11.4	<.001	.04	MA>AC,PR > CO
SD	13.4	15.6	17.5	17.4	14.0				
Decisional balance /Pro									
M	15.3	15.4	14.9	14.1	13.9	8.5	<.001	.03	MA,AC,PR>CO,PC
SD	2.5	2.7	2.8	2.9	3.4				
Decisional balance/Con									
M	13.7	13.7	13.6	13.3	12.8	2.4	=.051	.01	MA,AC,PR,CO>PC
SD	2.3	2.7	2.7	2.7	3.4				
Self-efficacy (long form)									
M	59.4	56.1	52.5	47.7	45.7	30.7	<.001	.10	MA,AC>PR>CO,PC
SD	13.7	12.8	12.7	12.6	16.0				
Health Promotional Model									
Enabling									
M	18.0	17.3	17.0	15.9	16.1	32.1	<.001	.10	MA>AC,PR>CO,PC
SD	2.7	2.2	2.0	2.0	2.0				
Predisposing									
M	31.9	30.9	30.0	28.9	28.8	43.1	<.001	.13	MA>AC>PR>CO,PC
SD	2.7	2.7	2.8	2.9	3.0				
Reinforcing									
M	17.4	16.7	16.5	15.8	15.5	23.1	<.001	.09	MA>AC,PR>CO,PC
SD	2.0	2.0	2.1	2.1	2.2				

Note. MA = maintenance; AC = action; PR = Preparation; CO = contemplation; PC = precontemplation.

Table 10. Univariate Summary of Stage of Change, Age, and BMI

Variable	MA	AC	PR	CO	PC	$F_{4,1127}$	p	η^2	Tukey Post Hoc Contrast
Age									
M	19.7	19.5	19.5	20.5	20.1	9.4	<.001	.03	MA,AC,PR>CO>PC
SD	1.7	5.5	1.9	1.5					
BMI									
M	23.2	22.8	20.1	21.6	21.1	7.7	<.001	.04	MA,AC,PR>CO>PC
SD	3.4	4.1	1.8	3.1	3.9				

Note. MA = maintenance; AC = action; PR = Preparation; CO = contemplation; PC – precontemplation.

DIRECT AND STEPWISE DISCRIMINANT FUNCTION ANALYSIS

Classification accuracy was examined using different combinations of TTM, PRE, and the following demographic variables: nationality, age, gender and BMI. In the TTM analysis, five out of eight predictor variables made significant and independent contributions to the discrimination among stages, Wilks' $\Lambda = .72$, $F(4,1125) = 107.92$, $p < .001$. In order of entry, the five predictors were behavior processes, nationality, the cognitive processes, gender, and self-efficacy (Tables 11 and 12). The overall accuracy in classification was 48.5% for TTM, with those in maintenance (66.8%) and in preparation (70.4%) having the most reliable profiles (Table 13).

Table 11. Structure Coefficients for Transtheoretical Model Constructs Alone

Predictor	Structure coefficients Function 1	Function 2	Function 3	Function 4
Behavior processes	.88*	.16	.36	.02
Decisional Balance (pros)	.25*	-.19	.15	.09
Decisional Balance (cons)	.21	-.22*	-.14	.08
Cognitive processes	-.28	.23	-.64	.56
Self-efficacy (Long form)	.49*	.09	.29	.46
Gender	.21	.04	-.65*	.38
Nationality	-.49*	.45	.30*	-.06
BMI	.22	-.11	-.30*	-.06
Age	-.26	-.01	-.02	.52*

*Signifies largest absolute correlation between each variable and any discriminant function.
ªThis variable is not used in the analysis.

Table 12. Summary of Stepwise Analysis for Transtheoretical Model Constructs Alone

Step	Variable	df	p	$1-\Lambda$	F	df
1.	Behavioral processes	4,1125	< .001	.28	107.9	4
2.	Nationality	4,1125	< .001	.11	33.8	8
3.	Cognitive processes	4,1125	< .001	.04	11.4	12
4.	Gender	4,1125	< .001	.02	6.3	16
5.	Self-efficacy	4,1125	< .001	.10	31.1	20

In the PRE analysis, three out of six predictor variables made significant and independent contributions to the discrimination among stages, Wilks' $\Lambda = .87$, $F(4,1125) = 4301$, $p < .001$. In order of entry, the three predictors were predisposing, nationality, and gender (Tables 14 and 15). The overall accuracy in classification was 45.0% for PRE, with those in maintenance (66%) and in preparation (65.6%) having the most reliable profiles (Table 16).

Table 13. Classification Matrix for Transtheoretical Model Constructs Alone

Observed classification % Correct		MA	AC	Predicted classification PR	CO	PC	Total
MA	66.8	**248**	0	120	0	3	371
AC	0.0	93	**0**	77	2	3	175
PR	70.4	103	0	**276**	5	8	392
CO	4.7	10	0	99	**6**	14	129
PC	28.6	3	0	34	8	**18**	63
Total	48.5	457	0	608	21	46	1,130

Note. MA = maintenance; AC = action; PR = preparation; CO = contemplation; PA = Precontemplation; values listed in bold signify agreement between observed and predicted classification.

Table 14. Structure Coefficients for Health Promotion Model Constructs Alone

Predictor	Function 1	Function 2	Structure Coefficients Function 3	Function4
Predisposing .	.74*	-.53	-.06	.41
Reinforcing .	.58*	-.08	.03	.18
Enabling	.65*	-.17	.01	.25
Gender	-.29	.09	.77*	.56
Nationality	.65	.75*	.09	.08
BMI[a]	-.24	-.26	.19	.07
Age	.34	.03	.67	-.67

*Signifies largest absolute correlation between each variable and any discriminant function. [a]This variable is not used in the analysis.

Table 15. Summary of Stepwise Analysis for Health Promotion Model Constructs Alone

Step	Variable	df	p 1-	Λ	F	df
1.	Predesposing	4,1125	< .001	.13	43.1	4
2.	Nationality	4,1125	< .001	.11	33.7	8
3.	Gender	4,1125	< .001	.02	6.3	12

In the TTM and PRE combined analysis, 5 out of 12 predictor variables made significant and independent contributions to the discrimination among stages, Wilks' $\Lambda = .72$, $F(4,1125) = 107.9$, $p < .001$. In order of entry, the five predictors were behavioral processes, predisposing, nationality, cognitive processes, and gender (Table 17 and 18). The overall accuracy in classification was also 49.0% for TTM and PRE combined, with those in maintenance (68%) and in preparation (69.9%) having the most reliable profiles (Table 19).

Table 16. Classification Matrix for Health Promotion Model Constructs Alone

Observed classification % Correct		Predicted classification					
		MA	AC	PR	CO	PC	Total
MA	66.0	**246**	0	127	0	0	373
AC	0.0	87	**0**	86	2	0	175
PR	65.6	132	0	**257**	3	0	392
CO	4.7	21	0	102	**6**	0	129
PC	0.0	10	0	47	6	**0**	63
Total	45.0	496	0	619	17	0	1,132

Note: MA = maintenance; AC = action; PR = preparation; CO = contemplation; PA = Precontemplation; values listed in bold signify agreement between observed and predicted classification.

Table 17. Structure Coefficients for Transtheoretical Model and Health Promotion Model Constructs Combined

	Structure coefficients			
Predictor	Function 1	Function 2	Function 3	Function 4
Behavior processes	.85*	.07	.45	-.04
Predisposing	-.54	-.25	.47	.57*
Reinforcing	-.50*	-.04	.27	.12
Enabling	-.47*	-.09	.39	.21
Self-efficacy (Long form)	.42*	.02	-.20	-.02
Decisional balance (pros)	.23*	-.22	.13	-.11
Decisional balance (cons)	.20	-.23*	.11	-.12
Cognitive processes	-.27	.23	.48	-.69
Gender	.21	.05	-.54*	.06
Nationality	-.47	.46	.37	-.54*
BMI[a]	.20	-.13	-.22*	.21*
Age	-.25	.02	-.07	-.42

*Signifies largest absolute correlation between each variable and any discriminant function.
[a]This variable is not used in the analysis.

Table 18. Summary of Stepwise Analysis for Transtheoretical Model and Health Promotion Model Constructs Combined

Step	Variable	df	p	1-Λ	F	df
1.	Behavioral processes	4,1125	<.001	.28	107.9	4
2.	Predisposing	4,1125	<.001	.13	43.9	8
3.	Nationality	4,1125	<.001	.11	33.8	12
4.	Cognitive processes	4,1125	<.001	.04	11.4	16
5.	Gender	4,1125	<.001	.02	6.3	20

**Table 19. Classification Matrix for Transtheoretical Model
and Health Promotion Model Constructs Combined**

Observed classification% Correct		Predicted classification					
		MA	AC	PR	CO	PC	Total
MA	68.0	**253**	0	115	0	4	372
AC	0.6	91	**1**	79	2	3	175
PR	69.9	103	0	**274**	9	7	392
CO	5.4	8	0	103	**4**	12	129
PC	30.2	3	0	29	11	**19**	63
Total	49.0	458	1	590	26	45	1,131

Note. MA = maintenance; AC = action; PR = preparation; CO = contemplation; PA = Precontemplation; values listed in bold signify agreement between observed and predicted classification.

DISCUSSION

This was the first comparative study of American and Chinese college students' stage of change for physical activity behavior on the basis of the full TTM, as well as the predisposing, reinforcing, and enabling (PRE) constructs from a health promotion model. The best predictive model was the one that combined the TTM and PRE constructs together, resulting in 49% accuracy in stage of change classification (versus 48.5% for TTM alone and 45% for PRE alone). This level of classification accuracy is similar to that reported in previous research, which has ranged from 50% to 69% (Cardinal, Kosma, and McCubbin, 2004; Cardinal, Tuominen, and Rintala, 2004; Gorely and Gordon, 1995; Hellman, 1997).

The variables that contributed the most to the participants' stage of change for physical activity classification in a stepwise analysis were, in order of entry, the behavioral processes of change, predisposing, nationality, cognitive processes of change, and gender. These were the five most important stage of change concomitants and resulted in each stage of change being distinguishable from the other in a manner consistent with theory (i.e., precontemplaton low through maintenance high).

Interestingly, nationality was a major contributor to stage of change classification, whereas other variables that are often considered in TTM studies (e.g., age and BMI) were not especially important. Also, in the only other true cross-cultural study of TTM, Cardinal, Tuominen and Rintala (2004) found that nationality (American versus Finnish) contributed 4% unique variance in an exploratory stepwise analysis. The present study suggests there may be a need for more non-Eurocentric research with TTM before concluding that it is a fully generalizable physical activity behavior change model. This is similar to the conclusion that Qi recently came to in her dissertation research of TTM in mainland China (Qi, Chung, and Hoon, 2005).

Some of the cultural differences in stage of change are actually observable in the overall classification rates. That is, the American participants were more likely to be in the maintenance stage and the Taiwan participants were more likely to be in the contemplation or precontemplation stages. Moreover, there were some participant characteristic differences with the Taiwan participants more likely to be older, have lower BMIs, and to spend more time sitting in comparison to their American counterparts.

The Chinese students spent more sitting time than the Americans and this may be because of cultural factors. Over thousands of years it is a Chinese virtue to be less physical and Chinese polite society promotes intellectual learning over physical activity. This observation supports other findings that suggest commonly held health beliefs and practices are important determinants of health behavior that are culturally specific (Hufford, 1997; Patchter, 1994; Jack, Harrison, and Airhienbuwa, 1994; Kramer, 1992; Huff and Kline, 1999). Future studies should more fully explore why these nationality or cultural differences exist and how such differences may be manifested at the intrapersonal, interpersonal, institutional, community, and policy levels.

Gender is another key concomitant, which is handled differently from one culture to the other (Wu and Jwo, 2005). The findings suggest that it may take Chinese female students the longest time to become physically active in comparison to Chinese male students, followed by American male students, and then American female students. Immediacy of stage of change of physical activity behavior may be different from culture to culture. For example, close to one third of American students work through their college years due to high college tuition costs whereas less than 10 % of Chinese students work through their college years.

While self-efficacy did contribute 10% unique variance in univariate analysis, it was not a key concomitant in the multivariate analysis. This is different than what has been observed in several previous TTM studies (Marshall and Biddle, 2001). Though speculative, there may be a conceptual problem with self-efficacy in this mixed culture sample. Specifically, even though self-efficacy is a widely used psychosocial term in the western world, it may have a different cultural meaning or relevance in the eastern world. For example, Chinese culture may focus more on group cohesion, whereas individuality may be emphasized more in American culture.

In the multivariate analysis, the maintenance and preparation stages were the most reliably predicted stages of change. It is understandable that the maintenance stage would be especially reliable, as one of its characteristics is sustaining a behavior change for greater than 6 months. Interestingly, however, the preparation stage was quite reliable, too, which suggests that this stage might be less transitory than previously thought. That is, people might get "stuck" in preparation. This confirms a previously novel finding made by Cardinal, Engels, and Smouter (2001) where they observed some preadolescent children were in "perpetual preparation" at the conclusion of an intervention study.

Beyond being the first cross-cultural study of TTM and PRE between Taiwan and the United States, another unique aspect of this study was establishing the construct validity of the stage of change measure on the basis of the IPAQ (Craig et al., 2003). This is the first application of IPAQ in Taiwan and the results of the present study support its continued use as a physical activity measure within a new country. Of course, this, too, should be the topic of future research, especially since both measures used in the current study were self-report measures. Using other, non-tautological approaches to establishing the concurrent validity of the IPAQ are warranted (e.g., accelerometers, pedometers, observation). Also, examining the IPAQ scale's stability over time would be a worthwhile psychometric contribution.

Although the questionnaires were translated using appropriate and systematic methodology, including back translation, the original questionnaires did, nonetheless, originate in the Unites States. Had the questionnaires originated in Taiwan, rather than the other way around, they may have captured some unique cultural relevance or conceptual meaning for the Taiwanese sample. Of course, this is one of the tremendous challenges of cross-cultural research, especially when the languages and customs themselves are so uniquely different.

The living circumstances of students at NTNU, which is located in Taipei, a city with a population of 2.6 million people, is very different than OSU, which is located in Corvallis, a small college town with a population of 50,000 people. Due to the geo-social difference, students' physical activity lifestyles may be different. In future studies it would be ideal to account for such geo-social differences. Likewise, while every attempt was made to recruit similar students at each respective university, the samples were, nonetheless, samples of convenience. In the future it would be ideal to obtain random samples of students from each respective university. This would increase the external validity of the study's findings.

Because this was a cross-sectional study, stage of change behavioral development trends could not be observed. To examine such trends, longitudinal studies are needed. It may also be interesting to incorporate qualitative approaches (e.g., interviews and observations) into such a study.

Similar to other findings, among all the scales and subscales employed in this study, the five most important factors indicated by the statistical analysis consistently reinforced the design principles of TTM, especially by the behavior and cognitive processes scales. This finding increases the external validity and the generalizability of these two scales.

The findings of this study favor the integration of the predisposing scale into TTM. Future studies should, therefore, consider integrating predisposing factor into TTM-based research and, possibly, physical activity interventions.

CONCLUSION

This was the first cross-cultural comparative study of American and Chinese college students' stage of change for physical activity behavior on the basis of the full Transtheoretical Model, as well as the predisposing, reinforcing and enabling constructs from a health promotion model. This study indicated that behavioral processes are the most important predictor, which is consistent with other TTM research findings. The predisposing construct from a health promotion model also contributed significantly to stage of change prediction, which is considered a unique finding and should be the topic of future research.

Behavioral processes of change, predisposing, nationality, cognitive processes of change, and gender were the five most important stage of change concomitants found in this study. The result was that each stage of change was distinguishable from the other in a manner consistent with theory.

It is understandable that the maintenance stage would be especially reliable. Interestingly, however, the preparation stage was quite reliable, too, which suggests that this stage might be less transitory than previously thought.

The construct validity of the stage of change measure on the basis of the IPAQ was established in this study as well. This is the first application of IPAQ in Taiwan and the results of the present study support its continued use as a physical activity measure within a new country.

As nationality was a key concomitant of stage of change classification, the present study suggests there may be a need for more non-Eurocentric research with TTM before concluding that behavior change strategies and techniques hypothesized in the model (e.g., behavioral and cognitive processes of change, decisional balance, and self-efficacy) are fully generalizable in physical activity behavior change interventions using mixed culture samples. Likewise, there may be some unique contributions to such interventions by incorporating constructs from a broader health promotion planning or intervention model.

ACKNOWLEDGEMENTS

This study was funded by an International Trade and Development Fellowship, Nippon Foundation of Japan awarded through the Oregon University System; the College of Health and Human Sciences' Research and Competitive Grants Program, Oregon State University; Corvallis Internal Medicine; Tung-Sung Art Culture Education Foundation, Taiwan; and the National Science Council, Republic of China (Grant No. NSC93-2314-B-242-012, C. H. Kao, Principal Investigator, Fooyin University).

REFERENCES

Armstrong, C.A., Sallis, J.F., Hovell, M.F., and Hofstetter, C.R. (1993). Stages of change, self-efficacy, and the adoption of vigorous exercise: a prospective analysis. *Journal of Sport and Exercise Psychology, 15*, 390-402.

Banville, D., Desrosiers, P., and Genet-Volet, Y. (2000). Translating questionnaires and inventories using a cross-cultural translation technique. *Journal of Teaching in Physical Education, 19*, 374-387.

Buckworth, J. (2001). Exercise adherence in college students: Issues and preliminary results. *Quest, 53*, 335-345.

Burbank, P. M., and Riebe, D. (Eds.). (2002). *Promoting exercise and behavior change in older adults: Interventions with the transtheoretical model*. New York, NY: Springer.

Buxton, K.E., Mercer, T.H., Wyse, J.P., and Hale, B.D. (1995). Assessing the stages of exercise behavior change and the stages of physical activity behavior change in a British worksite sample. *Journal of Sport Sciences, 13*, 50-51.

Cardinal, B. J. (1995). The stages of exercise scale and stages of exercise behavior in female adults. *Journal of Sport Medicine and Physical Fitness, 35*, 87-92.

Cardinal, B. J., Engels, H-J., and Smouter, J. (2001). Changes in preadolescents' stage of change for exercise behavior following "Healthy Kids 2000 - Get with it." *American Journal of Medicine and Sports, 3*, 272-278.

Cardinal, B. J., Engels, H-J., and Zhu, W. (1998). Application of the Transtheoretical model of behavior change to preadolescents' physical activity and exercise behavior. *Pediatric Exercise Science, 10*, 69-80.

Cardinal, B. J., Jacques, K. M., and Levy, S. S. (2002). Evaluation of a university course aimed at promoting exercise behavior. *Journal of Sports Medicine and Physical Fitness, 42*, 113-119.

Cardinal, B. J., Levy, S. S., John, D. H., and Cardinal, M. K. (2002). Counseling patients for physical activity. *American Journal of Medicine and Sports, 4,* 364-371.

Cardinal, B. J., Tuominen, K. J., and Rintala, P. (2003). Psychometric assessment of Finnish versions of exercise-related measures of Transtheoretical model constructs. *International Journal of Behavioral Medicine, 10,* 31-44.

Cardinal, B. J., Tuominen, K. J., and Rintala, P. (2004). Cross-cultural comparison of American and Finnish college students' exercise behavior using transtheoretical model constructs. *Research Quarterly for Exercise and Sport, 75,* 92-101.

Chakravarthy, M. V., Joyner, M. J., and Booth, F. W. (2002). An obligation for primary care physicians to prescribe physical activity to sedentary patients to reduce the risk of chronic health conditions. *Mayo Clinic Proceedings, 77,* 1-8.

CSFII The Continuing Survey of Food Intakes by Individuals in the United States, by race, Table set 11, 1993-96.

Corbin, C. B., and Lindsey, R. (1994). *Concepts of fitness and wellness*. Dubuque, IA: WCB Brown and Benchmark.

Craig, C. L., Marshall, A. L., Sjöström, M., Bauman, A. E., Booth, M. L., Ainsworth, B. E., Pratt, M., Ekelund, U., Yngve, A., Sallis, J. F., and Oja, P. (2003), International Physical Activity Questionnaire (IPAQ): 12-country reliability and validity. *Medicine and Science in Sports and Exercise, 35,* 1381-1395.

Craig, C. L., Marshall, A. L., Sjöström, M., Bauman, A. E., Booth, M. L., Ainsworth, B. E., Pratt, M., Ekelund, U., Yngve, A., Sallis, J. F., and Oja, P. (2003). *CSFII, The Continuing Survey of Food Intakes by Individuals in the United States, by race, Table set 11,* 1993-96.

Cullen, K. W., Koehly, L. M., Anderson, C., Baranowski, T., Prokhorov, A., Basen-Engquist, K., Wetter, D., and Hergenroeder, A. (1999). Gender differences in chronic disease risk behaviors through the transition out of high school. *American Journal of Preventive Medicine, 17,* 1-7.

Duda, J. L., and Allison, M. T. (1990). Cross-cultural analysis in exercise and sport psychology: A void in the field. *Journal of Sport and Exercise Psychology, 12,* 114-131.

Duda, J. L., and Hayashi, C. T. (1998). Measurement issues in cross-cultural research within sport and exercise psychology. In J. L. Duda (Ed.), *Advances in sport and exercise psychology measurement* (pp. 471-483). Morgantown, VA: Fitness Information Technology.

Dunn, A. L.. Andersen, R. E.. and Jakicic, J. M. (1998). Lifestyle physical activity interventions: History, short- and long-term effects, and recommendations. *American Journal of Preventive Medicine. 15, 398-412.*

Fleiss, J.L. (1981). *Statistical methods for rates and proportions* (2nd ed.). New York: John Wiley and Sons,

Gorely, P., and Gordon, S. (1995). An examination of the Transtheoretical model and exercise behavior in older adults. *Journal of Sport and Exercise Psychology, 17,* 312-324.

Green, L. W., and Kreuter, M. W. (1991). *Health promotion planning: An educational and environmental approach* (2nd Ed.). Mountain View, CA: Mayfield.

Hellman, E. A. (1997). Use of the stages of change in exercise adherence model among older adults with a cardiac diagnosis. *Journal of Cardiopulmonary Rehabilitation, 17,* 145-155.

Hensley, L. D. (2000). Current status of basic instruction programs in physical education at American colleges and universities. *Journal of Physical Education, Recreation and Dance, 71*(9), 30-36.

Huang, Y.W., Chiang. I.C., Lan, C.F. Fang, C.I., and Kwei, E.L. (1991). The adult health behavior in Taipei County, Taiwan. *Public Health Quarterly, 18(2), 133-147.*

Huff, R. M. and Kline, M. V. (1999). *Promoting health in multicultural populations: A handbook for practitioners.* Thousand Oaks, CA: Sage.

Hufford, D.J. (1997). Complementary and alternative therapies in primary care: Folk medicine. *Primary Care; Clinics in Office Practice, 24*(4), 724-741.

Jack, L., Harrison, I. E., and Airhihenbuwa, C. O. (1994). *Ethnicity and the health belief systems.* In Matiella, A.C. (Ed.). The multicultural challenge in health educations. Santa Cruz, CA: ETR Associations.

Janis, I., and Mann, L. (1977). *Decision making: A psychological analysis of conflict, choice, and commitment.* London: Cassel and Collier Macmillan.

Kearney, J. M., Graal, C. D., Damkjaer, S., and Engstrom, L. M. (1999). Stages of change towards physical activity in a nationally representative sample in the European Union. *Public Health Nutrition, 2,* 115-124.

Killoran, A. J., Fentem, P., and Caspersen, C. (1994). *Moving on: International perspectives on promoting physical activity.* London: Health Education Authority.

Kosma, M., Cardinal, B. J., and Rintala, P. (2002). Motivating individuals with disabilities to be physically active. *Quest, 54,* 116-132.

Kramer, B. (1992). Health and aging of urban American Indians. *Western Journal of Medicine, 157,* 281-25.

Kraemer, H.C., and Thiemann, S. (1987). *How many subjects? Statistical power analysis in research.* Newbury Park, CA: Sage.

Leslie, E., Sparling, P.B., and Owen, N. (2001). University campus setting and promotion of physical activity in young adults: Lessons from research in Australia and the USA. *Health Education, 101,* 116-25.

Liu, T.W. (1995). *The influential determinants of exercise behavior of students in a junior college.* Unpublished master's thesis, National Taiwan Normal University, Taipei, Taiwan.

Marcus, B. H., Banspach, S.W., Lefebvre, R.C., Rossi, J.S., Carleton, R. A., and Abrams, D.B. (1992). Using the stages of change model to increase the adoption of physical activity among community participants. *Research Quarterly for Exercise and Sport, 63,* 60-66.

Marcus, B. H., Bock, B. C., Pinto, B. M., Forsyth, L.H., Roberts, M. B., and Traficante, R. M. (1998). Efficacy of an individualized, motivationally-tailored physical activity interventions. A*nnals of Behavioral Medicine, 20,* 174-180.

Marcus, B. H., and Owen, N. (1992). Motivational readiness, self-efficacy and decision making for exercise. *Journal of Applied Social Psychology, 22,* 3-16.

Marcus, B.H., Rakowski, W., and Rossi, J. S. (1992). Assessing motivational readiness and decision-making for exercise. *Health Psychology,* 11, 257-261.

Marshall, S. J., and Biddle, S. J. H. (2001). The Transtheoretical model of behavior change: A meta-analysis of applications. *Annals of Behavioral Medicine, 23,* 229-240.

NHSIT, First Nutrition and Health Survey in Taiwan, 1993-1996

Nigg, C. R., and Courneya, K. S. (1998). Transtheoretical model: Examining adolescent exercise behavior. *Journal of Adolescent Health, 22*, 214-224.

Nigg, C. R., and Riebe, D. (2002). The Transtheoretical Model: Research Review of Exercise Behavior and Older Adults. In P.M. Burbank and D. Riebe (Ed.), *Promoting Exercise and Behavior Change in Older Adults*, (pp. 153-154). Springer Publish Company.

National Vital Statistic Report in the United States. (2002).

Patcher, L.M. (1994). Culture and clinical care: Folk illness beliefs and behaviors and their implications for health care delivery. *Journal of the American Medical Association, 271*, 690-694.

Plotnikoff, R.C., Blanchard, C., Hotz, S.B., and Rhodes, R. (2001). Validation of the decisional balance scales in the exercise domain from the transtheoretical model: A longitudinal test. *Measurement in Physical Education and Exercise Science, 5*(4), 191-206.

Prochaska, J. O., Velicer, W. F., DiClemente, C. C., and Fava, J. (1988). Measuring processes of change: Applications to the cessation of smoking. *Journal of Consulting and Clinical Psychology, 56*, 520-528.

Qi, S., Chung, C., and Hoon, S. (2005). *Stages of change in exercise for Chinese undergraduate students*. Unpublished manuscript.

Reed, G. R., Velicer, W. F., Prochaska, J. O., Rossi, J. S., and Marcus, B. H. (1997). What makes a good staging algorithm? Examples from regular exercise. *American Journal of Health Promotion, 12*, 57-66.

Reynold, K.D., Killed, J.D., Bryson, S.W., Maron, D.J., Taylor, C.B., Maccoby, N. and Farquhar, J. W. (1990). Psychosocial predictors of physical activity in adolescents. *Preventive Medicine, 19*,541-551.

Robert Wood Johnson Foundation and American Association of Retired Persons. (2003). Active for Life Program. Accessed Nov. 20. 2003. <<*http://www.rwjf. org/newsEvents/activelifeIndex.jhtml*>.

Rosen, C. S. (2000). Integrating stage and continuum models to explain processing of exercise messages and exercise initiation among sedentary college students. *Health Psychology, 19*, 172-180.

Rossi, J. S., Benisovich, S.V., Norman, G. J., and Nigg, C. R. (2000). *Development of a hierarchical multidimensional measure of exercise self-efficacy*. Cancer Prevention Research Center, Department of Psychology, University of Rhode Island, Stanford University, and Stanford School of Medicine.

Sparling, P.B. (2003). College physical education: An unrecognized agent of change in combating inactivity-related diseases. *Perspectives in Biology and Medicine, 46*, 579-587.

Sparling, P.B., and Snow, T. K. (2002). Physical activity patterns in recent college alumni. *Research Quarterly, Exercise Sport. 73*, 200-205.

Stone, E. J., McKenzie, T.L., and Booth, M.L. (1998). Effects of physical activity interventions in youth: Review and synthesis. *American Journal of Preventive Medicine, 15*, 298-315.

Traub, R. (1994). *Reliability for the social sciences, theory and applications*. Thousand Oaks, CA: Sage.

United States Department of Health and Human Services. (2000). *Healthy people 2010* (Conference edition in 2 volumes). Washington, DC: U.S. Government Printing Office.

Wright, J. W. (Ed.). (2001). *The New York Times almanac*. New York: Penguin.

Walton, J., Hoerr, S., Heine, L., Frost, S., Roisen, D., and Berkimer, M. (1999). Physical activity and stages of change in fifth and sixth graders. *Journal of School Health, 68*, 285-289.

Wu, T.Y., Pender, N., and Noureddine, S. (2003). Gender differences in the psychosocial and cognitive correlates of physical activity among Taiwanese adolescents: A structural and equation modeling approach. *International Journal of Behavioral Medicine, 10*, 93-105.

Wu, T.Y., and Jwo, J.L. (2005). A prospective study on changes of cognitions, interpersonal influences, and physical activity in Taiwan youth. *Research Quarterly for Exercise and Sport, 76, 1-10.*

Wyse, J., Mercer, T., and Ashford, B. (1994). *Stages of exercise behavior change and biomedical status.* Paper presented at the Cardiovascular Disease Prevention Conferences, II, London.

Zeigler, E. F. (2000). Global issues in the profession of physical education and sport. In J. R. Polidoro (Ed.), *Sport and physical activity in the modern world* (pp. 157-185). Boston, MA: Allyn and Bacon.

In: Weight Loss, Exercise and Health Research
Editor: Carrie P. Saylor, pp. 179-194

ISBN 1-60021-077-5
© 2006 Nova Science Publishers, Inc.

Chapter 8

PHYSICAL ACTIVITY AND CARDIOVASCULAR RISK FACTORS IN CHINA

Gang Hu and Zhijie Yu

Department of Epidemiology and Health Promotion, National Public Health Institute,
Helsinki and Department of Public Health, University of Helsinki, Finland;
Institute for Nutritional Sciences, Shanghai Institute for Biological Sciences, Chinese
Academy of Science, Shanghai, PR China.

ABSTRACT

There is good evidence that regular physical activity has a protective effect against several chronic diseases, including coronary heart disease, hypertension, obesity, diabetes, osteoporosis, colon cancer, depression and anxiety. Physical activity levels, including occupational and commuting physical activity, have decreased in recent years in China. Physical activity among Chinese urban people is very different in comparison to the Western populations. Walking or cycling to and from work and school constituted a large component of daily activities among the majority of Chinese urban population. Low level of leisure time physical activity was common in Chinese urban population. People with more daily walking or cycling to and from work and leisure time physical activity had lower levels of cardiovascular risk factors, including low levels of body mass index, blood pressure, total and low-density lipoprotein cholesterol, and triglyceride, high level of high-density lipoprotein cholesterol, and low prevalence of overweight, hypertension, and smoking. Regular leisure time physical activity reduced the risk of total, cancer, respiratory and cardiovascular deaths and daily walking or cycling to and from work also decreased the risk of colon cancer.

Sedentary lifestyle is an important lifestyle-related public health problem in the world [1]. Physical inactivity is not only associated with a number of health-related risk factors, including hypertension, lipid abnormalities, and obesity, but also seems to be an independent risk factor for cardiovascular disease (CVD), type 2 diabetes, the metabolic syndrome, and several types of cancers [1-14]. The prevalence of inactivity and its negative health consequences are rapidly increasing in both developed and developing countries [1, 4-6]. A recommendation from the Centers for Disease Control and Prevention (CDC)/the American College of Sports Medicine (ACSM) and National Institutes of Health Consensus Development Conference on Physical Activity and Cardiovascular Health concluded that intermittent or shorter bouts of activity (at least 10 minutes), including occupational, nonoccupational, or tasks of daily living, also have similar cardiovascular and health benefits if performed at a level of moderate intensity (such as brisk walking, cycling, swimming, home repair, and yard work) with an accumulated duration of at least 30 minutes per day [1, 15].

In recent twenty years, following the rapid economic development Chinese people have gradually changed their lifestyles. Lifestyle change in Chinese populations has led to a transition of the disease pattern [16, 17]. Cardiovascular disease has become the major cause of death in China [18, 19]. Hypertension, smoking, overweight, obesity, dyslipidemia, diabetes and the metabolic syndrome as the main CVD risk factors have become major public health problems in China [20-23]. The Fourth China Nutrition and Health Survey (4th CNHS) which was carried out between August and December 2002 among population-based samples of 272,023 individuals from 31 provinces, showed that 7.1% of Chinese adults aged 18 years and older were obesity (body mass index $\geq$30 kg/m^2), 22.8% of adults were overweight (body mass index $\geq$25), 18.8% of adults had hypertension (blood pressure $\geq$90/140 mm Hg, or using antihypertensive drugs), and 18.6% had dyslipidemia (one of the following: high-density lipoprotein cholesterol < 0.91 mmol/l; total cholesterol $\geq$5.21 mmol/l; or triglecerides $\geq$1.7 mmol/l) [23]. The prevalence of diabetes was reported to be 6.4% among urban subjects aged 25 years or more [23]. In Beijing, the second largest city in China, the prevalence of diabetes in the 1998 survey was 14% among men and 16% among women aged 40-89 years [21]. A cross-sectional study with 2048 subjects aged 20-74 years in Shanghai (the first largest city in China) compared the prevalence of the metabolic syndrome according to the World Health Organization (WHO) and the National Cholesterol Education Program Expert Panel (NCEP) definitions and indicated that the age-adjusted prevalence of the metabolic syndrome was higher by using WHO definition (17.1%) than by using NCEP definition (11.0%) [22].

Physical activity levels, including occupational and commuting physical activity, have decreased in recent years [23]. Commuting physical activity among Chinese urban people is very different in comparison to the Western populations. Walking or cycling to and from work and school constituted a large component of daily activities among the majority of Chinese urban population [24, 25]. In this chapter, we describe the physical activity level and its relationship to demographic and health-related characteristics and CVD risk factors among the Chinese population.

PHYSICAL ACTIVITY IN CHINA

In 1996 a cross-sectional survey of 2002 males and 1974 females was carried out in urban areas of Tianjin, the third largest city in China [24]. Table 1 describes commuting physical activity and leisure time physical activity in urban Tianjin. In this population, absence of leisure time physical activity was reported by 61% of the males and 67% of the females. Leisure time physical activity lasting 1-30 minutes per day was performed by 29%

of the males and 24% of the females, and about 10% of the participants reported more than 30 minutes of such activity per day. The mean duration of leisure time physical activity was 10 minutes for males and 8 minutes for females. Only 4% of females and 9% of males reported that they went to and from work by bus or performed no physical activity associated with commuting. A total of 50% of the males and 55% of the females reported 1-30 minutes of commuting physical activity on foot or by bicycle; 30% of the males and 34% of the females performed 31-60 minutes of such activity, and 11% of the males and 7% of the females cycled for more than 1 hour to and from work. The mean commuting time on foot or by bicycle was 31 minutes for males and 30 minutes for females, respectively. The total time of commuting physical activity plus leisure time physical activity was about 40 minutes in both genders [24].

Table 1. Physical activity among study subjects aged 15-69 years, Tianjin, China [24]

Type of physical activity	Males (%) (N = 2002)	Females (%) (N = 1974)
Leisure time (times per month)		
0	61	67
1-4	6	6
5-9	7	5
10-19	5	4
≥20	21	18
Leisure time (minutes/day)		
0	61	67
1-30	29	24
>30	10	9
Commuting on foot or by bicycle (minutes/day)		
0*	9	4
1-30	50	55
31-60	30	34
>60	11	7
Combined commuting and leisure time (minutes/day)		
0	7	3
1-30	38	44
31-60	32	36
>60	23	17

*Using motorized transport, or no commuting physical activity.

Recently, Fu and his colleague investigate the CVD health of residents in three major metropolitan cities in China, namely, Beijing, Hong Kong and Shanghai [26]. About 84% of residents in Beijing, and 80% residents in both Hong Kong and Shanghai reported less than 90 minutes/week in leisure time physical activity (Table 2). The mean duration of leisure time physical activity was 18 minutes/week in Beijing, 54 minutes/week in Hong Kong, and 49 minutes/week in Shanghai (Table 3) [26]. In another population-based, case-control study in

Shanghai assessing the association between physical activity, particularly commuting physical activity, and its joint effects with body mass index on colon cancer risk used 48.3 and 94.3 metabolic equivalent (MET)-hours/week as the cutpoints for low, medium, and high levels of commuting physical activity [25]. Since the cutpoint for the lowest level of commuting physical activity (48.3 MET-hours/week) was equivalent to about 7 hours of general jogging or playing tennis per week, the level of active commuting in this study population was relatively high.

Table 2. Number and percentage of subjects participating in leisure time physical activity per week in three cities, China [26]

City	Male (%)	Female (%)	Total (%)
Beijing			
≥90 minutes	41 (17)	25 (14)	66 (16)
<90 minutes	194 (83)	150 (86)	344 (84)
Hong Kong			
≥90 minutes	88 (23)	81 (17)	169 (20)
<90 minutes	292 (77)	385 (83)	677 (80)
Shanghai			
≥90 minutes	88 (19)	95 (20)	183 (20)
<90 minutes	374 (81)	383 (80)	757 (80)

Table 3. Mean values (SD) of leisure time physical activity (minutes/week) among subjects from three cities, China [26]

City	Male	Female	Total
Beijing	19 (34)	16 (32)	18 (33)
Hong Kong	68 (115)	43 (76)	54 (97)
Shanghai	50 (109)	49 (106)	49 (108)
Total	50 (102)	41 (87)	45 (94)

In 2000, one study also assessed the levels of sedentary lifestyle and leisure time physical activity among 4739 urban adults in Shanghai [27]. A total of 58% of the adults reported their sitting time at work/school or at home more than 5 hours per day, of them 34% reported their sedentary time more than 7 hours per day. About 65% of the adults participated in leisure time physical activity and 21% met the recommendation level from CDC and ACSM [1].

Kim and his colleagues compared lifestyle index, integrating diet, physical activity, smoking, and alcohol use between China and the US using the 1993 China Health and Nutrition Survey (N=8352) and the 1994–1996 US Continuing Survey of Food Intakes by Individuals (N=9750) [28]. In China, people were categorized into five levels of physical activity based mainly on work activity. The levels of work activity were grouped into very active, active, moderate, light, and sedentary. In the US, the frequency of vigorous exercise was categorized into five groups: daily or five to six times per week as 'very active', two to four times per week as 'active', once per week as 'moderate', one to three times per month as 'light', and rarely or never as 'sedentary'. The physical activity index showed a wide range of scores with great variation among the populations. The prevalences of people engaged in very active, active, moderate, light and sedentary levels of activity were 0.8%, 51.6%, 18.2%, 17.1%, and 12.4% in Chinese, and 26.7%, 21.4%, 7.4%, 5.2%, and 39.3% in Americans, respectively [28].

In 1997 the China Health and Nutrition Survey described physical activity and inactivity levels among Chinese school children aged 6-18 years [29]. Approximately 84% of Chinese youth actively commute to school for a median of 100-150 minutes/week. A total of 72% of Chinese youth engage in moderate/vigorous physical activity for a median of 90-110 minutes/week at school. Relatively few children (about 8%) participate in any moderate/vigorous physical activity outside school. A total of 72% of children engage in study-related activities outside school for a median of 420 minutes/week. Only 8% of Chinese school children, regardless of gender, watch television ≥2 hours/day; less than 1% watch ≥4 hours/day [29].

ASSOCIATIONS BETWEEN PHYSICAL ACTIVITY AND SELECTED HEALTH CHARACTERISTICS

In Tianjin Project [24], we also examined the association between physical activity and demographic and health-related characteristics among the urban population. Persons aged 35-49 years were less likely to participate in leisure time physical activity than those aged 15-34 years (Table 4). On the other hand, women aged 50-69 years were more likely than women aged 15-34 years to participate in such activity. Highly educated people, persons with high incomes, white-collar workers, and married people were significantly more likely to participate in leisure time physical activity than people in the reference group. Non-smokers, and persons going to and from work on foot or by bicycle were much more likely to engage in leisure time physical activity than smokers or people who went to and from work by bus [24].

Men aged 50-69 years were more likely to perform over 30 minutes of commuting physical activity on foot or by bicycle than males aged 15-34 years (Table 5). Persons with comparatively low incomes or who were married were significantly more likely to engage in commuting physical activity lasting 30 minutes or more than those who had higher incomes or were unmarried. Male blue-collar workers were more likely to perform over 30 min of commuting physical activity than male white-collar workers [24].

In the Shanghai survey assessing the levels of sedentary lifestyle and leisure time exercise, Gu and his colleagues found that adults with elder ages, with high level of education, and with high level of body mass index were significantly more likely to participate in leisure time exercise than adults with younger ages, with lower level of education, and with more normal body weight. Employed adults were less likely to participate in leisure time exercise than un-employed ones [27].

Table 4. Adjusted odds ratios (95% confidence interval) for leisure time physical activity by selected characteristics of male and female study subjects aged 15-69 years, Tianjin, China*[24]

Characteristic	Males	Females
Age (years)		
15-34	1.00	1.00
35-49	0.67 (0.51-0.88)	0.68 (0.52-0.90)
50-69	1.07 (0.79-1.45)	1.62 (1.13-2.31)
P value for trend	<0.001	<0.001
Education (years)		
0-6	1.00	1.00
7-12	1.03 (0.78-1.39)	1.30 (1.01-1.64)
>12	1.77 (1.23-2.54)	2.15 (1.48-3.12)
P value for trend	<0.001	<0.001
Income (yuan)†		
<300	1.00	1.00
300-500	1.52 (1.20-1.92)	1.48 (1.17-1.88)
>500	2.01 (1.53-2.63)	2.32 (1.76-3.06)
P value for trend	<0.001	<0.001
Married (yes versus no)	2.45 (1.86-3.23)	2.48 (1.92-3.20)
Occupation (blue-collar versus white-collar)‡	0.65 (0.48-0.87)	0.52 (0.38-0.73)
Current smoker (yes versus no)	0.66 (0.53-0.81)	0.62 (0.42-0.89)
Commuting physical activity (minutes/day)		
0	1.00	1.00
1-30	2.52 (1.67-3.81)	1.39 (0.76-2.53)
31-60	3.06 (2.00-4.69)	1.62 (0.88-2.96)
>60	3.14 (1.94-5.07)	2.08 (1.05-4.10)
P value for trend	<0.001	<0.001

*Association between personal characteristics and physical activity adjusted by age and three other socio-economic indicators, and association between smoking and physical activity adjusted by age, education, income, marital status and occupation.
†US $ 1 = 8.3 yuan.
‡Including only working subjects.

Table 5. Adjusted odds ratios (95% confidence interval) for more than 30 minutes of commuting physical activity by selected characteristics of male and female study subjects aged 15-69 years, Tianjin, China*[24]

Characteristic	Males	Females
Age (years)		
15-34	1.00	1.00
35-49	1.09 (0.84-1.41)	0.91 (0.71-1.16)
50-69	1.78 (1.34-2.37)	1.23 (0.88-1.71)
P value for trend	<0.001	NS†
Education (years)		
0-6	1.00	1.00
7-12	1.03 (0.75-1.14)	1.00 (0.73-1.39)
>12	0.94 (0.63-1.40)	1.29 (0.83-2.00)
P value for trend	NS	NS

Table 5 Continued

Characteristic	Males	Females
Income (yuan)‡		
<300	1.00	1.00
300-500	0.91 (0.73-1.14)	0.77 (0.63-0.96)
>500	0.74 (0.57-0.96)	0.78 (0.60-1.00)
P value for trend	<0.05	<0.05
Married (yes versus no)	2.45 (1.86-3.23)	2.48 (1.92-3.20)
Occupation (blue-collar versus white-collar)§	1.47 (1.09-1.98)	0.93 (0.69-1.26)
Current smoker (yes versus no)	0.96 (0.78-1.18)	0.92 (0.67-1.26)

*Association between personal characteristics and physical activity adjusted by age and three other socio-economic indicators, and association between smoking and physical activity adjusted by age, education, income, marital status and occupation.

†NS, not significant.

‡US $ 1 = 8.3 yuan.

§Including only working subjects.

PHYSICAL ACTIVITY AND CARDIOVASCULAR RISK FACTORS

Physical Activity and Cardiovascular Risk Factors in Tianjin Project

Time spent on commuting, leisure time, or commuting plus leisure time physical activity daily was inversely related to body mass index (P <0.05 for trends) and positively related to systolic blood pressure (P <0.05 for trends) among men in urban Tianjin in 1996 (Table 6) [30]. Duration of daily commuting physical activity was inversely associated with body mass index among women (P <0.05 for trend). The lowest mean values of systolic and diastolic blood pressure occurred in women reporting 31-60 minutes of commuting, or commuting plus leisure time physical activity daily. The highest mean values of systolic and diastolic blood pressure were seen in those having more than 60 minutes of these activities daily (P <0.01 for trend).

Table 7 shows the associations between physical activity and prevalences of overweight, hypertension, and smoking in both genders in urban Tianjin [30]. After adjustment for age, education, smoking, alcohol consumption, body mass index and occupational physical activity, the duration of commuting, leisure time, or combined commuting and leisure time physical activity in men was inversely associated with prevalence of overweight. The lowest prevalence of hypertension was seen in both genders who spent 31-60 minutes of commuting or commuting combined with leisure time physical activity, and the highest prevalence of hypertension was shown in those who did more than 60 minutes of the above-mentioned activity as compared to the reference group (P <0.05 for trend). Time spent on leisure time physical activity was positively associated with the prevalence of hypertension among men (P <0.05 for trend). The prevalence of smoking was consistently and inversely related to physical activity among both genders, although the commuting physical activity group did not reach statistical significance.

Table 6. Comparison of the adjusted mean (SE) of cardiovascular risk factors by physical activity (minutes/day) of male and female aged 15-69 years, Tianjin, China†[30]

	Men			Women		
	BMI (kg/m^2)	DBP (mm Hg)	SBP (mm Hg)	BMI (kg/m^2)	DBP (mm Hg)	SBP (mm Hg)
Commuting on foot or by bicycle						
0	23.8 (0.2)	81.2 (0.7)	124.0 (1.1)	23.5 (0.3)	79.0 (1.2)	122.9 (1.1)
1-30	23.0 (0.1)‡**	81.5 (0.3)	126.2 (0.5)‡**	23.2 (0.1)	79.0 (0.3)	122.7 (0.5)
31-60	23.3 (0.1)‡*	81.3 (0.4)	126.2 (0.7)	23.5 (0.1)	78.6 (0.4)	121.0 (0.6)
>60	23.2 (0.2)‡*	82.5 (0.6)	128.2 (1.0)‡**	22.6 (0.3)§**	82.0 (0.6)§**	125.2 (1.4)§*
P value for trend	*	NS	*	*	**	
Leisure time physical activity						
0	23.4 (0.1)	81.2 (0.3)	125.7 (0.4)	23.3 (0.1)	78.9 (0.3)	122.0 (0.5)
1-30	23.2 (0.1)	81.8 (0.4)	126.8 (0.7)	23.3 (0.2)	79.1 (0.5)	122.3 (0.8)
>30	22.7 (0.2)‡‖**	82.6 (0.7)‡*	127.7 (1.5)‡**	23.3 (0.3)	80.4 (0.8)	123.7 (1.3)
P value for trend	*	NS	NS	NS	NS	NS
Commuting plus leisure time physical activity						
0	23.9 (0.3)	81.3 (0.8)	124.4 (1.2)	23.4 (0.3)	79.6 (0.7)	122.6 (1.3)
1-30	23.1 (0.1)‡*	81.3 (0.3)	126.3 (0.5)	23.2 (0.1)	79.0 (0.3)	122.5 (0.6)
31-60	23.2 (0.1)‡*	81.3 (0.4)	125.5 (0.6)	23.4 (0.1)	78.5 (0.4)	120.7 (0.7)
>60	23.1 (0.2)‡*	82.3 (0.4)	127.9 (1.0)‡§*	23.3 (0.2)	80.8 (0.4)§**	124.3 (0.9)§*
P value for trend	*	NS	*	NS	**	*

†Adjusted for age, education, smoking, alcohol consumption, BMI (except with BMI as dependent variable), and occupational activity; BMI, body mass index; DBP, diastolic blood pressure; SBP, systolic blood pressure.

‡Significantly different from the lowest activity.

§Significantly different between 31-60 minutes activity and >60 minutes activity.

‖ Significantly different between 1-30 minutes activity and >30 minutes activity.

P<0.05; **P<0.01; NS, not significant

In another cross-sectional survey of 1786 men and 1992 women carried out in 1989 in urban area of Tianjin, we also clarified the association between physical activity and serum lipids levels [31]. Men commuting to and from work on foot or by bike had lower mean values of total cholesterol (P <0.01 for trend), low-density lipoprotein cholesterol (P <0.001 for trend) and triglyceride levels (P < 0.05 for trend) compared with those traveling to work by bus (Table 8). Women commuting to and from work on foot or by bike had higher mean value of high-density lipoprotein cholesterol (P <0.05 for trend) compared with those commuting to and from work by bus. There were no substantial relationships between leisure time physical activity and serum lipids. Occupational physical activity had also been found to be inversely associated with the prevalence of overweight in both genders in urban Tianjin [32].

Table 7. Adjusted odd ratios (95% confidence interval) for the association between physical activity (minutes/day) and overweight, hypertension and smoking among male and female aged 15-69 years, Tianjin, China† [30]

	Men			Women		
	Overweight	Hypertension	Smoking	Overweight	Hypertension	Smoking
Commuting on foot or by bicycle						
0	1.00	1.00	1.00	1.00	1.00	1.00
1-30	0.70 (0.49-0.99)*	1.13 (0.76-1.71)	0.72 (0.51-1.04)	0.86 (0.50-1.48)	0.91 (0.47-1.73)	0.60 (0.29-1.21)
31-60	0.84 (0.58-1.22)	0.86 (0.56-1.32)	0.71 (0.49-1.04)	1.03 (0.60-1.80)	0.74 (0.38-1.42)	0.59 (0.28-1.20)
>60	0.88 (0.57-1.37)	1.61 (0.99-2.62)	0.68 (0.43-1.06)	0.80 (0.42-1.54)	1.59 (0.74-3.40)	0.58 (0.23-1.49)
P value for trend	NS	**	NS	NS	*	NS
Leisure time physical activity						
0	1.00	1.00	1.00	1.00	1.00	1.00
1-30	0.89 (0.70-1.13)	1.33 (1.03-1.72)*	0.62 (0.50-0.80)***	1.04 (0.61-1.81)	1.02 (0.74-1.41)	0.55 (0.35-0.87)*
>30	0.64 (0.45-0.91)*	1.57 (1.10-2.25)*	0.53 (0.39-0.74)***	1.10 (0.70-1.89)	1.14 (0.76-1.72)	0.62 (0.37-1.05)
P value for trend	*	*	***	NS	NS	*
Commuting plus leisure time physical activity						
0	1.00	1.00	1.00	1.00	1.00	1.00
1-30	0.71 (0.48-1.03)	1.22 (0.78-1.89)	0.89 (0.60-1.33)	0.91 (0.53-1.56)	1.02 (0.50-2.09)	0.51 (0.24-1.09)
31-60	0.73 (0.49-1.08)	0.83 (0.53-1.31)	0.71 (0.48-1.07)	1.07 (0.62-1.86)	0.79 (0.38-1.03)	0.40 (0.18-0.86)*
>60	0.65 (0.43-0.98)*	1.66 (1.05-2.62)*	0.62 (0.41-0.94)*	0.95 (0.56-1.70)	1.32 (0.63-2.79)	0.33 (0.15-0.75)**
P value for trend	*	*	*	NS	*	*

† Adjusted for age, education, smoking, alcohol consumption, body mass index (except with overweight as dependent variable), and occupational activity; overweight was defined as body mass index ≥25; hypertension was defined as diastolic blood pressure ≥90 mm Hg and/or systolic blood pressure ≥140 mm Hg, or using ant hypertensive drugs.

• P<0.05; **P<0.01; ***P<0.001; NS, not significant.

Table 8. Adjusted means of serum lipids (mmol/l) by commuting and leisure time physical activity of male and female aged 20-49 years, Tianjin, China† [31]

	Total cholesterol		HDL cholesterol‡		LDL cholesterol‡		Triglycerides§	
	Men	Women	Men	Women	Men	Women	Men	Women
Commuting to and from work								
By bus	4.50	4.22	1.26	1.36	2.84	2.47	1.50	1.11
By foot <30 minutes or by bicycle <15 minutes	4.26 ‖**	4.19	1.25	1.37	2.62***	2.44	1.33*	1.05
By foot ≥30 minutes or by bicycle 15-60 minutes	4.25***	4.20	1.28	1.41*	2.59***	2.42	1.30*	1.07
By bicycle >60 minutes	4.33*	4.18	1.30	1.39	2.65**	2.42	1.31*	1.03
P value for trend	**	NS	NS	*	***	NS	*	NS
Leisure time physical activity								
<1 time or no/week	4.29	4.21	1.27	1.39	2.63	2.43	1.32	1.07
1-2 times/week	4.37	4.22	1.32	1.39	2.65	2.45	1.37	1.08
>2 times/week	4.26	4.09	1.26	1.33	2.61	2.40	1.28	1.00
P value for trend	NS	NS	NS	NS	NS	NS	NS	NS

†Adjusted for age, education, smoking, body mass index, and occupational activity.

‡HDL cholesterol, high-density lipoprotein cholesterol; LDL cholesterol, low-density lipoprotein cholesterol.

§Logarithmically transformed value was used in the analyses.

‖ Significantly different from going to and from work by bus.

*P<0.05; **P<0.01; ***P<0.001; NS, not significant.

Physical Activity and Cardiovascular Risk Factors in Other Studies in China

An early Chinese study evaluated the association between leisure time physical activity and CVD risk factors among 1,206 subjects in rural Shanghai [33]. It found that physical activity was inversely associated with hypertension, total cholesterol, body mass index and heart rate in men, and hypertension, blood pressure, body mass index and heart rate in women. High-density lipoprotein cholesterol and current smoking were not related to physical activity [33].

Another Chinese study investigated the relationship between different types and levels of physical activity (including occupational, leisure time, household and total physical activity) and CVD risk factors, including oxidative stress, blood lipids and insulin resistance, in a healthy female population in China [34]. The adjusted mean values of total cholesterol and apolipoprotein B were the lowest, whereas apolipoprotein A was the highest, in the moderate group of total physical activity. The serum apolipoprotein B level was higher in the low physical activity group during total, occupation, leisure time, and household. Triglycerides concentration was the highest in the low physical activity during total, occupation, and household [34].

Changes in Physical Activity and Changes in Body Mass Index

The China Health and Nutrition Survey assessed 8 year weight change between 1989 and 1997 in Chinese adults, and also determined the baseline characteristics of those who gained weight [35]. Overweight (body mass index ≥ 25 kg/m^2) doubled in females (10.5 % in 1989 and 20.7% in 1997) and almost tripled in males (5.0% in 1989 and 14.1% in 1997). Low physical activity at work was a strong predictor of weight gain. Compared to those whose weight remained stable (±2 kg/8 years), males and females who experienced greater weight gain (>5 kg/8 years) were 3 and 1.8 times more likely to engage in light rather than heavy work-related physical activity [35]. Moreover, they also found that 14% of households owned a motorized vehicle between 1989 and 1997. Compared with those without motorized vehicle, men who owned a vehicle experienced a 1.8-kg greater weight gain (p < 0.05) and had 2 to 1 odds of becoming obese [36].

Physical Activity and Mortality

Using a case-control study of 24079 dead cases and 13054 live controls, Lam and colleagues examined the relationship between leisure time physical activity and all-cause and cause-specific mortality in Hong Kong [37]. After adjustment for age, education, smoking status, alcohol consumption, and physical demand at work, leisure time physical activity had a strong, independent, and inverse association with total, cancer, respiratory, cardiovascular and other cause deaths (Table 9) [37].

Table 9. Adjusted odds ratios (95% confidence interval) for major categories of death by leisure time physical activity level in Hong Kong* [37]

Causes of death	Odds ratio (95% confidence interval)					
	Male			Female		
	<1 episode/ month	1 episode/month to 1-3 episodes/ week	≥4 episodes/week	<1 episode/ month	1 episode/month to 1-3 episodes/ week	≥4 episodes/week
All causes	1.00	0.60 (0.54-0.67)	0.66 (0.60-0.73)	1.00	0.81 (0.74-0.88)	0.71 (0.66-0.77)
Malignant neoplasms	1.00	0.62 (0.55-0.71)	0.75 (0.67-0.84)	1.00	0.76 (0.68-0.86)	0.79 (0.71-0.87)
Respiratory	1.00	0.48 (0.41-0.57)	0.54 (0.47-0.62)	1.00	0.61 (0.50-0.75)	0.55 (0.47-0.65)
Cardio-vascular	1.00	0.65 (0.56-0.75)	0.67 (0.60-0.76)	1.00	0.89 (0.78-1.03)	0.71 (0.63-0.80)
Others†	1.00	0.60 (0.51-0.71)	0.59 (0.51-0.69)	1.00	0.86 (0.74-1.01)	0.69 (0.60-0.79)

*Model adjusted for age, education level, smoking status, alcohol consumption and physical demand at work.
†Causes of death other than malignant neoplasms, respiratory, or cardiovascular.

Another population-based, case-control study in Shanghai assessed the effect of various physical activities on colon cancer risk [25]. Colon cancer risk generally declined with increasing levels of each type of physical activity, including occupational, leisure time, and commuting physical activities, in both men and women (Table 10). After adjusting the three physical activity variables for each other, age, education, family income, marital status, total energy intake, intake of red meat, carotene, and fiber, these trends remained significant only for commuting physical activity in both men (p <0.001) and women (p =0.007), and among women also for occupational physical activity (p =0.009) [25].

Table 10. Gender-specific risk of colon cancer by levels of lifetime commuting, occupational, and leisure physical activity, Shanghai, China [25]

Physical activity	Odds ratio (95% confidence interval)*			Odds ratio (95% confidence interval)†			P for trend‡
	Low physical activity	Medium physical activity	High physical activity	Low physical activity	Medium physical activity	High physical activity	
Men							
Occupational physical activity§	1.00	1.19 (0.90-1.59)	0.77 (0.55-1.15)	1.00	1.23 (0.93-1.64)	0.81 (0.59-1.19)	0.10
Leisure time physical activity§	1.00	0.97 (0.65-1.45)	0.64 (0.57-0.97)	1.00	1.17 (0.13-1.95)	0.72 (0.41-1.07)	0.06
Commuting physical activity§	1.00	0.98 (0.34-1.24)	0.56 (0.32-0.91)	1.00	1.11 (0.31-1.23)	0.52 (0.27-0.87)	<0.001
Women							
Occupational physical activity§	1.00	0.93 (0.68-1.13)	0.52 (0.32-0.91)	1.00	0.96 (0.69-1.16)	0.64 (0.39-1.02)	0.009
Leisure time physical activity§	1.00	0.97 (0.62-1.62)	0.79 (0.54-1.34)	1.00	1.03 (0.41-1.59)	0.84 (0.13-2.25)	0.15
Commuting physical activity§	1.00	0.92 (0.51-1.57)	0.58 (0.24-0.94)	1.00	0.87 (0.42-1.52)	0.56 (0.21-0.91)	0.007

*Adjusted for age, education, family income, marital status, total energy intake, intake of red meat, carotene, and fiber for both men and women and additionally for number of pregnancies and menopausal status for women.

†In addition to the adjustment for the variables mentioned in footnote*, adjusted also for the other two physical activity variables.

‡P for trend from the odds ratio described in the *footnote.

§The corresponding cutpoints for low, medium, and high levels of commuting physical activity were <48.3, 48.3–94.3, and >94.3 metabolic equivalent (MET)-hours/week; those for leisure time physical activity were <9.2, 9.2–13.6, and >13.6 MET-hours/week. The cutpoints for occupational physical activity measured by lifetime average energy expenditure were low (<8 kJ/minute), moderate (8–12 kJ/minute), and high (>12 kJ/minute).

Matthews and his colleagues also evaluated the effects of overall physical activity in adolescence and adulthood, and changes in activity over the lifespan on the risk of breast cancer in a case-control study of 1459 women newly diagnosed with breast cancer and 1556 age-matched controls in urban Shanghai [38]. Physical activity from leisure time exercise and sports, household, and transportation (walking and cycling) was assessed in adolescence (13-19 years) and adulthood (last 10 years), as was lifetime occupational activity. Leisure time exercise and sports in adolescence, in adulthood, and changes in exercise behaviour between adolescence and adulthood were separately associated with a decreased risk of breast cancer. Lifetime occupational activity was also inversely related to the risk of breast cancer. There was no significant evidence for a beneficial effect of household activity, and walking or cycling during commuting activity [38].

From the mid-1980s, Chinese economy experienced a strong growth with an average 8.3% increase in the gross national product per capita. At the same time, CVD became the leading cause of death, especially in urban areas. Following the rapid economic development in the last two decades, Chinese people have gradually changed and will further change their life habits in the present decade. The dietary pattern of high energy, high fat, high cholesterol and low carbohydrate, and decreased occupational and commuting physical activity and low leisure time physical activity have been observed and will be seen in Chinese populations [16, 17, 23]. Cardiovascular risk factors, such as overweight, obesity, hypertension, lipid abnormalities, diabetes and the metabolic syndrome will also most probably increase. Epidemiological evidence has shown that regular physical activity is one of medical benefits for cardiovascular health and quality of life [1, 4-6, 39, 40]. Regular physical activity is an important component of health lifestyle for all of us. Public health messages, health care professionals, and health care system should aggressively promote physical activity during occupation, commuting, and leisure time.

REFERENCES

[1]   Pate R. R., Pratt, M., Blair, S. N., Haskell, W. L., Macera, C. A., Bouchard, C., Buchner, D., Ettinger, W., Heath, G. W., King, A. C., Kiska, A., Leon, A. S., Marcus, B. H., Morris, J., Paffenbarger, R. S., Patrick, K., Pollock, M. L., Rippe, J. M., Sallis, J. and Wilmore, J. H. (1995). Physical activity and public health. A recommendation from the Centers for Disease Control and Prevention and the American College of Sports Medicine. *Jama*, 273, 402-407.

[2]   Lakka T. A., Venalainen, J. M., Rauramaa, R., Salonen, R., Tuomilehto, J. and Salonen, J. T. (1994). Relation of leisure-time physical activity and cardiorespiratory fitness to the risk of acute myocardial infarction. *N Engl J Med*, 330, 1549-1554.

[3]   Manson J. E., Hu, F. B., Rich-Edwards, J. W., Colditz, G. A., Stampfer, M. J., Willett, W. C., Speizer, F. E. and Hennekens, C. H. (1999). A prospective study of walking as compared with vigorous exercise in the prevention of coronary heart disease in women. *N Engl J Med*, 341, 650-658.

[4]   Blair S. N., Cheng, Y. and Holder, J. S. (2001). Is physical activity or physical fitness more important in defining health benefits? *Med Sci Sports Exerc*, 33, S379-399.

[5]   Wannamethee S. G. and Shaper, A. G. (2001). Physical activity in the prevention of cardiovascular disease: an epidemiological perspective. *Sports Med*, 31, 101-114.

[6]   Dubbert P. M., Carithers, T., Sumner, A. E., Barbour, K. A., Clark, B. L., Hall, J. E. and Crook, E. D. (2002). Obesity, physical inactivity, and risk for cardiovascular disease. *Am J Med Sci*, 324, 116-126.

[7]   Laaksonen D. E., Lakka, H. M., Salonen, J. T., Niskanen, L. K., Rauramaa, R. and Lakka, T. A. (2002). Low levels of leisure-time physical activity and cardiorespiratory fitness predict development of the metabolic syndrome. *Diabetes Care*, 25, 1612-1618.

[8] Tanasescu M., Leitzmann, M. F., Rimm, E. B., Willett, W. C., Stampfer, M. J. and Hu, F. B. (2002). Exercise type and intensity in relation to coronary heart disease in men. *Jama*, 288, 1994-2000.

[9] Hu G., Qiao, Q., Silventoinen, K., Eriksson, J. G., Jousilahti, P., Lindstrom, J., Valle, T. T., Nissinen, A. and Tuomilehto, J. (2003). Occupational, commuting, and leisure-time physical activity in relation to risk for type 2 diabetes in middle-aged Finnish men and women. *Diabetologia*, 46, 322-329.

[10] Barengo N. C., Hu, G., Lakka, T. A., Pekkarinen, H., Nissinen, A. and Tuomilehto, J. (2004). Low physical activity as a predictor for total and cardiovascular disease mortality in middle-aged men and women in Finland. *Eur Heart J*, 25, 2204-2211.

[11] Hu G., Barengo, N. C., Tuomilehto, J., Lakka, T. A., Nissinen, A. and Jousilahti, P. (2004). Relationship of Physical Activity and Body Mass Index to the Risk of Hypertension: A Prospective Study in Finland. *Hypertension*, 43, 25-30.

[12] Hu G., Lindstrom, J., Valle, T. T., Eriksson, J. G., Jousilahti, P., Silventoinen, K., Qiao, Q. and Tuomilehto, J. (2004). Physical activity, body mass index, and risk of type 2 diabetes in patients with normal or impaired glucose regulation. *Arch Intern Med*, 164, 892-896.

[13] Hu G., Tuomilehto, J., Silventoinen, K., Barengo, N. and Jousilahti, P. (2004). Joint effects of physical activity, body mass index, waist circumference and waist-to-hip ratio with the risk of cardiovascular disease among middle-aged Finnish men and women. *Eur Heart J*, 25, 2212-2219.

[14] Barengo N. C., Hu, G., Kastarinen, M., Lakka, T. A., Pekkarinen, H., Nissinen, A. and Tuomilehto, J. (2005). Low physical activity as a predictor for antihypertensive drug treatment in 25-64-year-old populations in Eastern and south-western Finland. *J Hypertens*, 23, 293-299.

[15] NIH Consensus Development Panel on Physical Activity and Cardiovascular Health. (1996). Physical activity and cardiovascular health. NIH Consensus Development Panel on Physical Activity and Cardiovascular Health. *Jama*, 276, 241-246.

[16] Popkin B. M., Keyou, G., Zhai, F., Guo, X., Ma, H. and Zohoori, N. (1993). The nutrition transition in China: a cross-sectional analysis. *Eur J Clin Nutr*, 47, 333-346.

[17] Paeratakul S., Popkin, B. M., Keyou, G., Adair, L. S. and Stevens, J. (1998). Changes in diet and physical activity affect the body mass index of Chinese adults. *Int J Obes Relat Metab Disord*, 22, 424-431.

[18] Murray C. J. and Lopez, A. D. (1997). Mortality by cause for eight regions of the world: Global Burden of Disease Study. *Lancet*, 349, 1269-1276.

[19] Cheng T. O. (2005). A preventable epidemic of coronary heart disease in modern China. *Eur J Cardiovasc Prev Rehabil*, 12, 1-4.

[20] Yu Z., Nissinen, A., Vartiainen, E., Song, G., Guo, Z. and Tian, H. (2000). Changes in cardiovascular risk factors in different socioeconomic groups: seven year trends in a Chinese urban population. *J Epidemiol Community Health*, 54, 692-696.

[21] Qiao Q., Hu, G., Tuomilehto, J., Borch-Johnsen, K., Ramachandran, A., Mohan, V., Iyer, S. R., Tominaga, M., Kiyohara, Y., Kato, I., Okubo, K., Nagai, M., Shibazaki, S., Yang, Z., Tong, Z., Fan, Q., Wang, B., Chew, S. K., Tan, B. Y., Heng, D., Emmanuel, S., Tajima, N., Iwamoto, Y., Snehalatha, C., Vijay, V., Kapur, A., Dong, Y., Nan, H., Gao, W., Shi, H. and Fu, F. (2003). Age- and sex-specific prevalence of diabetes and impaired glucose regulation in 11 Asian cohorts. *Diabetes Care*, 26, 1770-1780.

[22] Jia W. P., Xiang, K. S., Chen, L., Lu, J. X., Bao, Y. Q., Wu, Y. M. and Jiang, S. Y. (2004). A comparison of the application of two working definitions of metabolic syndrome in Chinese population. *Zhonghua Yi Xue Za Zhi*, 84, 534-538.

[23] Ministry of Public Health, *Nutrition and health status among Chinese: result from the Fourth China Nutrition and Health Survey*, Beijing, 2004.

[24] Hu G., Pekkarinen, H., Hanninen, O., Yu, Z., Huiguang, T., Zeyu, G. and Nissinen, A. (2002). Physical activity during leisure and commuting in Tianjin, China. *Bull World Health Organ*, 80, 933-938.

[25] Hou L., Ji, B. T., Blair, A., Dai, Q., Gao, Y. T. and Chow, W. H. (2004). Commuting physical activity and risk of colon cancer in Shanghai, China. *Am J Epidemiol*, 160, 860-867.

[26] Fu F. H. and Fung, L. (2004). The cardiovascular health of residents in selected metropolitan cities in China. *Prev Med*, 38, 458-467.

[27] Gu K., Shen, X. Z., Sun, J. M., Lin, J., Li, X. J., Li, D. L. and Wang, Z. G. (2002). Physical activity in Shanghai. *Sh J Pre Med*, 14, 444-446 (Chinese).

[28] Kim S., Popkin, B. M., Siega-Riz, A. M., Haines, P. S. and Arab, L. (2004). A cross-national comparison of lifestyle between China and the United States, using a comprehensive cross-national measurement tool of the healthfulness of lifestyles: the Lifestyle Index. *Prev Med*, 38, 160-171.

[29] Tudor-Locke C., Ainsworth, B. E., Adair, L. S., Du, S. and Popkin, B. M. (2003). Physical activity and inactivity in Chinese school-aged youth: the China Health and Nutrition Survey. *Int J Obes Relat Metab Disord*, 27, 1093-1099.

[30] Hu G., Pekkarinen, H., Hanninen, O., Yu, Z., Guo, Z. and Tian, H. (2002). Commuting, leisure-time physical activity, and cardiovascular risk factors in China. *Med Sci Sports Exerc*, 34, 234-238.

[31] Hu G., Pekkarinen, H., Hanninen, O., Tian, H. and Guo, Z. (2001). Relation between commuting, leisure time physical activity and serum lipids in a Chinese urban population. *Ann Hum Biol*, 28, 412-421.

[32] Hu G., Pekkarinen, H., Hanninen, O., Tian, H. and Jin, R. (2002). Comparison of dietary and non-dietary risk factors in overweight and normal-weight Chinese adults. *Br J Nutr*, 88, 91-97.

[33] Hong Y., Bots, M. L., Pan, X., Wang, H., Jing, H., Hofman, A. and Chen, H. (1994). Physical activity and cardiovascular risk factors in rural Shanghai, China. *Int J Epidemiol*, 23, 1154-1158.

[34] Ma J., Liu, Z. and Ling, W. (2003). Physical activity, diet and cardiovascular disease risks in Chinese women. *Public Health Nutr*, 6, 139-146.

[35] Bell A. C., Ge, K. and Popkin, B. M. (2001). Weight gain and its predictors in Chinese adults. *Int J Obes Relat Metab Disord*, 25, 1079-1086.

[36] Bell A. C., Ge, K. and Popkin, B. M. (2002). The road to obesity or the path to prevention: motorized transportation and obesity in China. *Obes Res*, 10, 277-283.

[37] Lam T. H., Ho, S. Y., Hedley, A. J., Mak, K. H. and Leung, G. M. (2004). Leisure time physical activity and mortality in Hong Kong: case-control study of all adult deaths in 1998. *Ann Epidemiol*, 14, 391-398.

[38] Matthews C. E., Shu, X. O., Jin, F., Dai, Q., Hebert, J. R., Ruan, Z. X., Gao, Y. T. and Zheng, W. (2001). Lifetime physical activity and breast cancer risk in the Shanghai Breast Cancer Study. *Br J Cancer*, 84, 994-1001.

[39] Erlichman J., Kerbey, A. L. and James, W. P. (2002). Physical activity and its impact on health outcomes. Paper 1: The impact of physical activity on cardiovascular disease and all-cause mortality: an historical perspective. *Obes Rev*, 3, 257-271.

[40] Katzmarzyk P. T., Janssen, I. and Ardern, C. I. (2003). Physical inactivity, excess adiposity and premature mortality. *Obes Rev*, 4, 257-290.

In: Weight Loss, Exercise and Health Research
Editor: Carrie P. Saylor, pp. 195-212

ISBN 1-60021-077-5
© 2006 Nova Science Publishers, Inc.

Chapter 9

INTENSE EXERCISE STIMULATES BLOOD NEUTROPHIL DEGRANULATION IN HUMANS AND RATS

Vladimir I. Morozov[1] and Michael I. Kalinski

Department of Biochemistry, Research Institute of Physical Culture,
Dynamo Ave. 2, St. Petersburg 197110, Russia
Exercise Physiology Laboratory, School of Exercise,
Leisure and Sport, Kent State University, Kent, Ohio 44242-0001, USA.

ABSTRACT

Objective. Changes in the neutrophil degranulation process induced by physical exercise have not been studied sufficiently. It is not clear how degranulation affects other neutrophil functions. The purpose of this study was to examine the effects of intensive physical activity on human athletes and rat blood neutrophil degranulation by determining activities of myeloperoxidase (MPO) and lysozyme, to investigate an oxidative burst activity in parallel with the dynamics of blood neutrophil degranulation in trained human subjects, and to evaluate the possible associations between degranulation intensity and the athlete's individual work capacity. *Methods.* Treadmill running and rowing were exercises used in human study. Animal model of exercise used was swimming with weight added to the body mass. The rat myeloperoxidase (MPO), human lysozyme and corticosterone concentrations were determined by radioimmunoassais. Enzymatic lysozyme activity was measured by a turbidimetric assay with Micrococcus lysodeicticus. *Results.* Acute exercise stimulated neutrophil degranulation. Significant increases of myeloperoxidase (MPO) (+67%) and lysozyme (+51%) contents were found in rat blood plasma after swimming. Blood plasma lysozyme concentration increased by 41% during treadmill exercise in athletes. Blood concentrations of neutrophil proteins normalized both in humans and animals during first hours of rest. An increase in neutrophil protein concentrations in plasma was accompanied by a decrease of their level in neutrophils. This association was observed as well when enzyme lysozyme activity was determined in both blood plasma and leukocytes. A degree of neutrophil secretory

---

[1] Corresponding author:Vladimir Morozov, Fax: (7-812) 247-03-41, E-mail: sakuta@mail.cytspb.rssi.ru

reaction in athletes depended on the mode of physical load: it was higher when rowers performed rowing exercise as compared to treadmill running. Data suggest an influence of glucocorticoid in the observed activation of neutrophil secretion. The neutrophil capacity for an oxidative burst was not changed by exercise, but decreased for the first 3-6 h of the post-exercise period. This suggests a lack of association between the oxidative burst activity and the degranulation process. *Conclusion.* Intense exercise in human athletes and animals leads to activation of blood neutrophil secretory degranulation. There is no association between degranulation process and the neutrophil oxidative burst activity. As a result of degranulation there is neutrophil protein concentration increase in plasma and its decrease in neutrophils. The neutrophil proteins appeared in blood during degranulation can be involved in enhancement of bactericidal potency of blood, activation of granulopoeisis, neutrophil efflux from bone marrow, and conditioning of blood endothelium for leukocyte extravasation.

Key words: exercise, neutrophil, degranulation, oxidative burst

INTRODUCTION

Intensive exercise load induces several changes in blood leukocytes, specifically, in the white blood cell count and function (See reviews: Sharp and Kautedakis 1992; Nieman and Henson 1994; Smith 1995; Smith and Pyne 1997; Nieman and Pedersen 1999; Peake 2002).

Neutrophil functional changes during exercise have been of focus of interest to researchers for some time. Over the past several years, the effects of exercise on neutrophil phagocytic activity, including adherence, chemotaxis, attachment, ingestion and killing of foreign agents have been well described and scrutinized (Ortega 1994; Smith 1997; Smith and Pyne 1997; Nieman and Pedersen 1999). The studies indicate that the effect of exercise on phagocytosis depends on the stage of the phagocytic process, but quite different responses have been observed in the adherence and chemotaxis capacities, depending both on intensity of exercise and on the type of the phagocyte studied (neutrophil or monocyte-macrophage). Earlier we demonstrated that repetitive bouts of swimming to exhaustion in rats resulted in neutrophil phagocytosis suppression and also in tissue injury of skeletal muscle (Morozov et al. 1991; 2001). Much less is known about the effects of physical activity on secretory function and oxidative burst activity of neutrophils. However these functions are important to uncover the antimicrobial capacity of these cells. Activation of the secretory function of neutrophils results in their degranulation and the efflux of granule content outside of the cell or into phagosome. Recent studies have shown that intense physical exercise can induce the degranulation of neutrophils that leads to increase of plasma concentration of marker neutrophil enzymes (elastase and myeloperoxidase - MPO) (Camus et al. 1998; Gleeson et al. 1998; Walsh et al. 2000). Further, degranulation response of neutrophils to bacterial stimulation in vitro was shown to be decreased after exercise (Robson et al. 1999; Walsh et al. 2000; Bishop et al. 2003). However, studies of oxidative burst activity of neutrophils under exercise have produced equivocal results (Robson et al. 1999; Walsh et al. 2000). Moreover, neutrophil respiratory burst activity can depend both on exercise intensity (Peake 2002) and methodology (Suzuki et al. 1996). Moderate intensity exercise may enhance respiratory burst activity but intense or long duration exercise may suppress both neutrophil degranulation and respiratory burst. Neutrophil degranulation studies failed to answer how rapid is the process of activation of the neutrophil degranulation during exercise. In addition, the dynamics of the appearance/disappearance of neutrophil proteins in plasma has been poorly investigated and this dynamic remains to be elucidated. It is also presently unclear whether there is an association between the degranulation intensity and the athlete's individual work capacity. Thus, alterations of neutrophil degranulation process by physical exercise has been insufficiently studied. At the same time there is no clarity about how degranulation affects the other neutrophil functions. Taking into consideration that neutrophil granular proteins are of interest as an object of the subsequent investigations planned on animals, it is important to compare the process of neutrophil degranulation by physical exercises in human and animal studies. This will give an advantage in studying an involvement of these proteins in some metabolic events taking place after physical exercise.

The purpose of this study was twofold: (1) to examine the effects of intensive physical activity on rat blood neutrophil degranulation by determining activities of myeloperoxidase (MPO) (azurophilic granules) and lysozyme (azurophilic + specific granules); (2) to investigate an oxidative burst activity in parallel with the dynamics of blood neutrophil degranulation in athletic human subjects, and evaluate the possible associations between the degranulation intensity and the athlete's individual work capacity.

MATERIALS AND METHODS

Subjects. The male rowers were tested on a treadmill, model 24-72 (Quinton Instruments, USA), using a stepwise lead up to exhaustion and in a "rowing test". The velocity of treadmill running was increased from 6.9 km/h till 12.0 km/h. Treadmill inclination at the beginning of running was 2.5°, after 3 min it was increased to 5.0° and in the following 3 min - to 7.5°.

Male rowers, aged 19 +/- 2.0 years (means +/- S.D.), were enrolled in the "degranulation" study. They were members of national rowing teams. Different athletes participated in the next three experiments. Fifteen rowers were participants of treadmill running (experiment 1). Exercise-altered plasma lysozyme concentrations and associations between individual duration of running and plasma lysozyme were studied. The mean duration of the running was 17 +/- 1.1 min, the mean work of the running was 171351 +/- 22259 J (means +/- S.D.).

Thirteen athletes participated in the second treadmill running (experiment 2). Exercise-altered plasma lysozyme concentrations, enzyme lysozyme activity and neutrophil content of lysosomal cationic proteins were investigated in parallel.

Eight rowers took part in a "rowing test" (experiment 3). Four 2-seat kayak teams were involved in this experiment. The rate of neutrophil secretory function alteration in specific for rowers "rowing test" was studied to compare it to treadmill running effect. The rowing load was 5-km kayak-paddling rounds. The time of the rowing was similar to running time in experiment 1. Finger blood samples were drawn during exercise at the 6th and 9th min, immediately after exercise, and at different time of recovery (30, 60, and 120 min). The indices of neutrophil degranulation - lysozyme concentration in the blood plasma and granulocytes, were measured by a radioimmunoassay (Pryatkin et al. 1988). Neutrophil lysosomal cationic proteins were stained by fast green in blood smears and color intensity was evaluated microscopically (Mazing and Staroselskaya 1981). Lysozyme activity was measured by a turbidimetric assay with Micrococcus lysodeicticus (Parry et al. 1965).

Ten male rowers, aged 17 +/- 1.5 years (means +/- S.D.) were involved in "oxidative burst" study (experiment 4). The mean time of treadmill running was 13.4 +/- 1.3 min. Capillary blood samples were drawn from fingers and transferred into tubes containing heparin (100 Units/ml) before, immediately after running, and at 1, 3, and 6 h of recovery. To evaluate the chemiluminescence response, the samples of the heparinized whole blood (0.02 ml) were mixed with Hanks' balanced solution without phenol red (0.9 ml) containing luminol (Serva; 10^{-4} mol L^{-1}). This mixture was thermostated for 5 min at 37°C. To initiate the reaction, 0.1 ml of zymosan (10 mg ml-1 Hanks' solution) was added and chemiluminescence response recorded in dynamics as cpm x 103. Maximum of this dynamics was considered to be a chemiluminescence response. When analyzing these data, it was taken into consideration that chemiluminescence response depends practically completely on neutrophils (Chusid and Shea 1986; Prasad et al. 1990). The leukocyte count also was determined in the chemiluminescence experiments. Subject treatment was consistent with the policies accepted for human studies in the Russian Federation.

Animal study. Adult male albino rats (5 months old) weighing 200-250 g, were housed in an animal room under a 12-h light, 12-h dark cycle with food and water available ad libitum. The model of exercise used was repetitive bouts of swimming with the added 8 % of body mass at the tail (the 1-min-long exercise alternated with rest for 1.5 min) until exhaustion. The swimming tank measured 85 x 90 x 100 cm (height x width x length). The temperature of water was 30-32°C. The average total duration of the exercise was about 40 min. In experiments with measuring MPO and lysozyme the animals were sacrificed before (pre-exercise), immediately after exercise, and at different times (2, 4, 8, 12, 24, 48, 72, and 120 h) during the recovery period (N = 3 per each point). In other experiments blood samples were drawn from rat tails.

The neutrophil myeloperoxidase (MPO) activity was determined by a radioimmunoassay (Tsyplenkov et al. 1988). The rat MPO was isolated from intraperitoneal leukocytes (Morozov et al. 1997). Human lysozyme was purchased from Calbiochem (USA). Antisera to both proteins were produced in rabbits. AntiMPO IgG was purified by the procedure described by Jaton et al. (1979). This IgG was conjugated with Sepharose 4B to precipitate MPO from plasma and leukocyte preparations. To evaluate the amount of precipitated MPO, affinitive IgG isolated on MPO-Sepharose 4B column was used. For the radioimmunoassay, this IgG was labeled with ^{125}I, using the Iodogen procedure (Paus et al. 1982). For enzyme quantitation in rat and human neutrophils, these cells were isolated by the Ficoll procedure (Böyum, 1968). Contaminated erythrocytes were lysed by hypotonic shock. Neutrophils were collected, washed, and suspended in 0.15 M NaCl.

Cell preparations (about 90 percent neutrophils) were submitted to lysis (a 6-fold freezing-melting) and centrifuged to sediment cell debris. The supernatants were used for analysis of the enzymes.

To characterize phagocyte secretion activity we have used an index of lysozyme secretion (IS). IS was calculated as a ratio plasma / neutrophils lysozyme content following the formula: $IS = Lys_{plasma} \bullet (1 - Hct) / [Lys_{blood} - Lys_{plasma} \bullet (1 - Hct)]$, where Lys_{plasma} and Lys_{blood} are plasma and whole blood lysozyme concentrations in pg per 1 µl samples and Hct is hematocrit. Using this approach lysozyme content in lysozyme-containing blood cells (neutrophils + monocytes) can be evaluated after measuring lysozyme concentration in whole blood and plasma, Hct and relative content of (neutrophils + monocytes): Lys (pg per cell) =

$[Lys_{blood} - Lys_{plasma} \bullet (1 - Hct)] / L(N + M)$, where L – total white blood cell count, N – neutrophils, M – monocytes. When testing this calculation during the treadmill experiment lysozyme concentrations were determined to be 1.26 +/- 0.24 pg/cell before and 0.86 +/- 0.30 pg/cell after exercise (N = 3). Lysozyme concentrations measured in isolated neutrophils and monocytes of the same subject were similar: 1.21 +/- 0.39 (N) and 1.18 +/- 0.24 (M) pg/cell before and 1.12 +/- 0.42 (N) and 0.83 +/- 0.38 (M) pg/cell after exercise. Plasma lysozyme concentration is in proportion to lysozyme-containing cells count (Hansen, 1973) but IS does not depend on number of cells and can be applied as a simple and convenient index for blood phagocyte secretory activity evaluation.

The data obtained were presented as means +/- S.E.M. The statistical significance of the results was determined using Student's t-test and Signs Test (Conover 1971). A $P < 0.05$ was required for the results to be considered statistically significant. One-way regression analysis was used to investigate correlations of work capacity and lysozyme secretion. Correlation ratio η was calculated because of non-linear dependency of work capacity and lysozyme secretion.

All treatments adhered to the guidelines for the care and treatment of animals and were performed in compliance with the current laws of the Russian Federation.

RESULTS

Human Study

Lysozyme neutrophil secretion. Experiment 1. After the first 6 minutes of treadmill running the lysozyme content was significantly increased by 41% (p < 0.05) and remained elevated by 20% at the end of exercise session compared to the pre-exercise level in blood plasma of athletes (Fig. 1). That time the neutrophil lysozyme concentration decreased by 26% (p < 0.05). During the 2-h recovery period the plasma lysozyme concentration returned to the initial level whereas neutrophil lysozyme content increased, although it did not reach the pre-exercise value.

Significant correlations were revealed between the individual duration of running (T_{max}) and 1) the plasma lysozyme concentration for 6 min - L_{6min} ($y = 11.0 + 9.3x - 5.0x^2$; $\eta = 0.70$; $P < 0.05$), 2) ($L_6 - L_0$) ($y = 15.3 - 0.8x - 3.5x^2$; $\eta = 0.88$; $P < 0.01$) and 3) ($IS_6 - IS_0$); ($y = 14.84 - 0.28x - 0.05x^2$; $\eta = 0.95$; $P < 0.001$), where y is T_{max}, x is lysozyme concentration and IS is index of lysozyme secretion, η is a correlation ratio.

Experiment 2. Additional evidence of neutrophil secretory function stimulation by exercise were obtained during parallel determinations of concentration and enzyme lysozyme activity in human athletes blood plasma and blood neutrophil total content of lysosomal cationic proteins (Table 1). Exercise resulted in 46 % and 33 % raising of plasma lysozyme concentration and activity correspondingly, while neutrophil content of lysosomal cationic proteins decreased 6 % (p < 0.05). There was a strong association between concentration and enzyme activity of lysozyme (r = 0.74; p < 0.05) and between neutrophil lysozyme concentration and neutrophil content of lysosomal cationic proteins (r = 0.84; p < 0.05).

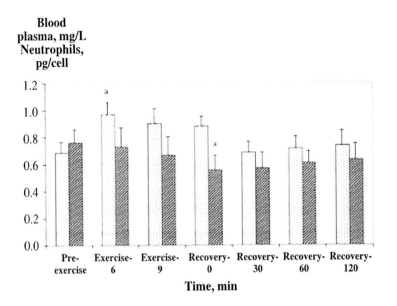

Fig. 1. Effects of treadmill running on lysozyme concentration in athletes blood plasma [image] and neutrophils [image] .N = 15; means +/- S.E.M.; a) P < 0.05; Signs Test. (With permission of Springer-Verlag).

Table 1.Effect of treadmill running to exhaustion on lysozyme efflux from blood phagocytes in athletes

Index	Before exercise	Post-exercise time, min			
		0	30	60	120
Plasma lysozyme concentration, mg/ml	1.11 +/- 0.08	1.62 +/- 0.12 [d]	1.40 +/- 0.1 [a]	1.18 +/- 0.24	1.27 +/- 0.14
Lysozyme activity, U/ml	4.8 +/- 0.4	6.4 +/- 0.5 [a]	5.6 +/- 0.5	5.2 +/- 0.5	4.7 +/- 0.9
Neutrophil lysosome cationic proteins	1.52 +/- 0.02	1.43 +/- 0.02 [c]	-	1.47 +/- 0.03	1.51 +/- 0.02

Means +/- S.E.M. N = 13. After exercise vs. before exercise: a) P < 0.05; c) P < 0.01; d) P < 0.001; t-Test. Neutrophil lysosome cationic proteins are presented in relative units.

Experiment 3. If rowers (N = 8; Sings test) executed specific load (5 km kayak-paddling) neutrophil secretion activity was higher as compared treadmill running. After rowing plasma lysozyme concentration was 52.6 % higher (p < 0.01) and its neutrophil content was 37.4 % lower (p < 0.05) compared to its pre-exercise level. At the 30 min of recovery period lysozyme concentration in plasma diminished but was 16.7 % higher the pre-exercise rate. Neutrophil lysozyme content changed poorly this time (-30.8 %). In 1 h there was the second 65.4 % increase of plasma lysozyme concentration (p < 0.01). Its neutrophil content grew but was still 15 % lower the pre-exercise rate. It is interesting that the neutrophil level increase in 1 h after the finish of rowing was remarkably higher (+221 %) when compared to treadmill running (+60 %). An important feature of rowing exercise was significant lysozyme concentration increase at 1 h of rest. Probably, this increase was connected with neutrophil mobilization from bone marrow to the blood that is evidenced as a 6-fold enhancement of young neutrophil forms and blood neutrophil lysozyme efflux intensification.

Oxidative burst. Neutrophil capability for oxidative burst was not changed in human athletes by physical activity, but decreased for the first 3-6 h thereafter (Table 2). The exercise led to an increase by 73% of the leukocyte number in blood. The 2nd leukocyte count increase was observed at three hours of recovery. The 1st peak was due to lymphocytes, the 2nd, to neutrophils. Chemiluminescence changed in parallel with the leukocyte/neutrophil count (r = 0.79/0.80; P < 0.05), while the correlation coefficients between the lymphocytes and chemiluminescence was only 0.55 (n.s.). This statistically significant correlation between the neutrophil count and blood chemiluminescence suggests that the neutrophils probably were the main components of the chemiluminescence response.

When the chemiluminescence intensity value was calculated per neutrophil, there were no changes immediately after the exercise and at the 1st h of recovery. However this value was reduced by 22% and 28% at the 3rd and 6th h of the post-exercise period, respectively (Table 2). Such dynamics of the neutrophil oxidative burst activity indicates no association of this activity with the degranulation process.

Table 2. Effect of treadmill running to exhaustion on chemiluminescence response of blood leukocytes in athletes

Index	Before exercise	Post – exercise time, hours			
		0	1	3	6
Leukocytes (x 10^{-6}/L)	5440±509 (100 %)	9405±748 [a] (173 %)	5110±406 (94 %)	8405±537 [a] (155 %)	7140±419 (131 %)
Lymphocytes (x 10^{-6}/L)	2254±211 (100 %)	5215±428 [a] (231 %)	1509±108 (67 %)	2988±367 (133 %)	2723±186 (121 %)
Neutrophils (x 10^{-6}/L)	2820±316 (100 %)	3685±386 (131 %)	3042±254 (108 %)	5227±428 [a] (185 %)	4021±312 [a] (143 %)
Chemiluminescence (cpm per sample)	66171 ± 6821 (100 %)	93057 [a] ± 9373 (141 %)	73479 ± 6225 (111 %)	105330 [a] ± 11369 (159 %)	69840 ± 7869 (106 %)
Chemiluminescence (cpm x 10^2/min per neutrophil)	122.70 ± 12.69 (100 %)	130.35 ± 10.40 (106 %)	121.76 ± 8.11 (100 %)	104.03 ± 10.55 (78 %)	87.35 [a] ± 7.48 (72 %)

Measurements were done in duplicates. Means +/– S.E.M. N = 10. After exercise vs. before exercise: a) P < 0.05; Signs Test.

Animal Study

Lysozyme and myeloperoxidase neutrophil secretion. Analysis of the neutrophil myeloperoxidase revealed that a significant elevation in the concentration of MPO (+67%) and lysozyme activity (+51%) in blood plasma of rat was observed after the rats swam to exhaustion (Fig. 2, A, B). After the swimming session the content of MPO in neutrophils and in lysozyme was decreased by 34% and 26% respectively. During recovery, concentrations of MPO and lysozyme returned relatively rapidly to basal values both in plasma and in neutrophils (Fig. 2, A, B).

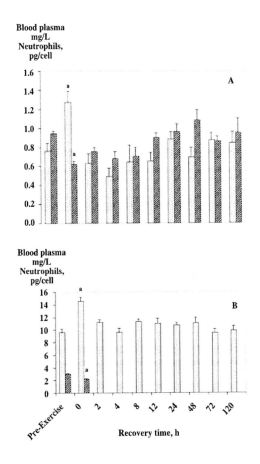

Fig. 2. Effects of swimming to exhaustion on myeloperoxidase (A) and lysozyme (B) concentrations in rat blood plasma [::::] and neutrophils [//////] . N = 3 (per point); means +/- S.E.M.; a) P < 0.05; b) P < 0.02; c) P < 0.01; d) P < 0.001; t-Test. (With permission of Springer-Verlag).

Secretion activation mechanism study. Treadmill running-induced blood cortisol alterations are presented on figure 3. At the moment of exercise completion hormone concentration was 77 % higher than it was before exercise. Thirty min later cortisol level reached its maximal value exceeded pre-exercise one by 85 %. There was a gradual decrease of cortisol concentration during next 1.5 h of recovery period but it remained 46 % higher than the pre-exercise level. Reliable association was found between cortisol and lysozyme concentrations during the first 6 min of exercise (r = 0.57; p < 0.05).

Considering the rapid exercise-stimulated cortisol enhancement into blood and the literature data on its involvement in count and function of leukocyte regulation, the animal study was closely reexamined to clarify the assumed glucocorticoid influence on neutrophil degranulation.

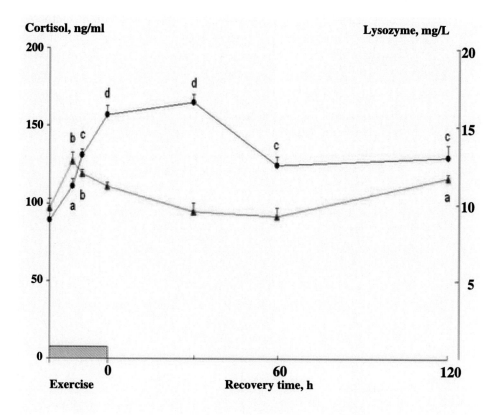

Fig. 3. Effects of treadmill running on cortisol (○) and lysozyme (●) concentrations in athlete blood plasma.N = 5; means +/- S.E.M.; a) P < 0.05; b) P < 0.02; c) P < 0.01; d) P < 0.001; t-Test.

Exercise-induced alterations of lysozyme activity, number of neutrophils and corticosterone concentration in blood are presented on figure 4. Under the influence of exercise, lysozyme activity increased by 51 %. During the first 4 h of the rest period lysozyme activity decreased to the basal rate but then it recovered again to 16-18 % during 8-48 h of rest. Then, lysozyme activity decreased and reached the basal level. Swimming-induced blood alterations of lysozyme activity, neutrophil count and corticosterone concentration are presented in figure 4. Exercise stimulated 2-phase leukocyte increase in blood (data are not shown). The 1st leukocyte peak observed immediately after exercise was mainly depended on lymphocytes. The 2nd peak found at 8-12 h of recovery consisted of neutrophils in the main. Maximum of blood neutrophil count (+ 81 %) was found at 8 h of the rest period (Fig. 4, A). Then neutrophil level gradually decreased and it was found 31-42 % lower than the pre-exercise rate after 3-5 days of recovery. Exercise resulted in 272 % increase of serum corticosterone concentration (Fig. 4, C). Then there was wave-like alterations of hormone rate and at 12 h it exceeded by 69 % the baseline.

Intramuscular corticosterone injection at the dose 1 mg per 100 g mass of animal resulted in 20 % lysozyme activity increase (p > 0.05) 30 min later (Fig. 5, B). Hormone injection was accompanied by neutrophil count decrease at the first 4 h and then it returned its resting level (Fig. 5, C).

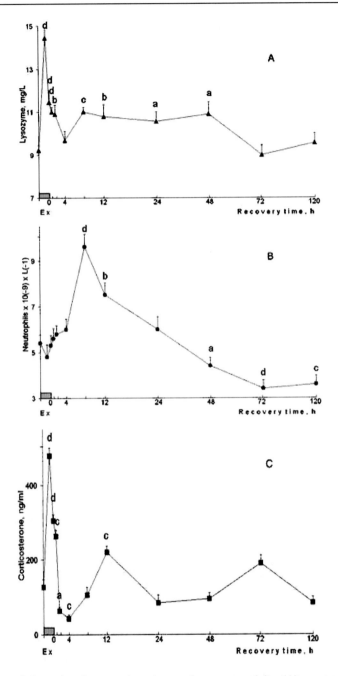

Fig. 4. The effect of the swimming to exhaustion on lysozyme activity (A), neutrophil count (B) and corticosterone concentration (C) in rat blood.N = 7; means +/- S.E.M.; a) P < 0.05; b) P < 0.02; c) P < 0.01; d) P < 0.001; t-Test.

When being delivered into defibrinated rat blood samples corticosterone stimulated increasing plasma lysozyme activity (Table 3). After 15 min of incubation with hormone plasma lysozyme activity was 15-22 % higher compared to control. The rate of activity increase was dependent on corticosterone concentration in samples. At 30 min of incubation enzyme secretion maximum was observed at minimal corticosterone concentration (+ 22 %). There was no significant differencies between samples at 1h.

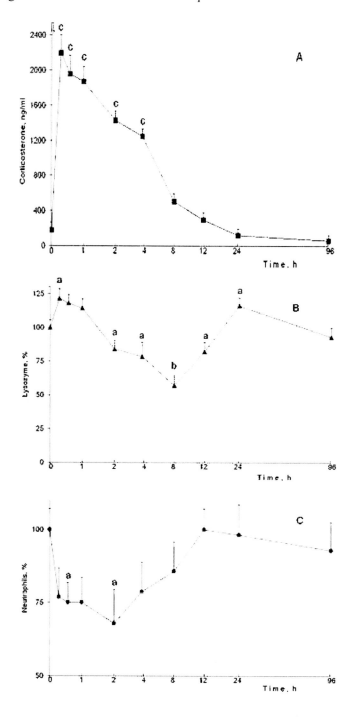

Fig. 5. The effect of intramuscular corticosterone injection on corticosterone concentration (A), lysozyme activity (B) and neutrophil count (C) in rat blood.N = 5; means +/- S.E.M.; a) P < 0.05; b) P < 0.01; c) P < 0.001; t-Test.

Table 3.Different corticosterone concentrations influence on lysozyme activity in blood plasma

Corticosterone concentration, μg/ml	Incubation time, min		
	15	30	60
0.125 (Control)	4.82 +/- 0.08	4.78 +/- 0.09	6.33 +/-0.09
0.45	5.54 +/- 0.06 [c]	6.33 +/- 0.06 [d]	6.62 +/- 0.07
0.90	5.69 +/- 0.08 [c]	5.56 +/ 0.05 [b]	6.70 +/- 0.08
2.00	5.89 +/- 0.09 [c]	5.54 +/- 0.07 [b]	5.91 +/- 0.10

Control - endogenous corticosterone concentration. Means +/- S.E.M. N = 5. b) $P < 0.02$; c) $P < 0.01$; d) $P < 0.001$; t-Test.

DISCUSSION

Exercise has been described to produce secretion of several neutrophil granule proteins in blood (Camus et al. 1998; Turton et al. 1998; Walsh et al. 2000; Morozov et al. 2003). These proteins are present either in individual types of granules (the specific granules that contain lactoferrin and elastase and the azurophilic granules that contain MPO) or in granules of both types (lysozyme). Blood monocytes also contain these proteins. Which of these cells are a basic source of the granule protein secretion induced by physical exercise remains unclear. Our present findings, as well as data from the literature (Jessup et al. 1985) suggest that monocyte involvement in leukocyte protein balance in plasma under exercise condition is insignificant. In the human study, we measured lysozyme concentration in blood neutrophils and monocytes as well as the ratio of these cells in the course of the experiment. The contents of lysozyme were similar in both types of the cells, amounting to 0.75 +/- 0.11 pg per neutrophil and to 0.81 +/- 0.19 pg per monocyte. The lysozyme content in monocytes decreased only 8 % after treadmill running. In our earlier experiments (unpublished data) we showed that the monocyte/neutrophil ratio was lower than 10% throughout the period of observation. Lysozyme balance calculated at the point "6 min" from the beginning of exercise has shown that observed lysozyme concentration in blood plasma for 0.3 μg/ml is in good compliance with its content decrease in neutrophils at the same time. In addition, the monocyte secretion activity is lower as compared to neutrophils (Jessup et al. 1985). Taken together, these data suggest that the neutrophils should be considered as the most predominant source of leukocyte granular proteins secreted to blood plasma during physical exercise.

Walsh et al. (2000) have shown that 2-h cycling at 60% VO_2 max causes an increase of plasma elastase concentration. The authors consider this fact to be evidence for neutrophil degranulation by exercise. It is of interest that prolonged exercise (triathlon) induced a statistically significant increase of the granulocyte MPO content in human plasma over the baseline levels both immediately after exercise and after a 1 h recovery period (Camus et al. 1998). Our findings are in good agreement with these data, despite the differences in exercise intensity and duration among these studies. In all of these studies a similar degranulation reaction of blood neutrophils in response to exercise was found.

It is important to compare secretion of different neutrophil protein markers. They were elastase (Walsh et al. 2000), lactoferrin (Suzuki et al. 2003; Inoue et al. 2004), MPO (Bury and Pirnay 1995; Camus et al. 1998), lysozyme (Morozov et al. 2003) in human studies and MPO and lysozyme in animal studies (Morozov et al. 2003). Besides, we have shown exercise-induced neutrophil content decrease of lysozyme and MPO in humans and rats (Table 1; figures 1,2). Data from our cytological approach (experiment 2), based on evaluation of total neutrophil lysosomal cationic proteins, gave reliable additional evidence of exercise-stimulated secretory degranulation of blood neutrophils. However, in the Bishop et al. study (2003) 2-h cycling resulted in the fall in LPS-stimulated elastase release by 47 % but the authors failed to find an exercise influence on total elastase content of neutrophils. Nonetheless, the above cited literature data and the results of our study suggest reasons for intense and rather prolonged exercises to stimulate secretory degranulation of blood neutrophils, followed by increase of neutrophil proteins in serum and their content in neutrophils.

Additionally, using treadmill running until exhaustion as a model of exercise in the human we found a close correlation between the intensity of the neutrophil degranulation process and the work capacity of the athletes. In fact, the values of the degranulation process intensity can be used for the prediction of work capacity, using the neutrophil index of secretion - IS (see section Materials and methods). The correlation with the work capacity was particularly close for ($IS_{6min} - IS_{0min}$) ($\eta = 0.95$; $P < 0.001$).

If rowers executed specific load (rowing), neutrophil secretion activity was higher when compared to treadmill running. Both loads were near exhaustive and similar regarding their duration. Nevertheless the effect of the rowing was reliably stronger: plasma and neutrophil lysozyme concentrations were 1.3-fold and 1.4-fold lower immediately after exercise correspondingly. We can only suppose that during specific activity the rowers can mobilize their efforts more effectively and complete more volume of the work compared to treadmill running.

Additional data obtained in our observations of humans indicate, that even moderate intensity exercise stimulates blood neutrophil degranulation, although to a lesser degree. At the end of one hour of exercise, the content of neutrophil proteins decreased from 1.58 +/- 0.02 to 1.52 +/- 0.03 (N = 15; $p < 0.05$; Signs test) threas their concentration in blood serum average increased ($p > 0.05$). These facts also suggest an association between the exercise intensity and the level of the neutrophil degranulation reaction.

It is known that neutrophils can secrete different types of proteins, depending on the intensity and, probably, the nature of activity (Klebanoff and Clark 1978). Normally, mobilization of specific granules unlike azurophilic ones takes place rapidly, usually within minutes. It is expected, that azurophilic MPO-containing granules would be mobilized later. Finding a statistically significant increase of the granulocyte MPO content in human plasma over the baseline levels immediately after exercise in both the present study and in the experiments of Camus et al (1998), indicates a strong effect of intensive loading on blood neutrophils, which causes degranulation of azurophilic granules.

As theorized by Camus et al (1998), the bacterial lipopolysaccharide (LPS) that is translocated to blood could be a stimulus that activates the secretory reaction involved in the process of the exercise-induced neutrophil activation (Camus et al. 1998). These authors did not find a statistically significant correlation (r = 0.26) between the MPO and plasma endotoxin levels in participants of a sprint triathlon at the end of competition and during the recovery. They concluded that endotoxemia was not involved in the process of the exercise-induced granulocyte degranulation.

According to our data, the degranulation reaction develops rapidly. The stimulus might be related to the actions of hormones, such as catecholamines or glucocorticoids.

We showed also that an elevation of glucocorticoids in rat and human blood during exercise coincided in time with an increase of lysozyme content (Fig. 3, 4). Moreover a reliable association was observed during the first 6 min of exercise in the human study. We have found in vitro a statistically significant increase of the plasma lysozyme level after a delivery of corticosterone in rat blood samples (Table 3).

These data suggest that increased concentration of glucocorticoids might stimulate the activating degranulation reaction of blood neutrophils. Assuming that physical activity stimulates blood neutrophil degranulation, it should result in a decrease of the determined protein content in neutrophils and a concomitant increase in blood plasma. From these assumptions, another two questions can be raised: a) what effect on neutrophils can the decrease of granule protein content have and b) what the functional significance of the proteins secreted by neutrophils? Previously, it was shown that degranulation occurring during 2 h cycling produces a decrease in the neutrophil LPS-stimulated in vitro degranulation response (Walsh et al. 2000). Our earlier observations support the notion that degranulation is a probable cause of a decrease of phagocytic potency of these cells (Morozov et al. 1991). To this point, the impairment of phagocytic activity can depend both on a decrease of proteins that provide normal rate of phagocytosis and also on the fact that both these reactions depend on ATP (Klebanoff and Clarck 1978). Thus, the neutrophil degranulation reduces the neutrophil capability required for normal phagocytosis by these cells.

To elucidate the possible interrelations between degranulation and oxidative burst intensity of blood neutrophils, we studied the neutrophil-stimulated chemiluminescence response. In the present investigation we failed to observe a relationship between neutrophil degranulation (lysozyme efflux) and the oxidative burst intensity (Table 2).

Walsh et al. failed to find any change in isolated neutrophil oxidative burst activity during the 2-h post-exercise recovery period (Walsh et al. 2000). Robson et al. (1999) compared effects of exhausting exercise at 80% VO_2max (1 h) with a more prolonged exercise at 55% VO_2max on blood neutrophil function. The mean cycling times to fatigue were 37 min and 164 min, respectively. Both exercise bouts caused statistically significant (p < 0.05) elevations of the blood leukocyte count and reductions in the in vitro neutrophil degranulation response to bacterial LPS and oxidative burst activity. The authors observed higher blood leukocyte and neutrophil counts at the lower work rate for a longer duration, while parameters of neutrophil functions were lower than those observed at 80% VO_2max. These data indicate that neutrophil function changes under exercise depend not only on the intensity of exercise but also its duration. Our findings do not support the hypothesis of concurrent interrelations between degranulation and oxidative burst intensity of blood neutrophils (Witko-Sarsat et al. 2000). A possible cause of the oxidative burst decrease might be efflux to blood of immature bone marrow neutrophils that have a lower capacity for the oxidative burst. Clearly, such a situation suggests a need for further study.

We observed that the post-exercise changes of plasma neutrophil proteins depend on the rapid decrease of these proteins in circulation. They can be involved in the regulation of some post-exercise events. We hypothesize (Fig. 6), that the link between neutrophil proteins and exercise stress could be related to three specific functions of these proteins. First, these proteins can promote a more pronounced blood bactericidal potency. The time of realization of this function might be limited by the duration of the increase of the cationic protein content in circulation. A similar point of view was formulated by Inoue et al. (2004). Taking into account the fast disappearance of these proteins from the blood, other possible functions must be considered to be more important. Second, these proteins can activate granulopoiesis in the bone marrow and influx to the circulation of neutrophils rich in lysosome cationic proteins. Several studies suggested that neutrophil proteins indeed are the factors, which stimulates the bone marrow granulopoiesis (Delforge et al. 1985; Metcalf 1997). Finally, the neutrophil cationic proteins can have a regulatory significance. For example, they are responsible for conditioning of vascular endothelium for the subsequent white cell extravasation, the first step of migration of these cells to the local skeletal muscle injury. This hypothesis is supported by the observation that cathepsin G and other neutrophil proteases can be important for transendothelial migration of leukocytes (Owen et al. 1995; Cepinskas et al. 1997).

It is of interest, that many granule neutrophil proteins are of cationic nature and can interact with endotheliocytes neutralizing their cell charge and, thus, facilitating neutrophil anchoring. These proteins can also promote the appearance of adhesion molecules on the surface of endotheliocytes. Such action can be an important event for the extravasation of leukocytes and their migration towards muscle tissue injury location (Morozov et al. 2001).

It is unknown whether the degranulation develops when activated neutrophils are fixed on the vessel endothelium to move across the vessel wall or if they drift into the blood stream. We expect that the most suitable place of degranulation is the vascular wall, as it provides a high local concentration of neutrophil enzymes and oxidants that can be involved in the mechanism of neutrophil extravasation. Degranulation and oxidant release by adherent human neutrophils in vitro can be stimulated by TGF-1 (Balazovich et al. 1996). Moreover, cytotoxic agents are not released until activated neutrophils have migrated into extravascular tissues (Rainger et al. 1998). These facts could account for an increased expression of the integrin adhesive receptor CD11b on granulocytes during intensive endurance exercise (Jordan et al. 1999). These authors consider this phenomenon to be partly responsible for the increased adhesion of granulocytes to endothelial cells and to be capable of facilitating their tissue infiltration after endurance exercise.

The presented data suggest that intensive physical exercise activates the secretory function (degranulation) of blood neutrophils. Both types of neutrophil granules (specific and azurophilic) appear to be involved in this process. Activation of degranulation develops rapidly, and similarly, the neutrophil proteins rapidly disappear from circulation. On the contrary, the neutrophil activity responsible for the oxidative burst was not changed by the exercise. From the biological point of view neutrophil secretory degranulation accompanied by granule content efflux into circulation is a part of adaptive organism response to intense external influence. To understand the meaning of this reaction, further studies are necessary.

These data suggest also that "rat swimming model" is a very useful tool for investigating the rat leukocyte reactions to exercise. The similarities in neutrophil reactions in humans and rats suggest that using the rat model can provide useful information in further investigations of events following the degranulation reaction of neutrophils.

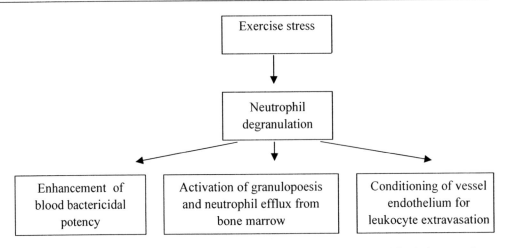

Fig. 6. Possible functions of lysosome cationic proteins released from blood neutrophils during exercise. (With permission of Springer-Verlag).

ACKNOWLEDGMENTS

This work was supported by the Russian Federation State Committee for Sports and Physical Culture. We thank Dr. Elena A. Pavlova (State Research Institute of Lake and River Fishery, Saint Petersburg) for her contribution to statistical calculations. We are very much obliged to Andrew Morozov (Student of Saint Petersburg Polytechnic State University) for his excellent technical assistance with figures and Galina Sakuta (Institute of Cytology RAS, Saint Petersburg) for her great help with microscopical evaluation of neutrophil cationic lysosomal proteins. We are indebted to Professor Christian W. Zauner (Greenville, NC) for his useful advises and helping during preparation of the manuscript.

The first version of this article was published in the European Journal of Applied Physiology (2003, volume 89: 257-262). It is reproduced with additions. Permission from Springer-Verlag is gratefully acknowledge.

REFERENCES

Balazovich K, Fernandez R, Hinkovska-Galcheva V, Suchard S, Boxer L (1996) Transforming growth factor-beta1 stimulates degranulation and oxidant release by adherent human neutrophils. *J Leukoc Biol* 60 : 772-777

Bishop N, Walsh N, Scanlon G (2003) Effect of prolonged exercise and carbohydrate on total neutrophil elastase content. *Med Sci Sports Exerc* 35 : 1326-1332

Böyum A (1968) Isolation of mononuclear cells and granulocytes from human blood. *Scand J Clin Invest* 12 : 77-89

Bury T, Pirnay F (1995) Effect of prolonged exercise on neutrophil myeloperoxidase secretion. *Int J Sports Med* 16 : 410-412

Camus G, Nys M, Poortmans J, Venneman I, Monfils T, Deby-Dupont G, Juchmes-Ferir A, Deby C, Lamy M, Duchateau J (1998) Possible in vivo tolerance of human polymorphonuclear neutrophil to low-grade exercise-induced endotoxaemia. *Mediators Inflamm* 7 : 413-415

Cepinskas G, Noseworthy R, Kvietys P (1997) Transendothelial neutrophil migration. Role of neutrophil-derived proteases and relationship to transendothelial protein movement. *Circ Res* 81 : 618-626

Chusid MJ, Shea ML (1986) Quantitation of corneal inflammation by chemiluminescense. *Arch Ophthalmol* 104:1540-1544

Conover W (1971) *Practical Nonparametric Statistics*. John Wiley, New York

Delforge A, Stryckmans P, Prieels J, Bieva C, Ronge-Collard E, Schlusselberg J, Efira A (1985) Lactoferrin: Its role as a regulator of human granulopoiesis. *Ann N Y Acad Sci* 459 : 85-96

Gleeson M, Walsh N, Blannin A, Robson P, Cook L, Donnelly A, Day S (1998) The effect of severe eccentric exercise-induced muscle damage on plasma elastase, glutamine and zinc concentrations. *Eur J Appl Physiol Occup Physiol* 77 : 543-546

Jaton J, Brandt D, Vassalli P (1979) Isolation and characteristics of immunoglobulines, antobodies and their polypeptide chains. In: Lefkovits I, Pernis B (eds) *Immunological methods*. Acad Press, New York

Jessup W, Leoni P, Dean R (1985) Costitutive and triggered lysosomal enzyme secretion. In: Dean RT, Stahl P (eds) *Developments in Cell Biology*. Secretory Process, Vol. 1. Butterworths, London, pp 38-57

Jordan J, Beneke R, Hutler M, Veith A, Luft F, Haller H (1999) Regulation of MAC-1 (CD11b/CD18) expression on circulating granulocytes in endurance runners *Med Sci Sports Exerc* 31 : 362-367

Inoue H, Sakai M, Kaida Y, Kaibara K (2004) Blood lactoferrin release induced by running exercise in normal volunteers: antibacterial activity. *Clin Chim Acta* 341 : 165-172.

Klebanoff S, Clarck R (1978) *The neutrophil: Function and Clinical Disorders*. North-Holland Publ. Co., Amsterdam

Mazing Y, Staroselskaya I (1981) Evaluation of reliability of lysosomal cationic test for laboratory diagnostics. *Lab Delo* 10 : 582-584 (In Russian)

Metcalf D (1997) The molecular control of granulocytes and macrophages. Ciba Foundation Symp 204: *The Molecular Basis of Cellular Defence Mechanisms*. John Wiley and Sons, Chichester, 40-56

Morozov V, Isotova E, Pryatkin S, Tsyplenkov P (1991) Effect of muscular activity on the blood neutrophil system. *Sechenov Fiziol Zh* USSR 77 : 53-61 (In Russian)

Morozov V, Pryatkin S, Kalinsky M, Rogozkin V (2003) Effect of exercise to exhaustion on myeloperoxidase and lysozyme release from blood neutrophils. *Eur J Appl Occup Physiol* 89 : 257-262

Morozov V, Tsyplenkov P, Kokryakov V, Volkov K, Vinogradova N (1997) Isolation and characterization of myeloperoxidase from leukocytes of rat peritoneal fluid. *Biochemistry* (Moscow) 62 : 623-630 (English version)

Morozov V, Usenko T, Rogozkin V (2001) Neutrophil antiserum response to decrease in proteolytic activity in loaded rat muscle. *Eur J Appl Occup Physiol* 84 : 195-200

Owen C, Campbell M, Boukedes S, Campbell E (1995) Inducible binding of bioactive cathepsin G to the cell surface of neutrophils. A novel mechanism for mediating extracellular catalytic activity of cathepsin G. *J Immunol* 155 : 5803-5810

Parry R, Chandan R, Schanani R (1965) Rapid and sensitive assay of muramidase. *Proc Soc Exper Biol* 199 : 384-394

Paus E, Bormer O, Nustad K (1982) Radioiodination of proteins with Iodogen method. In: Proceeding of the Symp "Radioimmunoassay and related procedures in medicine", Part 1. *IAEA*, Vienna, pp 161-171

Peake J (2002) Exercise-induced alterations in neutrophil degranulation and respiratory burst activity: possible mechanisms of action *Exerc Immunol* Rev 8 : 49-100

Nieman D, Henson D (1994) Role of endurance exercise in immune senescence. *Med Sci Sports Exerc* 26 : 172-181

Nieman D, Pedersen B (1999) Exercise and immune function. Recent developments. *Sports Med* 27 : 73-80

Peake J (2002) Exercise-induced alterations in neutrophil degranulation and respiratory burst activity: possible mechanisms of action. *Exerc Immunol* Rev 8 : 49-100

Prasad K, Kalra J, Chaudhary AK, Debnath D (1990) Effect of polymorphonuclear leukocyte-derived oxygen free radicals and hypochlorous acid on cardiac function and some biochemical parameters. *Am Heart J* 119 : 538-550

Pryatkin S, Nazarov I, Morozov V, Rogozkin V (1988) Radioimmunoassay for human lysozyme. *Vopr Med Khimii* 34 : 74-78 (in Russian)

Rainger G, Rowley A, Nash G (1998) Adhesion-dependent release of elastase from human neutrophils in a novel, flow-based model: specificity of different chemotactic agents. *Blood* 92 : 4819-4827

Robson P, Blannin A, Walsh N, Castell L, Gleeson M (1999) Effects of exercise intensity, duration and recovery on in vitro neutrophil function in male athletes. *Int J Sports Med* 20 : 128-135

Sharp N, Kautedakis Y (1992) Sport and overtraining syndrome: immunological aspects *Br Med Bull* 48: 518-533

Smith J (1997) Exercise immunology and neutrophils. *Int J Sports Med* 18 Suppl 1 : S46-55

Smith J, Pyne D (1997) Exercise, training, and neutrophil function. *Exerc Immunol Rev* 3 : 96-116

Suzuki K, Nakaji S, Yamada M, Liu Q, Kurakaka S, Okamura N, Kumae T, Umeda T, Sugawara K (2003) Impact of a competitive marathon race on systemic cytokine and neutrophil responses. *Med Sci Sports Exerc* 35 : 348-355

Suzuki K, Sato H, Kikuchi T, Abe T. Nakaji S, Sugawara K, Totsuka M, Sato K, Yamaya K (1996) Capacity of circulating neutrophils to produce reactive oxygen species after exhaustive exercise. *J Appl Physiol* 81 : 1213-1222

Tsyplenkov P, Morozov V, Rogozkin V, Kokryakov V (1988) Immunoradiometric assay for rat myeloperoxidase. *Ukrain Biokem* J 60 : 72-75 (in Russian)

Turton E, Spark J, Mercer K, Berridge D, Kent P, Kester R, Scott D (1998) Exercise-induced neutrophil activation in claudicants: a physiological or pathological response to exhaustive exercise? *Eur J Vasc Endovasc Surg* 16 : 192-196

Walsh N, Blannin A, Bishop N, Robson P, Gleeson M (2000) Effect of oral glutamine supplementation on human neutrophil lipopolysaccharide-stimulated degranulation following prolonged exercise. *Int J Sport Nutr Exerc Metab* 10 : 39-50

Witko-Sarsat V, Rieu P, Descamps-Latscha B, Lesavre P, Halbwachs-Mecarelli L (2000) Neutrophils: Molecules, functions and pathophysiological aspects. *Lab Invest* 80 : 617-653

In: Weight Loss, Exercise and Health Research
Editor: Carrie P. Saylor, pp. 213-230

ISBN 1-60021-077-5
© 2006 Nova Science Publishers, Inc.

Chapter 10

PREGNANCY AND EXERCISE – SHOULD HEALTHY PREGNANT WOMEN ACTIVELY TRAIN?

Jouko Pirhonen[1], Elisabeth Rettedal*, Tom Hartgill* and Pelle Lindqvist#*

*University of Oslo, Oslo, Norway
#University of Lund, Malmö, Sweden

ABSTRACT

Background: The aim of this review article is to examine the evidence in the literature with regard to the safety of exercise in pregnancy.

Material and methods: A literature search revealed fourteen randomised controlled trials which were systematically reviewed. The outcome measures looked at were both short and long term consequences of training in healthy pregnant women.

Results: The methodology of all included studies was qualitatively evaluated, though few were graded as good. The majority were small and had variable compliance from the volunteers. There was a lack of standardisation of the training schedules: the frequency ranged from 3 - 5 times per week, training intensities varied from age related maximal heart rates of 50 - 75% and exercise periods ranged from 20 – 60 minutes in length. Overall however, the exercise could be classified as moderate.

The literature revealed neither the fetus nor the mother derived harm from moderate exercise in pregnancy. Pregnant women who exercised in the above manner delivered normal healthy infants. With increasing intensity of exercise it appears the children are born with a lower percentage of body fat and thereby a lower birth weight, though still within normal range. This form of training does not appear to increase the incidence of preterm birth or caesarean section. The low number of studies and small patient numbers make it difficult to draw any conclusions with regard to teratogenic effects of hyperthermia. The exclusion of women who developed obstetric complications means it is not possible to draw any conclusions as regards exercise and the risk of placental abruption or bleeding.

---

[1] Corresponding author: Jouko Pirhonen, Department of Obstetrics and Gynaecology, Ullevaal University Hospital University of Oslo, Kirkeveien 166, N-0407 Oslo, NORWAY TEL: +47-22118911
Email: tiina_jouko_pirhonen@hotmail.com, Jouko.Pirhonen@medisin.uio.no

Conclusion: Moderate exercise seems to have positive effects on pregnancy by way of improved physical well being. Moderate exercise also appears to increase psychological well being – the women feel better. Children born to mothers who exercised regularly showed no significant difference to those born to sedentary mothers in either a positive or a negative way. There was no apparent positive or negative effect on the infant at birth. From currently available data it appears that regular exercise of moderate intensity is both safe and commendable in pregnancy.

Further research in this area is required to assess whether physical activity can increase the risks of obstetric complications or cause significant effects from hyperthermia, particularly where exercise intensity is greater than as described here.

INTRODUCTION

Whether women can train or not during pregnancy is debated amongst healthcare professionals and lay folk, many studies have been carried out but results are not consistent. Only a few studies are large and of good quality, there are only two metanalysis (1, 2) which concluded with further research being required in this area.

There are few studies on exercise in pregnancy in Norway. Nordhagen found in one study, 70% of pregnant Norwegian women were physically active in at least two of three trimesters (3). For information regarding physical activity in pregnancy women seek advice from their Primary Healthcare Centres, General Practitioners or the internet. It is important therefore for healthcare workers to have access to accurate information on what type and intensity of exercise is acceptable in pregnancy for mother and child. Currently there is no consensus of opinion on whether or not pregnant women can train or to what intensity they can exercise which reflects a general lack of knowledge.

Pregnancy is a major physiological stress on a woman; physical activity produces some of the same physiological changes. The main concern related to exercise and pregnancy is of potential harm caused to the fetus. Harmful effects on the fetus may be caused by hyperthermia which is a known teratogen, hypoxia due to reduce blood flow to the uterus, fetal growth restriction and trauma. Potential negative effects on the pregnant woman are increased risk of obstetric complications such as bleeding, preterm labour and an increased risk of caesarean section. However, one would also expect physical activity during pregnancy to be beneficial, particularly for the women, for example reducing the risk of depression and gestational diabetes. On a smaller scale physical activity may improve self esteem and thereby their work capacity and could reduce complications during labour.

There are many women who stop training when they become pregnant, though exercise had been a positive experience and one can only speculate as to the reasons for stopping. It is likely this is due to a relative uncertainty with regard to safety for both mother and baby; whether there are any positive gains is also important.

In this article we have undertaken a qualitative, systematic review of randomised controlled trials concerning exercise and pregnancy. The aim of this review is to investigate whether or not there is evidence in the literature on the safety of exercise in pregnancy and secondly whether aerobic exercise should be recommended to pregnant women.

EXPLANATION OF TERMS

- **Healthy Pregnancy:** A pregnancy without known obstetric or medical complications (for which physical activity would increase the risks to the fetus or pregnant woman).
- **Exercise:** In the context of this review means aerobic physical activity with a minimum heart rate increase of 50% of the age related maximum.

LITERATURE SEARCH

The literature search was done in 2002-2003. Search terms used were "pregnancy + exercise + consequences/effects" in the Medline/Pubmed database and the Cochrane Library. Reference lists and related literature were used, authors were not contacted and only published data was used. The results of the literature search gave 14 randomised controlled trials concerned with exercise and pregnancy.

THE TYPE OF PUBLICATION

The main criterion for inclusion of a study was randomisation. When investigating whether a factor has an effect (positive or negative) the most important question is whether subjects were allocated randomly to the intervention or control group. Randomisation is the only technique which without bias gives comparable groups. In studies with sufficient participants randomisation ensures balance of known and unknown confounding or prognostic factors (4). Chalmers (5) showed that not blinding which category participants were allocated to often lead to uneven distribution of prognostic factors, which may have a greater effect on the study than the intervention itself (6). The literature search revealed many studies on exercise and pregnancy though only in a minority was randomisation performed. In most studies women who were already physically active were selected to the intervention group, then the control group selected based on known prognostic factors without taking into account the many unknown prognostic factors.

The second inclusion criterion was a physical activity level leading to a rise in the heart rate at a minimum of 50% of the age related heart rate. Many of the potentially harmful effects of exercise, particularly to the fetus, would be expected to occur when a significant proportion of the maternal blood flow was diverted to skeletal muscle, away from the uterus and fetus. Sufficient energy expenditure is also required to raise maternal body temperature to a level that may be harmful to the fetus.

The third criterion was a healthy pregnant woman, with no known obstetric or medical complications prior to inclusion in the study.

The fourth criterion was parameters measured looked at the effects of exercise on the pregnant woman or the fetus.

There were no limits as to the size, date or language of the studies though only English language studies were found. In areas where the selected publications could not reach conclusions, the literature was reviewed to show where current research stands today. This is meant as a perspective for readers and not a definitive answer.

EXAMINATION OF METHODOLOGY FOR INCLUDED STUDIES

Studies were scored in relation to the randomisation procedure and information on participant drop out. The scoring method used was developed by Jadad et al (7), with scoring from 0-3 where 3 is the highest score. Thereafter the methodological quality of the included studies were assessed using the "12 questions to help assess a randomised controlled study" developed by the Critical Appraisal Skills Programme (CASP, Oxford). The CASP system categorises the studies as "very good, good, average or poor." The studies with their CASP scores are presented in Table I.

(For abbreviations used in Table I see footnote 1)

Table I: Included studies – method assessment

Study	Year published	Method	Scoring (Jadad) QA
Bell, Palma (8)	2000	Randomised, only 52% of the women agreed to randomisation. All the women included in the study wished to train 5 times/week or more. With allowances for dropouts. Poor compliance 61 women randomised, 33 continued to train 5 times/week, 28 reduced it to 3 times/week.	Jadad:2 QA: average
Carpenter, Sady, Sady Haydon, Thompson, Coustan (9)	1990	Randomised, further details not given No info with regards to dropouts or compliance. EG – 7, CG - 7	Jadad:1 QA: Average
Clapp, Kim, Burciu, Lopez (10)	2000	Randomised by use of anonymised envelopes. Participants included pre-pregnancy. Originally 50, 4 dropouts – 2 from EG non-compliant, 1 premature birth in each group. Compliance excellent EG – 22, CG – 24,	Jadad:3 QA: good
Clapp, Kim, Burciu, Schmidt, Petry, Lopez (11)	2002	Randomised by use of anonymised envelopes. Participants included in the study pre-pregnancy. Originally 80, 5 dropouts – 2 non-compliance, 2 premature births, 1 IUGR and bleeding. Unclear which groups these belonged to. Dropouts excluded from analysis. Compliance excellent. 3 training groups: Hi-Lo – 26, Mod-Mod – 24, Lo – Hi – 25	Jadad:3 QA: good
Collings, Curet, Mullin (12)	1982	The first 5 self-selected which group, the remaining 15 were randomised. Dropouts not taken into account. EG – 12, CG – 8	Jadad:1 QA: average
Erkkola (13)	1976	Randomised, not explained further. Originally 83, 7 did not want to participate, 14 drop outs, 3 moved in both groups, 1 spontaneous abort in EG, 1 threatened abortion in both groups, 2 premature deliveries in CG, 1 in EG, 1 termination in EG, 1 unknown dropout. EG – 31, CG – 31. Primigravidae.	Jadad:2 QA: average

Table I: Included studies – method assessment (Continued)

Study	Year published	Method	Scoring (Jadad) QA
Kulpa, White, Visscher (14)	1986	Randomised, not explained further. Originally 141, 56 dropouts- spontaneous abortion (n=8), non-compliance (n=2) those who stopped (n=20) were eliminated from study. Serious obstetric complications analysed separately (n=26, 10 from EG and16 from CG). Studied over 2,5 years. EG – 17 primigravidae, 21 multigravidae CG – 20 primigravidae, 27 multigravidae	Jadad:2 QA: average
Lee (15)	1996	Randomised by randomisation table Originally 370, 19 dropouts Variable compliance; 15,4% did not participate, 27,4% minimum participation. 1/week for 1-5 weeks, 34,3% 1/week for 6-15 weeks, 22,9% 1/week for minimum16 weeks EG – 176, CG – 177.	Jadad:3 QA: good
Marquez-Sterling, Kaplan, Halberstein, Signorlie, Perry (16)	1997	Randomised, not explained further Originally 20, 5 dropouts– 1 in EG moved, 2 in CG due to work, 2 in CG lost contact EG – 9 primigravidae, CG – 6 primigravidae	Jadad:2 QA: average
Pijpers, Wladimiroff, McGhie (17)	1984	Randomised, not explained further Primigravidae. No dropouts. EG – 14, CG – 14	Jadad:2 QA: good
Prevedel, Calderon, Abadde, Borges, Rudge (18)	2001	Randomised, not explained further No information on dropouts or compliance EG – 22, CG – 19.	Jadad:1 QA: average
Sibley, Ruhling, Cameron-Foster, Christensen, Bolen (19)	1981	Randomised, not explained further No dropouts and good compliance EG – 7, CG – 6	Jadad:2 QA: average
South-Paul, Rajagopal, Tenholder (20)	1988	Randomized, not explained further Originally 23, 6 dropouts – 3 (2 from EG) due to work, 1 had twins(EG), 1 appendicitis (EG), 1 placenta previa (EG). EG – 10, CG – 7, primi- og multigravidae.	Jadad:2 QA: good
Varassi, Bazzano, Edwards (21)	1988	Randomised, not explained further Originally 36. Multips. 4 excluded from CG for other medical intervention, 2 excluded from EG unwilling to train. EG – 13, CG – 17	Jadad:2 QA: average

EG: Exercise Group, CG: Control Group, QA: Qualitative Assessment
Hi-Lo: reducing from 60-20min exercise in week 24, Mod-Mod: exercised 40 min throughout pregnancy, Lo-Hi: increased from 20-60 min in week 24

Overall none of the studies were of "very good" quality, of the 14 studies included only 5 were of "good" quality with the rest being of "average" quality. When applying Jadad's criteria: 3 studies scored 3 points, 8 scored 2 points and 3 scored 1 point. The process of randomisation used is important in assessing if the procedure itself was adequately performed; an important part of the randomisation process is concealed random allocation, whereby those who are carrying out the study do not know which group a participant is in, this principle (blinding) should also be extended to those who are analysing the results. Lee (15) specified that he used a randomisation table; Clapp (10, 11) used anonymous envelopes without further clarification in both studies. None of the other studies specified how the randomisation was performed or whether any form of blinding was used.

Several of the studies included details of participants withdrawing from the studies, though only Lee (15) included these in the analysis. If one wishes to have robust data it is best to include the participants who withdrew in their group, when analysing the data. Such "intention to treat" analysis strengthens the results (4). This type of study allows one to analyse these results even though they were not a parameter originally planned for investigation. The complications which the participants develop may be a result of exercise and thus need to be included in order to advise women on exercise in pregnancy.

The limited randomised studies available indicate this is a difficult area to investigate, in Bell's study (8) only 51% of participants wanted to be randomised, the remainder did not want to risk limiting their physical activity. Lee's study (15) was the only large study with 351 participants. Bell (8), Clapp (10), Erkkola (12) and Kulpa (14) were studies with over 60 participants. The other studies were small, making it difficult to infer anything from the results, unless there is a large and / or statistically significant difference.

In order to establish an effect from an intervention it is necessary to minimise other variables, a good starting point is to study the groups at the beginning in order to assess their baseline physical fitness and ensure equality between the groups. Only a few of the studies compared the groups at the start of the study. It is important that the groups are otherwise treated similarly (4), however this is difficult to achieve in this type of study. By treating the groups with a similar follow-up and ensuring blinding of the investigators it is possible to reduce bias, though several studies actually had more frequent monitoring of the intervention group.

Instructions (or lack of) given to the control groups are also of importance; knowing or limiting the extent of physical activity undertaken during the study period allows some control over the study. In 4 studies the women were asked to continue their normal daily activity (10, 11, 12 and 15) and Kulpa (14) allowed them to train a maximum of once a week. Some of the studies gave diaries for participants to fill in with physical activity and other variables such as diet to record.

In most studies the training regime was organised and undertaken with an instructor making it easier to ensure participants followed the programme. Four studies (8, 10, 11 and 13) allowed participants to do their own training regime, documenting the exercises in a diary. Intuitively, one would expect organised training regimes to give better compliance, though Lee's study (15) demonstrated poor compliance despite organised training. A few studies gave information on compliance varying from very good to poor, though many studies did not give information on compliance. Where compliance with an exercise regime is poor it makes interpreting the results difficult: if participants have not completed the regime the results may be misinterpreted.

LITERATURE REVIEW AS A METHOD

In a systematic review, one aims to use all available information from around the world on a subject. This entails searching all relevant databases, reference lists and contacting authors with regard to unpublished data (4). In this article we have searched for all randomised controlled studies on the subject, though cannot exclude that others may exist in other databases or unpublished. Authors were not contacted directly, which could have increased the quality of this study certainly with regard to precise questions surrounding methods and results of the included studies but also of unpublished data. Within exercise and pregnancy there are many studies though few were randomised controlled. Other criteria for selection in the literature could have been used such as number of participants, however we wanted to look at the effect of exercise during pregnancy so only chose randomised controlled studies where the groups were comparable.

The author's assessment of the included studies is important, there is an advantage in several people have looked at the articles critically. In this study only the principle author has reviewed the articles using a scoring system developed by Jadad et al (7) and the checklist developed by CASP. Few studies were of "good" quality though none were assessed as "poor" quality. An exclusion criterion that could be used were on those studies which excluded participants who developed obstetric complications but this would have left only one study. There were large variations in method quality and number of participants, those studies assessed as "good" were given greater weight.

The studies under examination should be homogenous in a systematic review (4), the studies included in this review examined the same phenomenon: physical activity in pregnancy, but they did not measure the same parameters and end points varied between studies making a meta-analysis difficult. In addition most of the studies were small and not of "very good" methodology so statistic analysis of the studies is not advisable. A meta-analysis would have improved the quality of the review as the results would be objective rather than subjective as in a qualitative review. In order to objectify the review as much as possible scoring systems such as those of Jadad (7) and CASP were used.

EMPIRICAL RESULTS OF INCLUDED STUDIES

Table 1 shows an alphabetical list of the 14 studies included, the type of exercise performed varied from walking, jogging, rowing, cycling, swimming, aerobics and cross country skiing. All the infants born were healthy at birth; preterm birth and caesarean section were the only obstetric complications used as an outcome measures. Lee (15) was the only investigator who did not exclude participants from the analysis when obstetric complications arose, the six other studies (8, 10, 11, 12, 13 and 16) which had recorded obstetric complication subsequently removed them from their analysis.

The training regimes in the different studies varied. Pijpers looked only at short term effects of 2 sessions lasting 5 minutes (17). The other studies had exercise programmes over longer time periods. Two studies investigated the consequences of different exercise intensities (8, 11) on participants who were all in physical training programmes at

Table II : Outcome measures – results

Outcome	Studies	Participants	Results
Premature birth(PB)	Bell	Dropout	1 PB in each of the groups
	Clapp (2000)	Dropout	1 PB in each of the groups
	Clapp (2002)	Dropout	2 PB in each of the groups
	Collings	20	No s.s difference
	Erkkola	Dropout	1 PB in EG, 2 PB in CG
	Lee	351	No s.s difference
	Marquez-Sterling	15	No s.s difference
Caesarean Section	Collings	EG 12/20	2 caesarean sections in CG, 0 in EG, no s.s difference
	Lee	EG 176/351	No s.s difference
	Marquez-Sterling	EG 9/20	1/3 caesareans in each of the groups
Apgar score (AS)1 and 5 min.after birth	Clapp (2000)	46	AS 8 or over in all, no s.s difference
	Clapp (2002)	75	AS 8 or over in all, no s.s difference
	Collings	20	AS 8 or over 5 min. postpartum, No s.s difference
	Kulpa	85	No s.s difference
	Lee	351	No s.s difference
	Marquez-Sterling	15	AS 9 or over 5 min. postpartum, no s.s difference
	Sibley	13	AS 8 or over, no s.s difference
Birth weight (average weight per group, in grams)	Bell	61	Increased birth weight in those that trained 5 times/week not s.s
	Clapp (2000)	46	EG – 3750, CG – 3490, s.s difference
	Clapp (2002)	75	Lo-Hi – 3370, s.s. lower (Mod-Mod 3430, Hi-Lo 3820)
	Collings	20	EG – 3600, CG – 3350, No s.s difference. (figures not given)
	Kulpa	85	EG – 3286, CG – 3325, no s.s difference
	Lee	351	EG – 3515, CG – 3722, no s.s difference
	Marquez-Sterling	15	
Ponderal Index	Clapp (2000)	46	No s.s difference
	Clapp (2002)	75	Lo-Hi og Mod-Mod groups s.s lower.

Table II : Outcome measures – results (Continued)

Outcome	Studies	Participants	Results
Fetal heart rate (FHR) during og 5 min. after training	Collings	20	FHR 120-160 bpm during and 5 min. after training
	Pijpers	28	FHR 120-160 bpm 5 min. after training
	Sibley	13	FHR over 160bpm in 2 cases during training, otherwise 137-160 bpm during and 5 min. after training
Placenta volume and growth rate	Clapp (2000)	46	Placental volume s.s increased in EG, less non-functional tissue
	Clapp (2002)	75	Placentas growth rate s.s. increased in the Hi-Lo group
	Collings	20	Placental volume increased in EG, not s.s.
Physical form objectively measured at beginning and end	Carpenter	14	Pulse oximetry s.s increased in EG, but not MVO2, SV, HR
	Collings	20	MVO2 s.s. increased in EG from 2nd to 3rd trimester
	Erkkola	62	PWC s.s. increased in EG in weeks 26 and 38. MVO2 s.s increased in EG
	Kulpa	85	EG s.s improved fitness
	Marquez-Sterling	15	EG s.s increased training capacity, reduction in CG
	Prevedel	41	MVO2 s.s. increased in EG
	Sibley	13	EG maintained their fitness, reduced in CG, not s.s
	South-Paul	17	Increased fitness in EG, not s.s.
Blood Pressure	Erkkola	62	Increased diastolic pressure in CG from 10th to 38th week, not s.s.
	Lee	351	Somewhat lower diastolic pressure in EG, not s.s.
	Sibley	13	
Weight gain during pregnancy (in kg)	Collings	20	EG – 15,8, CG – 14, No s.s difference EG – 15,7, CG – 16,3, No s.s difference
	Clapp (2000)	46	
	Clapp (2002)	75	The Lo-Hi group put on less weight s.s less (12 vs. 14,6 og15,5)
	Kulpa	85	Multigravida in CG put on s.s more
	Marquez-Sterling	15	EG – 16,2, CG – 15,7, No s.s difference
	Prevedel	41	EG – 14,5, CG – 12,5, No s.s difference
Duration of second stage	Collings	20	No s.s difference Primips in EG s.s shorter duration
	Kulpa	85	No s.s difference
	Lee	351	

Table II : Outcome measures – results (Continued)

Outcome	Studies	Participants	Results
Pain during birth	Lee	351	No s.s difference EG expressed s.s. less pain experienced during birth
	Varassi	20	
Experience of physical and psychological well-being	Lee	351	S.s higher in EG
	Marquez-Sterling	15	S.s higher in EG
	Sibley	13	S.s higher in EG
Post-natal depression	Lee	351	No s.s difference
Post-partum incontinence	Lee	351	No s.s difference

[2] EG: Exercise Group, CG: Control Group,

Hi-Lo: reducing from 60-20min exercise in week 24, Mod-Mod: exercised 40 min throughout pregnancy, Lo-Hi: increased from 20-60 min in week 24

SS: statistical significance, MVO2: maximal oxygen uptake, PWC: physical work capacity, BPM: beats per minute, HR: heart rate, SV: stroke volume, O2puls: pulse oximetry recruitment. Bell (8) started with a regime of 5 times per week, reducing to 3 times per week at 25 weeks in 28 0f 61 participants. Clapp (11) had 3 groups : Lo-Hi increased from 20 to 60 minutes in week 24, Mod-Mod exercised for 40 min throughout pregnancy and Hi-Low reduced from 60 to 20 minutes in week 24. All three groups exercised 5 times per week.

The remaining 11 studies looked at sedate women who were randomly allocated to the exercise group or control group. Exercise intensity, length of training times and number of training sessions per week varied: Intensity varied from 50% to 80% of maximal age related heart rate, some studies gave heart rates for the participants to achieve varying from 120 to 156 beats per minute. Sibley (19) chose individual intensities for each participant without giving further explanation. Two studies (9, 15) did not give information on the intensity of the exercise regimes. Length of regimes varied from 20 to 60 minutes, three studies (14, 18 and 20) did not give this information. In the majority of studies the participants trained 3 times per week, Clapp's (10) study trained 3 to 5 times per week, whereas Kulpa's (14) study did not state how often participants trained.

The studies also varied in relation to when the intervention started and stopped in the pregnancy. Bell (8), Clapp (10, 11), Erkkola (12) and Kulpa (14) started in the first trimester, the others in the second trimester. Most continued to delivery though Carpenter (9), Erkkola (13), Prevedel (18), Sibley (19) and South-Paul (20) terminated their studies in the third trimester.

Table II shows the results of different outcome measures. Results for individual studies in relation to a given outcome measure reads directly from the same line as the study is placed. All studies used the student's t-test for statistical analysis; P values for statistical significance were mostly $P < 0.05$ though some were as low as $P < 0.001$. For abbreviations in Table II see footnote 2.

Only three studies had preterm labour as an outcome measure, but four other studies recorded how many delivered preterm though excluding them from the analysis. None of these studies (8, 10, 11, 12, 13, 15 and 16) showed a statistically significant difference in the number of preterm births. Frequency of caesarean section was an outcome measure in three studies (12, 15, 16), but no statistically significant difference was found. Half of the studies (10, 11, 12, 14, 15, 16 and 19) looked at the Apgar scores which were all over 8 for all the children at birth.

Seven studies also looked at birth weight; all the children weighed over 3kg. Clapp (10) found in fact children born to mothers who exercised weighed significantly more, though the other six studies found no significant difference. Bell (8) who compared two exercising groups found those women who continued to train 5 times per week gave birth to bigger children but the difference was not significant. Clapp (11) comparing three training regimes found again significant differences: women in the Lo-Hi group (increasing from 20 -60 minutes at week 24) gave birth to children with significantly lower birth weight. In both of Clapp's studies (10, 11) he also compared the ponderal index, in the control group study there was no difference but in the study with 3 training regimes the ponderal index was significantly lower in the Lo-Hi and Mod-Mod groups.

Pijpers (17) looked at only short term effects of exercise including fetal heart rate five minutes after exercise; the heart rate was between 120-160 beats per minute. Two other studies (12, 19) compared fetal heart rates, Colling's (12) found a significant increase during exercise though within normal range (120-160) and five minutes after exercise. Sibley (19) found two of the seven participants in the exercise group had fetal heart rates over 160 beats per minute during training, though all were within normal (120-160) range five minutes after exercise again.

Two studies comparing an exercise group with a control group looked at the placental volume. Clapp (10) found the placentas in the exercise group had significantly larger volume, more villi and less non functional tissue. In his study with 3 training regimes (11) Clapp also found significant increase in growth rate in those who reduced training at 24 weeks (Hi-Lo group). Colling's study (12) showed a larger placental volume in the exercise group, though this was not statistically significant.

Eight studies investigated whether participants in the exercise groups got the improvement in their physical condition. Several parameters were used to measure physical fitness such as work capacity, estimated maximal oxygen uptake and aerobic capacity. In order to collectively review the results, the term objectively measured physical fitness is used. In Sibley's study (19) the exercise group maintained their fitness levels, whereas in the control group it fell, the results were not significant. Results from Collings (12), Erkkola (13) and Prevedel (18) demonstrated a significant rise in maximal oxygen uptake in the exercise groups; Carpenter (9), Kulpa (14), Marquez-Sterling (16) and South-Paul (20) also showed improvement in physical fitness in the training groups.

Blood pressure was measured at different stages of the pregnancy and was an outcome measure in three of the studies. Erkkolas (13) study showed an increase in diastolic pressures from 10th to 38th week of gestation in the control group, whereas Sibley (19) found lower diastolic pressures in the exercise group (not statistically significant). Lee (15) found no differences between their groups.

Weight gain during the pregnancy was an outcome measure in six studies, the five studies comparing exercise with control group found only small changes (10, 12, 14, 16 and 18). Kulpa (14) found multigravida in the control group increased their weight significantly more than in the other three groups. In his study with three exercise regimes (11) there was a significantly lower increase in the group which increased their training regime (Lo – Hi group).

Kulpa (14) and Lee (15) examined the duration of the second stage of labour. Lee found no difference between the exercise and control groups; though by distinguishing between primigravida and multigravida, Kulpa found significantly shorter second stages in the primigravidae as compared to the control group. Personally experienced pain (as measured by pain score questionnaires) during labour was an outcome measure in two studies; Varassi (21) found women in the exercising group experienced less pain whereas Lee (15) saw no difference between the groups. The way in which exercise effected the women's physical and psychological well being was an outcome measure in three studies: all three found a significant increase in the parameters measured (15, 16 and 19).

DISCUSSION

Extensive physiological changes occur in pregnancy, for a majority of which, hormones appear to be a prerequisite. Major cardiovascular changes occur which affect the ability to exercise; Cardiac output increases in the first trimester, reaching its nadir (a 30-50% increase) in the second trimester. This increase is due to a fall in total peripheral vascular resistance and concomitant increase in stroke volume and heart rate. The diastolic blood pressure falls by 5-10 mmHg through the second trimester and the systolic pressure either falls slightly or shows no change. The blood pressure then rises again towards term eventually reaching pre-pregnancy levels. Blood volume gradually increases by 40-50% through the first and second trimester, though the increase is greater in plasma volume than erythrocytes leading to the physiological anaemia of pregnancy (22). Blood flow distribution is also significantly altered, increasing flow to the visceral organs ensuring good flow to the uterus and thereby securing blood flow to the feto-placental unit (23). Respiration is also altered in pregnancy: tidal volume increases 50% and maximal oxygen uptake increases by 10-20%. This increased ventilation reduces the arterial carbon dioxide tension (paCO2) inducing a mild maternal alkalosis which in turn facilitates gas exchange across the placenta so hindering fetal acidosis (23). The hormonal changes can cause mechanical alterations by relaxation of ligaments which in turn lead to greater joint instability (24). Basal metabolic rate and heat production increase also in pregnancy; pregnant women require circa 300 kcal extra per day and the fetal body temperature is approximately 1°C higher than maternal (25) allowing heat transfer from fetus to mother (26).

Physical activity gives similar changes to a woman's physiology as a pregnancy. The changes that occur are increased heart rate, a fall in peripheral resistance and unlike pregnancy a raised blood pressure (greater systolic change than diastolic); these changes lead to an increase in cardiac output (27). With increasing work intensity core body temperature may also rise, though this is not scientifically proven in humans. A 20 minute exercise regime at 70% intensity can theoretically increase core body temperature by 1.5°C (28). Physical activity leads to a redistribution of the blood supply moving it from visceral organs and skin, to the exercising skeletal muscle, as intensity increases so does the redistribution (23). Respiratory changes are increased respiratory rate and tidal volume (27); physical activity also raises the basal metabolic rate as the exercising muscle requires energy. Over time regular aerobic training will increase oxygen uptake, raise stroke volume, lower the resting pulse rate and may help lower blood pressure (29).

In the studies included in this review, the exercise groups trained aerobically 3 – 5 times per week for 20 – 60 minutes with a work intensity of between 50 – 75% of maximal age related heart rate. The extent to which the participants reached the desired training effect was looked at in eight of the studies (9, 12, 13, 14, 16, 18, 19 and 20). The majority found the exercising group gained a significant improvement in physical fitness. A few found the women merely maintained fitness whereas the control groups fell in fitness; this may be due to the effects being masked by the changes of pregnancy.

Theoretical risks to the fetus from the combination of the physiological changes of aerobic exercise and pregnancy are fetal hypoxia, growth restriction, hyperthermia and trauma. The redistribution of blood flow during training can be great enough to cause a reduction in blood flow to the placenta thereby inducing fetal hypoxia. Active skeletal muscle may be able to alter the energy substrate accessibility to such a degree as to cause fetal growth restriction. Hyperthermia is a known teratogen leading to increased risk of neural tube defects (30). Fetal trauma is of particular risk in contact sports where there is a risk of a blow to the uterus. Trauma was not investigated by the included studies and will therefore not be discussed further in this review.

Fetal oxygen deprivation is difficult to measure in utero and carries a risk of preterm labour, though indirectly the fetal heart rate and its variability can be used. Those studies which did assess fetal heart rate patterns (11, 17 and 18) demonstrated normal parameters 5 minutes after training. In only one study did the fetal heart rate rise above 160 beats per minute during the training regime in two of seven participants otherwise fetal heart rate recordings were unremarkable.

Physical exercise tends to direct blood flow away from the visceral organs, including the placenta, thus a possible cause of reduced transport of oxygen and nutrients to the fetus. Three studies investigated the placental volume (10, 11 and 12) of which two compared with a control group (10, 12), both studies showed larger placental volume in the exercise group though only one was statistically significant. Clapp (10) demonstrated a larger proportion of functional and villous tissue in the placentas of exercising groups. The third study (11) looking at three training regimes demonstrated a significant increase in placental growth rate in the reducing exercise (Hi-Lo) group. These results suggest the placenta adapts to regular exercise by increasing its volume and quantity of functional tissue, thereby compensating for the reduction in blood flow during exercise.

Birth weight is an indicator of fetal growth restriction (22) and among the five studies (10, 12, 14, 15 and 16) with a control group comparison only one study showed the exercise group delivered significantly larger babies (10). The other studies had no significant differences in birth weight, in fact all studies where birth weight was recorded, these were within the normal ranges. Significantly smaller babies were born in the group where exercise was increased (Lo-Hi, 11), these children had significantly less body fat, and ponderal index suggested symmetrical growth thus not growth restricted. Maternal weight gain in pregnancy is a poor, non-specific measure of pregnancy wellbeing (22), those studies measuring this parameter (10, 12, 14, 16 and 18) found small differences all within the normal range. Clapp's study (11) found those who increased their training regime (Lo-Hi group) showed a significant lack of weight gain. Overall the results indicate moderate training has little effect on the babies' birth weight but that increasing exercise intensity can lead to a reduction in birth weight principally through reduced body fat.

Birth weight is an important predictor of fetal morbidity, if physical exercise led to an increased risk of preterm birth, perinatal complications would also be expected to rise. None of the studies found an increase in preterm deliveries and all who measured, had Apgar scores of 8 or over. The Apgar score indicates fetal vitality and scores of 8 – 10 of 10 suggests normal vital functions at birth. The results were consistent through all the studies included in this review.

Maternal body temperature was not measured during exercise; however a teratogenic effect might become apparent through an increase in children born with anatomical abnormalities to women in the exercise groups. Approximately 3% of all babies born have this type of abnormality (22), therefore a large cohort is required in order to test this hypothesis. No babies in these studies were born with abnormalities. A recently published longitudinal study (31) investigating core body temperature in an exercising group where work intensity was 85% of age related maximum showed a fall in maternal core body temperature, which may assist in protecting the fetus from hyperthermia.

Healthcare workers are most concerned with possible harmful effects of physical activity on the pregnant woman and their unborn child. Obstetric complications such as abruptio placenta, gestational diabetes, pre-eclampsia, preterm delivery, increasing the incidence of caesarean section or direct injury to ligaments and joints of the women caused by the changes in connective tissue and altered posture which occurs in pregnancy. Injuries were not reported in any of the studies and cannot be commented on further in this review. The obstetric complications which occurred during the pregnancy, in many of the studies lead to the exclusion of that person, whereas complications arising in labour were an outcome measure. Those studies (8, 10, 11, 12, 13, 15 and 16) which used preterm labour and caesarean section as outcome measures found no differences between exercising or control groups. Some complications, such as first trimester spontaneous miscarriage could not be assessed as most studies started in the second trimester.

Three studies (13, 15 and 19) followed blood pressure changes during the exercise periods, when compared to control groups the differences were small and insignificant. Had a positive effect of exercise (as might be expected) been apparent, this would have been interesting for those who develop pre-eclampsia. Regular aerobic exercise can lower blood pressure (29), though none of the reviewed studies demonstrated this effect.

The incidence of obesity and diabetes mellitus during pregnancy is increasing in westernised societies (22), even though in pregnancy fasting blood sugar levels tend to be lower (32). An indirect and rough guide to whether exercise affects blood sugar regulation and thereby appetite would be changes in weight. The studies in which weight was an outcome measure (10, 12, 14, 16 and 18) showed normal weight gain in all groups, only the study (11) with three exercise regimes demonstrated a significantly smaller weight gain in those who increased their training (Lo-Hi). Other studies (33, 34) not included in this review of gestational diabetes have shown exercise, diet control and insulin use all have a similar effect on lowering blood sugar levels. Regular aerobic exercise gives lower, more stable blood sugar and can therefore form part of a treatment regime. There is no information on the incidence of gestational diabetes in the studies reviewed, and a large population (greater than all the 14 studies reviewed here put together) would need to be investigated to see a significant difference. Further investigation in this area is required.

The myth that women who maintain physical fitness have shorter, easier deliveries compared with their more sedate counterparts is popular, only one of the studies (14) investigating the length of the second stage of labour found a difference. The primigravida who exercised had a shorter second stage of labour; the two other studies (12, 15) found no difference. Two studies looked at pain scores during labour (15, 21), one found lower pain scores in those who exercised (21) whereas the other found no difference.

Regular exercise during pregnancy could also have other positive effects, for example less risk of depression. Many women experience postnatal depression. Exercise increases serotonin levels in the brain, which may have a protective effect against depression. Nordhagen (3) found lower levels of depressive symptoms in physically active pregnant women than in sedate women, in his retrospective study. Lee (15) found no difference in rates of postnatal depression between exercising and control groups.

Longstanding exercise regimes could also reduce the risks of incontinence after delivery; Lee's study (15) showed no differences between their groups though none of the studies employed pelvic floor training in their exercise regimes. Pelvic floor exercises have been shown to reduce the frequency of incontinence after delivery in other studies (35).

The most consistent positive outcome measure found in the studies was the personally experienced effect of exercise on physical and psychological wellbeing of the women. All the studies investigating this parameter demonstrated a significant improvement in the exercise group, though in medical terms this is not the most important, for the women to feel better was very important.

None of the studies in this review followed the children postpartum; there are retrospective studies looking at morphometry and neuropsychological development of children in mothers who actively trained in pregnancy (36, 37). These children had similar if not higher scores on neuropsychological testing. The studies included in this review all delivered healthy children and it would be interesting to have follow up studies of their development. None of the studies in this review showed a direct positive effect on the fetus or child of physically active women.

REFERENCES

[1]   Lokey EA, Tran ZV, Wells CL, Myers BC, Tran AC Effects of physical exercise on pregnancy outcomes: a meta-analytic review. *Medicine and Science in Sports and Exercise* 1991; Vol. 23, No. 11; 1234-9

[2]   Kramer MS. Aerobic exercise for women during pregnancy (Cochrane review) In: *the Cochrane Library*, Issue 2, 2002

[3]   Nordhagen IH, Sundgot-Borgen J. Fysisk aktivitet hos gravide i relasjon til svangerskapsplager og depressive symptomer. *Tidsskrift for den Norske Lægeforening nr.* 5, 2002; 122: 470-4

[4]   Bjørndal A, Flottorp S, Klovning A. Medisinsk kunnskapshåndtering. *Gyldendal Akademisk* 2000

[5]   Chalmers TC, Celano P, Sacks HS, Smith H. Bias in treatment assignment in controlled clinical trials. *New England Journal of Medicine* 1983; 309:1358-61

[6]   Kuns R, Oxman AD. The unpredictability paradox: review of empirical comparisons of randomised and non-randomised clinical trials. *British Medical Journal* 1998; 317: 1185-90

[7]   Jadad AR, Moore RA, Carroll D, Jenkinson C, Reynolds JM, Gavaghan DJ, McQuay HJ. Assessing the quality of reports of randomised clinical trials: is blinding necessary? *Controlled Clinical Trials* 1996; 17: 1-12

[8]   Bell R, Palma S. Antenatal exercise and birth weight. *Australian and New Zeeland Journal of Obstetrics and Gynaecology* 2000; 40; 1: 70-73

[9]   Carpenter MW, Sady Sp, Sady MA, Haydon BB, Coustan DR, Thompson PD. effects of exercise training in midpregancy: a randomised controlled trial. *Annual meeting – society for gynaecologic investigation* 1990; 497

[10]   Clapp JF, Kim H, Burciu B, Lopez B. Beginning regular exercise in early pregnancy: effect on fetoplacental growth. *American Journal of Obstetrics and Gynaecology* 2000; 183: 1484-8

[11]   Clapp JF, Kim H, Burciu B, Schmidt S, Petry K, Lopez B. Continuing regular exercise during pregnancy: effect of exercise volume on fetoplacental growth. *American Journal of Obstetrics and Gynaecology* 2002; 186: 142-7

[12]   Collings CA, Curet LB, Mullin JP. Maternal and fetal responses to a maternal aerobic exercise program. *American Journal of Obstetrics and Gynaecology* 1983; 145: 702-707

[13] Erkkola R. The influence of physical training during pregnancy on physical work capacity and circulatory parameters. *Scandinavian Journal of Clinical Laboratory Investigations* 1976; 36: 747-54

[14] Kulpa PJ, White BM, Visscher R. Aerobic exercise in pregnancy. *American Journal of Obstetrics and Gynaecology* 1987; 156: 1395-403

[15] Lee G. Exercise in pregnancy. Modern Midwife 1996; 6: 28-33

[16] Marquez-Sterling S, Perry AC, Kaplan TA, Halberstein A, Signorlie JF. Physical and psychological changes with vigorous exercise in sedentary primigravidae. *Medicine and Science in Sports and Exercise* 2000; 32 (1): 58-62

[17] Pijpers L, Wladimiroff JW, Mcghie J. effect of short-term maternal exercise on maternal and fetal cardiovascular dynamics. *British Journal of Obstetrics and Gynaecology* 1984; 91: 1081-6

[18] Prevedel TTS, Calderon IMP, Abadde JF, Borges VTM, Rudge MVC. Maternal effects of hydrotherapy in normal pregnant women. *Journal of Perinatal Medicine* 2001; 29 (Suppl 1, part 2): 665-6

[19] Sibley L, Ruhling RO, Cameron-Foster J, Christensen C, Bolen T. Swimming and physical fitness during pregnancy. *Journal of Nurse Midwifery* 1981; 26, 3-12

[20] South-Paul JE, Rajagopal KR, Tenholder MF. The effect of participation in a regular exercise program upon aerobic capacity during pregnancy. *Obstetrics and Gynaecology* 1989; 71; 175-9

[21] Varassi G, Bazzano C, Edwards T. Effects of physical activity on maternal plasma beta-endorphin levels and perception of labour pain. *American Journal of Obstetrics and Gynaecology* 1988; 71: 175-9

[22] Bergsjø P, Maltau JM, Molne K, Nesheim BI. Obstetrikk. *Gyldendal Akademisk* 2000, 3. utgave

[23] Artal R. Exercise and pregnancy. *Clinics in Sports Medicine* 1992; 11; 2; 363-76

[24] Calguneri M, Bird HA, Wright V. Changes in joint laxity occurring during pregnancy. *Ann Rhem Dis* 1982; 41; 126-8

[25] Hytten FE, Chamberlain G. *Clinical Physiology in Obstetrics*. Oxford. Blackwell, 1980

[26] ACOG Technical Bulletin Number 189. Exercise during pregnancy and the postpartum period. *International Journal of Gynaecology and Obstetrics* 1994; 45: 65-70

[27] Berne RM, Levy MN. Principles of physiology. *Mosby* 2000, 3. edition

[28] Artal R, Wiswell RA, Drinkwater BL. *Exercise in pregnancy*. Baltimore; Williams and Wilkins 1991, 2. edition

[29] Halbert JA, Silagy CA, Finucane P, Withers RT, Hamdorf PA, Andrews GR. The effectiveness of exercise training in lowering blood pressure: a meta-analysis of randomised controlled trials of 4 weeks or longer. *Journal of Human Hypertension* 1997; 11 (10): 641-9

[30] Edwards MJ. Hyperthermia as a teratogen: a review of experimental studies and their clinical significance. *Teratogenesis Carcinog Mutagen* 1986; 6: 563-82

[31] Lindqvist PG, Marsal K, Merlo J, Pirhonen JP. Thermal response to submaximal exercise before, during and after pregnancy: a longitudinal study. *Journal of Maternal and Fetal Neonatal Medicine* 2003 Mar; 13 (3): 152-6

[32] Clapp JF, Seaward BL, Sleamaker RH, Hiser L. Maternal physiologic adaptations to early human pregnancy. *American Journal of Obstetrics and Gynaecology* 1988; 159; 1456-60

[33]   Bung P, Artal R, Khodiguian N. Regular exercise therapy in disorders of carbohydrate
       metabolism in pregnancy – results of a prospective, randomised longitudinal study.
       Journal of Perinatal Medicine 1993 Mar; 53 (3): 188-93

[34]   Jovanovic-Peterson L, Durak Ep, Peterson CM. Randomised trial of diet versus diet
       plus cardiovascular conditioning on glucose levels in gestational diabetes. *American
       Journal of Obstetrics and Gynaecology* 1989; 161: 415-9

[35]   Harvey MA. Pelvic floor exercises during and after pregnancy: a systematic review of
       their role in preventing pelvic floor dysfunction. *Journal of Obstetrics and
       Gynaecology* Canada 2003 Jun; 25 (6): 487-98

[36]   Clapp JF, Simonian S, Lopez B, Appelby-wineberg S, Harcar-sevcik R. The one-year
       morphometric and neurodevelopmental outcome of the offspring of women who
       continued to exercise regularly throughout pregnancy. *American Journal of Obstetrics
       and Gynaecology* 1998; 178; 594-9

[37]   Clapp JF, Capeless El. Neonatal morphometrics after endurance exercise during
       pregnancy. *American Journal of Obstetrics and Gynaecology* 1990; 163: 1805-11

In: Weight Loss, Exercise and Health Research
Editor: Carrie P. Saylor, pp. 231-247

ISBN 1-60021-077-5
© 2006 Nova Science Publishers, Inc.

Chapter 11

ESTROGEN INFLUENCE ON SKELETAL MUSCLE DAMAGE, REPAIR AND FUNCTION

Peter M. Tiidus[1]

Department of Kinesiology and Physical Education
Wilfrid Laurier University

ABSTRACT

Recent research, primarily in rodent models, has demonstrated that estrogen can diminish post-exercise skeletal muscle leukocyte infiltration, as well reduce a number of indices of muscle damage. Data on estrogen influence in humans, primarily based on male versus female comparisons, has produced more conflicting results. There are several mechanisms by which estrogen can potentially influence muscle damage and inflammatory responses following exercise-induced disruption. However, more research is necessary to determine the role of these mechanisms in estrogenic effects on skeletal muscle. Although some preliminary data is available, the physiological significance of the potential influence of estrogen on muscle damage and inflammatory responses has also yet to be characterized. In particular, the potential effects of estrogen on muscle repair mechanisms are just beginning to be explored. In addition, several human and animal studies have suggested that estrogen may also influence skeletal muscle strength, fatigue and function and that there may be interactive effects of estrogen and progesterone in these effects. This review will provide an overview and summary of these estrogen and skeletal muscle related controversies. It will also discuss the potential implications of estrogenic influence on skeletal muscle damage, repair and function in humans. These issues are particularly relevant to post-menopausal females and relate to the health controversies associated with post-menopausal hormone replacement therapy.

---

[1] Corresponding author: Peter M. Tiidus, Ph.D.Professor and Chair Department of Kinesiology and Physical Education Wilfrid Laurier University Waterloo ON Canada N2L 3C5 ptiidus@wlu.ca , 519-884-0710 ext. 4157, 519-747-4594 (fax)

Key words: Estrogen, skeletal muscle, muscle damage, muscle repair, muscle strength, post-menopausal females

INTRODUCTION

While the effects of testosterone on skeletal muscle are fairly well known, the potential influence of estrogen on skeletal muscle has not yet received the same amount of attention. Nevertheless, there is a growing body of research evidence, which suggests that estrogen can have significant effects on a number of aspects of skeletal muscle function, development and physiology. This chapter will specifically highlight the potential for estrogen to affect skeletal muscle damage, inflammation and repair processes following intense exercise or other damaging insult and the potential effects of estrogen on skeletal muscle function in a relevant female human model.

GENERAL EFFECTS OF ESTROGEN ON SKELETAL MUSCLE

Estrogen is an important hormone with a range of functions associated primarily with female sexual characteristics and function. However estrogen also has a significant number of other important effects on many other tissues including skeletal muscle. Specifically, in skeletal muscle, estrogen has been shown to reduce carbohydrate utilization and increase fat utilization in skeletal muscle during exercise (D'eon et al. 2002). In addition, estrogen can influence muscle cell growth (Kahlert et al. 1997) and possibly the maintenance of muscle mass in post-menopausal women (Sipilä et al. 2001). Estrogen can also influence skeletal muscle fatigue and twitch characteristics (Hatae 2001, McCormick et al. 2004) and the expression of muscle proteins such as myosin heavy chains associated with fast and slow skeletal muscle characteristics (Kadi et al. 2002). Estrogen will also have indirect effects on skeletal muscle in rodent models by influencing the spontaneous activity levels of rats as assessed by wheel running and open field movement (Ogawa et al. 2001).

The presence of estrogen receptors on skeletal muscle has been repeatedly demonstrated (Kahlert et al. 1997, Lemoine et a. 2002. Lemoine et al. 2003). However it is likely that the full effects of estrogen on skeletal muscle may be influenced by both receptor mediated and other non-receptor mediated mechanisms (Nadal et al. 2001).

ESTROGEN EFFECTS ON TISSUE DAMAGE AND INFLAMMATION

While this chapter focuses on the influence of estrogen on skeletal muscle damage, inflammation and repair, it is instructive to note that estrogen has been demonstrated to attenuate damage and inflammatory responses in a number of other tissues as well. Specifically, a number of studies have demonstrated that estrogen can significantly diminish post-insult damage and inflammatory responses in neurological tissue and the brain (Sribnick et al. 2004, Moosman and Behl 1999), the vascular endothelium (Karas et al. 2001), liver

(Harada et al. 2001), skin (Ashcroft et al. 1999) and cardiac muscle (Squadrito et al. 1997) among others.

The various mechanisms by which estrogen may be acting in these tissues to diminish damage and inflammation and to aid repair may be ubiquitous to numerous tissues (Dubey and Jackson 2001, Sribnick et al. 2004) and generally correspond, with some exceptions, with mechanisms by through which estrogen may act on skeletal muscle (Bär and Amelink 1997, Tiidus 2001). These mechanisms will be discussed in greater detail later in this chapter. Hence, the potential ability of estrogen to influence skeletal muscle damage, inflammation and repair in skeletal muscle is not unique, but is instead a general effect of estrogen which is manifest in many other tissues. As will be detailed in this chapter, the question of whether estrogen can influence post-exercise skeletal muscle damage, inflammation and repair is not one of, if; but rather to what degree this is possible in humans and to what extent is this ability physiologically and functionally significant.

ESTROGEN INFLUENCE ON SKELETAL MUSCLE DAMAGE

A considerable body of evidence has accumulated which demonstrates the attenuating influence of estrogen on indices of damage in cardiac muscle following ischemia-reperfusion injury both in isolated and whole body animal and human models (i.e Dubey and Jackson 2001, Xu et al. 2004, Node 1997). The effects of estrogen on indices of skeletal muscle damage, particularly following exercise or eccentric muscle contractions are less extensively documented.

A common clinical measure of exercise induced muscle disruption is the elevation of circulating levels of creatine kinase (CK) (Clarkson and Sayers 1999). Creatine kinase is a metabolic enzyme which is prone to unintended transversal of the sarcolemma membrane when muscle or membrane damage occurs. Although circulating CK level has been used as an indirect marker of skeletal muscle damage, it is a relatively poor quantitative indicator of actual muscle structural disruption. Nevertheless, post-exercise changes in circulating CK level can be a relatively sensitive indicator of muscle sarcolemma membrane perturbation (Clarkson and Sayers 1999).

A series of roden- based studies clearly demonstrated an attenuating effect of estrogen on post-exercise muscle CK leakage. Bär et al. (1988) reported that ovariectomized female rats and male rats had significantly greater elevations in circulating CK activity than normal female rats following exercise. They further found that treating ovariectomized female rats and male rats with estrogen prevented post-exercise elevations in circulating CK activities and were similar to the results seen in normal female rats. To further bolster the relationship between estrogen and the loss of muscle CK via sarcolemma disruption, Amelink et al (1990) electrically stimulated isolated muscles from male, female and ovariectomized female rats with or without estrogen replacement. In all cases, estrogen replacement greatly diminished in vitro CK loss from isolated muscles following electrical stimulation. Other more recent studies have also reported that estrogen replacement would significantly diminish post-exercise or post-injury elevations in serum CK activity in rodents (Tiidus et al. 2001, Sotiriadou et al. 2003, Feng et al. 2004). These studies provide compelling evidence for an effect of estrogen in stabilizing muscle sarcolemma membranes and attenuating exercise induced muscle sarcolemma disruption, at least in animal models.

Few human studies have directly examined the influence of estrogen or estrogen supplementation on indices of post-exercise muscle sarcolemma disruption on CK release. However, it has been well documented that adult human females will typically have lower serum CK elevations following muscular exercise than males (Shumate et al. 1979, Tiidus and Ianuzzo 1983, Stupka et al. 2000). This has been interpreted as an effect of estrogen on membrane stabilization (Amelink and Bär 1986).

Other indirect evidence of the potential for estrogen to influence post-exercise muscle disruption is its effects on heat shock proteins (HSP). HSPs are rapidly synthesized in tissues in response to various forms of stress, including exercise and muscle damage. Their primary function is to act a "chaperones" for protein folding following synthesis and they are important assistants for protein synthesis and assembly during recovery from exercise (Paroo et al. 2002). Two studies (Paroo et al. 1999, Paroo et al. 2002) have demonstrated that estrogen can attenuate specific HSP (HSP70) expression in skeletal muscle of rodents following exercise. This has been interpreted as a protective effect of estrogen on exercise induced muscle disruption since HSP70 is induced by exercise stress and muscle disruption. Estrogen has also been demonstrated to attenuate indices of oxidative stress in injured muscles of rats, suggesting a potential for reduction in free radical induced damage (Feng et al. 2004). However, not all studies have found direct evidence for estrogenic attenuation of indices of oxidative stress following exercise in rodents (Tiidus et al. 1998).

Evidence for estrogen influence on post-exercise muscle structural disruption is also not yet complete. Only a limited number of animal studies have examined gender differences on muscle structural damage and have not always produced consistent results. Few studies have directly examined the effects of estrogen on these parameters. Using a downhill running model, Komulainen et al. (1999), found that for up to 96 hours following downhill running, male animals generally experienced greater and earlier histo-pathological indices of damage to muscle structural proteins (desmin, dystrophin actin etc.) and a greater degree of muscle fibre swelling. They also noted much higher muscular activities of beta-glucuronidase (a lysosomal enzyme activated in response to muscle damage) in male than female animals (Komulainen et al. 1999). Another, earlier study had also noted greater disruption of histochemically determined muscle banding patterns in male than in female rats at 2 days following intense exercise (Amelink et al. 1991). However, Van der Meulen et al. (1991) did not note any histologically determined differences in muscle damage in male and female rats following exercise of greater intensity and duration than that employed by Amelink et al (1991).

A recent study examined the effects of gender on muscle lesions and damage in mdx mice (mice with inherited Duchenne muscular dystrophy) (Salimena et al. 2004). This study concluded that female hormones were at least partially responsible for the lower levels of muscle damage indicators and lesions seen in female compared to male mdx mice (Salimena et al. 2004).

Hence, although relatively few studies that have examined gender or direct estrogen effects on differences in susceptibility to muscle damage in rodents, the majority of these studies have suggested a protective effect of estrogen, based primarily on gender differences, on various forms of damage. However, more research is needed using models, which directly manipulate estrogen levels to confirm these tentative conclusions.

Human studies comparing gender differences in susceptibility to muscle damage have tended to use indirect measures of muscle damage such as muscle swelling, stiffness, soreness and loss of muscle force (Clarkson and Sayers 1999). These studies have generally not found major gender differences in the degree of muscle damage induced by unaccustomed exercise (as determined by the above indirect indicators of damage) (Sayers and Clarkson 2001, Clarkson and Hubal 2001).

Ayers et al. (1998) did report higher indices of lipid peroxidation (which may be related to the degree of muscle or muscle membrane disruption) in amenorrheic female athletes than in normal female athletes following exercise, which they attributed to differences in circulating estrogen levels. Dernbach et al (1993) also reported that female rowers had lower blood indices of oxidative stress than male rowers during an intense 30 day training cycle. In contrast, Chung et al. (1999) did not find any differences in indices of oxidative stress following exercise in females during different phases of the menstrual cycle.

Stupka et al. (2000, 2001) examined histochemical indices of muscle damage in biopsy samples from eccentrically exercise quadriceps muscles from males and females and did not consistently find gender based differences in the degree of damage observed. However, the large variability inherent in biopsy assessments of human muscle damage following eccentric exercise may mask any subtle gender based differences.

Taken together the limited number of studies examining gender differences in susceptibility to exercise induced muscle damage do not yet suggest that there are major differences present in humans. However, studies directly examining the potential for estrogen to diminish exercise induced muscle damage have yet to be performed. The potential effects of estrogen on muscle damage and post-exercise recovery could have particular relevance for post-menopausal females where estrogen levels have been drastically reduced (Tiidus 2003). It may be likely that pre- and post-menopausal women would manifest greater estrogen based differences in susceptibility to muscle damage than seen in human gender based differences. Indeed, Roth et al (2000) reported greater evidence of ultra-structural muscle damage in older (65-75 years) than younger (20-30 years) females following strength training, while no such differences were found between older and younger males. They attributed the differences in training-induced muscle damage between older (post-menopausal) and younger females at least partially to differences in circulating estrogen levels. These possibilities need to be addressed with more targeted research involving this population.

ESTROGEN INFLUENCE ON POST-EXERCISE MUSCLE INFLAMMATORY RESPONSES

Exercise induced muscle damage and membrane disruption is typically followed by leukocyte infiltration seen as an early neutrophil influx and a later macrophage influx (Tiidus 1998, Malm et al. 2000). Neutrophils and macrophages are important in assisting in the clearance of damaged tissue and in the activation of muscle satellite cells and repair processes (Tiidus 1998, Chalmers and McDermott 1996). Since, neutrophils in particular have been demonstrated to increase inflammation related damage following injury in skeletal muscle as well as other tissues (Walden et al. 1990, Tiidus 1998, Sribnick et al. 2004), the attenuation of their infiltration may be associated with reduced injury (Squadrito et al. 1997, Tiidus et al.

2001). Alternatively, macrophages are critical in activating muscle satellite cells and repair processes (Anderson and Wozniak 2004). Hence, attenuation or delay in their infiltration could also delay skeletal muscle repair (St. Pierre-Schneider et al. 1999, Tiidus 2001).

As previously noted, estrogen has been shown to diminish post-damage leukocyte infiltration in a number of other tissues including cardiac muscle, brain and neurological tissues, liver and vascular endothelium (Sribnick et al. 2004, Moosman and Behl 1999, Karas et al. 2001, Harada et al. 2001, Squadrito et al. 1997). Hence it is not surprising that several studies have also reported the attenuating effect of estrogen on post-damage leukocyte infiltration in skeletal muscle (Tiidus and Bombardier 1999, St. Pierre-Schneider et al. 1999, Tiidus et al. 2001, Stupka and Tiidus 2001, Tiidus et al. 2005).

Tiidus and Bombardier (1999) where the first to report that female rats exhibited significantly attenuated neutrophil infiltration into skeletal muscles at 24 hours following running exercise compared to male rats. When male rats where administered daily estrogen injections for 14 days prior to exercise they also exhibited the same blunted increase in post-exercise muscle neutrophil infiltration as female rats. Subsequently, this finding was confirmed using overiectomized female rats with or without estrogen replacement and assessing muscle neutrophil infiltration one hour post-exercise via histochemical and biochemical methods (Tiidus et al. 2001). Estrogen administration to ovariectomized female rats also attenuated neutrophil infiltration into skeletal muscle at 2 hours following ischemia-reperfusion induced injury (Stupka and Tiidus 2001).

It is possible that the effects of estrogen on mitigating post-exercise increases in muscle neutrophil infiltration may be influenced by muscle fibre type. The above studies all examined plantaris muscle, which is of mixed fibre type. A subsequent study (Tiidus 2005) found that estrogen administration to male rats continued to diminish elevations in neutrophil infiltration following downhill running in a primarily type I fibre population muscle (soleus) but not in a primarily type II fibre population muscle (white vastus). This finding needs to be confirmed with further research.

No studies have yet directly reported on the influence of estrogen on other leukocyte (specifically macrophages) infiltration of skeletal muscle following damage. St. Pierre-Schneider et al. (1999) reported delayed macrophage infiltration in female mouse muscle relative to males following eccentric contraction induced injury. They attributed this finding to possible influences of estrogen. Further studies are warranted to more definitively document any influence of estrogen on post-damage skeletal muscle macrophage infiltration.

As with measures of muscle damage, no studies to date have attempted to directly examine the effects of estrogen on post-exercise leukocyte infiltration into human skeletal muscle following exercise. Three studies have reported on gender-based differences, possibly attributable at least in part to estrogen, on leukocyte infiltration into quadriceps muscles following eccentric exercise (Stupka et al. 2000, MacIntyre et al. 2000, Stupka et al. 2001). Using a non-specific histochemical marker for leukocytes, Stupka et al. (2000) reported relatively greater increases in indices of leukocyte infiltration of the quadriceps muscles in males versus females at 48 hours post-exercise. However, a subsequent study by the same group reported no attenuation of either neutrophil or macrophage infiltration into quadriceps muscle of females relative to males following either one or two bouts of eccentric muscle contractions (Stupka et al. 2001). Both of these studies relied on muscle biopsy samples and immuno-histochemistry to assess muscle leukocyte infiltration. As previously noted, the potentially large variability in determining muscle leukocyte infiltration from biopsy samples may have confounded some of these results.

Using radioactive labeling of neutrophils and nuclear imaging of the thigh region, MacIntyre et al. (2000) also assessed gender differences in muscle neutrophil infiltration at 2 and 4 hours post-eccentric exercise. In apparent contrast to the rodent studies (i.e. Tiidus et al. 2001) and one of the above human studies (Stupka et al. 2000) they reported significantly greater elevations in neutrophil presence in post-exercise muscles of females relative to males (MacIntyre et al. 2000).

There are as of yet to few studies, with too many methodological differences and limitations to adequately assess the potential effects of estrogen on post-damage muscle leukocyte infiltration in humans. However, the consistent, albeit limited, evidence from rodent models which has examined skeletal muscle and other tissues, strongly suggests that estrogen does exert a meaningful attenuating effect on the leukocyte infiltration phase of inflammatory responses to damage in skeletal muscle. The extent and physiological significance of this effect in humans remains to be determined.

A confounding variable that may influence gender-based comparisons of post-exercise leukocyte infiltration is the potential antagonizing effects of progesterone on estrogen influence on inflammation. Recently, Xing et al. (2004) reported that estrogen diminished leukocyte infiltration into the vascular endothelium of ovariectomized female rats following injury and progesterone had no independent effect on leukocyte infiltration. However, when both estrogen and progesterone were provided to the ovariectomized rats, the presence of progesterone completely negated the attenuating influence of estrogen on post-damage leukocyte infiltration into the vascular endothelium. This possibility could also explain some of the variability found in the limited number of human studies that have looked at gender differences in post-exercise muscle leukocyte infiltration.

ESTROGEN INFLUENCE ON POST-EXERCISE MUSCLE REPAIR

If estrogen does have a significant effect on muscle damage and inflammation, can it also influence skeletal muscle repair? Until recently very few studies have attempted to assess the potential for estrogenic influence on skeletal muscle repair. Activation and proliferation of skeletal muscle satellite cells are critical in the regeneration process of muscle (Charge and Rudnicki 2004). Three recent studies using rodent models (Feng et al. 2004, Salimena et al. 2004, Tiidus et al. 2005) provide some preliminary evidence for the potential of estrogen to significantly influence skeletal muscle repair and regeneration mechanisms involving muscle satellite cells.

As previously noted, Salimena et al (2004) used mdx mice (mice with inherited Duchenne muscular dystrophy) to examine, among other things, gender differences in muscle degeneration and regeneration processes. Their findings suggested that greater muscle regeneration, as determined by immuno-histochemical detection of markers for activated muscle satellite cells, was occurring in the female mdx mice than in the males. This resulted in significantly less dystrophic necrosis in the female mice than in the male mice and suggested that female hormones such as estrogen played an important role in up-regulating muscle repair mechanisms and satellite cell activation and suppressing inflammation in mdx mice. This suggestion was further supported by findings that ovariectomized and older female mdx mice did not enjoy the same muscle regeneration or satellite cell activities as seen in younger female mice with higher estrogen levels (Salimena et al. 2004).

In a study more relevant to normal humans, Feng et al. (2004) also reported on muscle regeneration, as determined by a histochemical marker of muscle satellite cell activation (desmin), following strain induced injury, in normal and ovariectomized female rats with low or high levels of estrogen supplementation. They suggested that increased activation of muscle satellite cells may have been occurring in injured muscles of normal and high-estrogen replaced ovariectomized females when compared to the low-estrogen ovariectomized females. This would suggest that estrogen could influence the degree of post-injury muscle satellite cell activation, possibly leading to greater repair potential. (Feng et al. 2004).

A very recent study from our laboratory (Tiidus 2005) also suggests an accentuating effect of estrogen on muscle satellite cell activation following eccentric exercise in rats. In this study, male rats with or without estrogen supplementation performed eccentrically biased exercise by running downhill on a treadmill. Three days later immuno-histochemical determination of muscle satellite cells found that male rats with estrogen supplementation had significantly greater numbers of activated satellite cells in both predominantly fast (white vastus) and slow (soleus) muscles than male rats without estrogen supplementation (Tiidus et al. 2005). This finding again suggested that higher estrogen levels would apparently stimulate greater increases in muscle repair mechanisms following exercise-induced muscle disruption and potentially enhance rate of muscle recovery.

Taken together, these studies suggest that estrogen may indeed be a factor in influencing muscle repair mechanisms and that further more comprehensive research is warranted to follow up on these preliminary results. To date, no human studies have addressed the issue of estrogen or gender influence on muscle repair or satellite cell activation and proliferation.

MECHANISMS OF ESTROGEN INFLUENCE ON SKELETAL MUSCLE DAMAGE

The above sections outlined the growing evidence for the ability of estrogen to influence skeletal muscle damage, inflammation and repair indices. While more research is required, particularly in humans, to firmly establish the parameters and physiological significance of estrogen influence on skeletal muscle damage and recovery, it is instructive to examine the potential mechanisms by which estrogen may be able to influence these processes.

A number of studies have established that estrogen is a strong in vitro antioxidant (Tiidus 1995). Unlike similar steroid hormones testosterone and progesterone, which have no antioxidant properties, estrogen possesses a hydroxyl group on their "A" steroid ring (analogous to that found on the antioxidant vitamin E) (Sugioka et al. 1987). By donating a hydrogen ion from the hydroxyl group, estrogen maybe able to terminate peroxidation chain reactions and thus act as an antioxidant (Sugioka et al. 1987). A number of studies have also noted the antioxidant potential for estrogen in various physiological in vivo situations (i.e. Hernandez et al. 2001). However, as noted earlier in this chapter, the evidence for a strong antioxidant effect of estrogen, which may protect muscle from oxidative stress induced damage during and following exercise is at best contradictory. Hence, the primary mechanisms by which estrogen may act in skeletal muscle may involve other avenues of action.

Since both estrogen apha- and beta- receptors are present in skeletal muscle (Lemoine et al. 2002, Wiik et al. 2003), it is also possible that some estrogen influence on muscle damage and membrane stability is receptor mediated.

Estrogen may also be able to act as a membrane stabilizer by being directly incorporated in muscle cell membranes (Tiidus 1995, Amelink and Bär 1997). Estrogen has been reported to have direct effects on membrane fluidity (Whiting et al. 2000). It may well be this property of estrogen, which can act to diminish sarcolemma disruption and the previously noted serum CK elevations, which are indicative of muscle membrane disruption (Tiidus 2003).

By diminishing sarcolemma disruption, estrogen could also help maintain cellular calcium homeostasis by dampening the damage induced extra-cellular calcium influx into muscle that characteristically occurs with exercise-induced muscle damage (Tiidus 2003). Loss of calcium homeostasis will activate phospholipases which can break down membrane phospholipids (Sribnick et al. 2004) and muscle proteolytic enzymes such as calpain, which will then aid in removing damaged proteins and perhaps occasion further inflammation related muscle disruption (Belcastro et al. 1998). By stabilizing muscle sarcolemma and thus maintaining, cellular calcium homeostasis, estrogen could diminish activation of muscle proteolytic enzymes such as calpain (Tiidus et al. 2001, Tiidus 2003). Indeed, we have demonstrated that estrogen will attenuate muscle calpain activity following exercise in ovariectomized female rats, possibly through such mechanisms (Tiidus et al. 2001).

Hence estrogen may diminish not only direct exercise induced damage but also secondary muscle damage associated with reactions to initial damage such as proteolysis or inflammation.

MECHANISMS OF ESTROGEN INFLUENCE ON SKELETAL MUSCLE INFLAMMATION

As previously noted, estrogen will likely also diminish neutrophil infiltration and thereby potentially reduce the secondary damage which neutrophils may cause in assisting to clear damaged muscle via oxidative reactions (Tiidus 1998, Tiidus 2001). Since neutrophils are clearly implicated in oxygen radical induced tissue damage during inflammation (Schlag et al. 2001), the attenuation of neutrophil infiltration by estrogen could clearly be a factor in reducing further muscle damage.

There are a number of potential mechanisms by which estrogen may be able to influence post-damage muscle neutrophil infiltration. One possibility is related to the potential for calpain proteolytic activity to produce neutrophil chemo-attractive peptides (Belcastro et al. 1998). By inhibiting calpain activity following exercise, as described above, estrogen may reduce the amount of calpain produced neutrophil chemo-attractants and thus the amount of neutrophil infiltration into damaged muscle (Tiidus 2003). We have previously demonstrated the correlation of such events in rodent muscles (Tiidus et al. 2001).

Other studies using other tissues have also linked estrogen to the attenuation of leukocyte infiltration by other mechanisms, which may also be factors in estrogen influence on leukocyte infiltration in skeletal muscle.

Estrogen has been shown to up-regulate nitric oxide synthase (NOS) in the endothelium and thereby mitigate leukocyte rolling, adhesion and infiltration in to injured endothelia, induced by ischemia-reperfusion injury (Prorock et al 2003). Tissues in female animals also have greater amounts of NOS than found in male animals (Laughlin et al. 2003). Increases in nitric oxide in skeletal muscle also can inhibit calpain activation and thereby also reduce secondary inflammation and damage (Koh and Tidball 2000). Increases in tissue NO production may occur through direct estrogen action on NOS or via estrogen receptor mediated influence on NO production (Harada et al. 2001). Several studies have also found that some tissues are protected from damage and leukocyte infiltration via estrogen receptor mediated mechanisms (Karas et al. 2001, Pare et al. 2002), possibly by influencing calcium activated potassium channels (Node et al. 1997).

Estrogen may also be able to limit the binding of the pro-inflammatory transcription factor NFκB to DNA, thereby limiting a number of inflammatory related responses in tissues (Sribnick et al. 2004). These responses could include the inhibition of the transcription of leukocyte chemoattractants such as monocyte chemoattractant protein 1 and matrix mettalloproteinase-9 (Sribnick et al. 2004). Studies have also suggested that estrogen can limit leukocyte infiltration by other mechanisms including, inhibition of TNF-α production and thereby limiting the ICAM-1 mediated binding of leukocytes to injured tissues (Squadrito et al. 1997).

The mechanisms by which estrogen may be able to influence leukocyte infiltration into skeletal muscle are not yet know, but will likely involve several of the above and possibly other mechanisms in multi-factoral ways. In addition, further research may be necessary to clarify the potential interactive and counteractive effects of the combination of estrogen and progesterone in influencing leukocyte infiltration (Xing et al. 2004). These interactions may be critical to understanding estrogen influence in real situations involving younger and post-menopausal human females.

MECHANISMS OF ESTROGEN INFLUENCE ON SKELETAL MUSCLE REPAIR

Most studies agree that inhibition of neutrophil infiltration into tissues and skeletal muscle will likely reduce secondary injury and thereby enhance repair (Tiidus 2001). However, the infiltration of macrophages are important for the activation of muscle satellite cells and subsequent muscle repair (Chargé and Rudnicki 2004). The potential inhibition of macrophages into skeletal muscle by estrogen may therefore theoretically inhibit skeletal muscle recovery (Tiidus 2001). However, as previously noted in this chapter, the overall effects of estrogen on muscle and other tissues tends to be to reduce damage and to speed regeneration. Hence, if estrogen does inhibit macrophage infiltration and their subsequent activation of satellite cells in skeletal muscle, other damage inhibiting and regenerative processes may be sufficient to outweigh this potential disadvantage.

A number of trophic factors from secreted from macrophages or generated within the damaged muscle itself have been demonstrated to stimulate satellite cell activation and muscle regenerative processes following muscle damage. These include, hepatic growth factor (HGF), insulin-like growth factor-1 (IGF-1) and interleukin-6 (IL-6) and other cytokine family growth factors (Chargé and Rudnicki 2004). The interaction of these and other regulatory factors in muscle satellite cell activation and muscle repair regulation are complex and not yet fully understood. Nevertheless, estrogen has been demonstrated to potentially influence at least some of these factors, particularly HGF and IGF-1 levels in skeletal muscle (Hawke and Garry 2001, Chargé and Rudnicki 2004) via influence over regulatory mechanisms such as NO production in muscle (Prorock et al. 2002). Hence while the mechanisms by which estrogen might influence muscle satellite cell activation and muscle repair are unknown, there are several theoretical mechanisms by which estrogen may be able to exert a positive influence. More research is needed to begin to tease out these possibilities. This is particularly important since some preliminary findings in animals (Tiidus et al. 2005, Salimena 2004) suggest that estrogen can indeed positively influence post-damage repair and muscle satellite cell numbers. The implication of these possibilities in humans, are as of yet unknown.

PRACTICAL IMPLICATIONS OF ESTROGEN INFLUENCE ON MUSCLE FUNCTION AND STRENGTH IN HUMANS

The previous sections have outlined the evidence for estrogenic influence on skeletal muscle damage, inflammation and repair. If estrogen can indeed significantly diminish muscle damage and aid recovery (something which particularly in humans is not yet certain), this could have a number of potential implications. Most applicably there could be significant implications for post-menopausal females who may now have noticeably greater potential to sustain muscle damage from trauma or exercise and be slower to heal. The controversial health effects of hormone replacement therapy (Grady 2003, Grodstein et al. 2003) in older females would also be factors in considering whether estrogen replacement alone or in combination with progesterone would ultimately show short or longer- term benefits for muscular health of older females.

In addition to potentially influencing muscle damage and repair mechanisms, there are also some suggestions that skeletal muscle strength, fatigue and trainability may also be influenced by estrogen in older females (Sipilä et al. 2001), perhaps via some of the mechanisms discussed in this chapter. As earlier pointed out, estrogen may be able to influence skeletal muscle growth and protein expression (Kahlert et al 1997, Kadi et al 2002) in animal models. The potential for estrogen supplementation to help maintain muscle mass and strength, particularly in older females is intriguing and potentially significant.

The evidence for estrogen influencing skeletal muscle mass, strength and fatigue in older females is generally positive. Several studies have suggested that hormone replacement may have helped preserve muscle strength or lean body mass over a period of months or years, in sedentary post-menopausal women relative to menopausal and aging related strength or lean body mass loss experienced by similar age women who were not hormone replaced (Phillips et al. 1993, Skelton et al. 1999, Greeves et al. 1999, Sorensen et al. 2001, Teixeira et al.

2002). Other studies have also found that training in combination with estrogen replacement in post-menopausal females enhanced strength gains more than strength training alone and that strength training may increase muscle strength more in post-menopausal females who are estrogen replaced than those that are not (Meeuwsen et al. 2000, Sipilä et al. 2001, Sipilä and Poutamo 2003, Tiidus et al. 2004). It is also possible that strength training induced strength gains in estrogen replaced post-menopausal females may result in functional improvements such as greater dynamic balance stability, and possibly lower risks of falls, than seen in non-estrogen replaced females (Tiidus et al. 2004). Still other studies have reported positive changes in muscle strength and fatigue rate in women in periods of their menstrual cycle during which estrogen levels were higher (Sarwar et al. 1996).

In contrast to these positive findings, a few studies have not shown a relationship between estrogen replacement and muscle strength in post-menopausal females. Two cross-sectional studies have found no significant differences in muscle size, strength or function between post-menopausal females who were on hormone replacement versus those that were not (Seeley et al. 1995, Bemben and Langdon 2002). The reasons for these differences in findings are not immediately clear. It may relate to differences in subject populations, ages, length of time on hormone replacement, study design or other variables. Nevertheless, the majority of studies do seem to point to a relationship between improved muscle strength and function and hormone replacement in post-menopausal women who undertake weight training and in better maintenance of strength in post-menopausal women who are sedentary.

Estrogen might influence skeletal muscle strength and size in post-menopausal females through a number of different mechanisms (Sipilä and Poutamo 2003). Some potential mechanisms include the positive effects of estrogen replacement in stimulating increases in other important anabolic hormones such as growth hormone and insulin-like growth factor-1 in post-menopausal females which would positively influence muscle mass (Kraemer et al. 1998, Sipilä and Poutamo 2003). In addition, it is likely that the influences of estrogen on skeletal muscle damage, inflammation and repair that are discussed in this chapter are significantly involved in these effects.

More research is still needed to establish the effectiveness and physiological significance of estrogen replacement in the maintenance and enhancement of muscle size, strength and function in post-menopausal females. However, if the promises of earlier research are born out, it may be prudent to further evaluate these potentially positive effects of estrogen replacement in post-menopausal females and the implications on their health and capacities for independent living and functioning as they age. These effects would need to be further counterbalanced with the newer data regarding the potential negative health impacts of estrogen replacement in this population (Grady. 2003). Ultimately, prudent, selective and limited use of estrogen replacement may assist in optimizing muscle function, strength and mass in aging female populations with the aim of optimizing their function and independent living capacities into old age.

CONCLUSION

Research, primarily in animal models has demonstrated the potential for estrogen to diminish post-exercise muscle damage and inflammation and enhance repair. These findings need to be further researched in humans, to better establish their actual physiological and practical significance and the physiological mechanisms by which they may act. Nevertheless, there is growing evidence that post-menopausal females in particular may benefit from prudent and selective estrogen replacement in optimizing muscle strength and limiting age related muscle mass loss and functional decline. Further research, is needed to more clearly establish the potential and limitations of estrogen replacement in optimizing the health and muscular function and independent living capacity of aging post-menopausal females.

REFERENCES

Amelink GJ and Bär PR (1986) Exercise-induced protein leakage in the rat: effects of hormone manipulation. *J Neurol Sci* 76: 61-66.

Amelink GJ, Koot RW, Erich W, Van Gijn J and Bär PR (1990) Sex-linked variation in creatine kinase release and its dependence on oestradiol can be demonstrated in and in-vitro rat skeletal muscle preparation. *Acta Physiol Scand* 128: 115-122.

Amelink GJ, Van der Waal W, Van Gijn J and Bär PR (1991) Exercise induced muscle damage in the rat: The effect of vitamin E deficiency. *Pflugers Arch* 412: 417-421.

Anderson JE and Wozniak AC (2004) Satellite cell activation on fibers: modeling events in vivo-an invited review. *Can J Physiol Pharmacol* 82: 300-310.

Ashcroft GS, Greenwell-Wild T, Horan MA, Wahl SM and Ferguson M (1999) Topical estrogen accelerates cutaneous wound healing in aged humans associated with and altered inflammatory response. *Am J Pathol* 155: 1137-1146.

Ayers S. Baer J, and Subbiah MTR (1998) Exercise-induced increase in lipid peroxidation parameters in amenorrheic female athletes. *Fertility Steril* 69: 73-77.

Bär PR and Amelink GJ (1997) Protection against muscle damage exerted by oestrogen: hormonal or antioxidant action? *Biochem Soc Trans* 25: 50-54

Bär PR, Amelink GJ, Oldenburg B and Blankenstein MA (1988) Prevention of exercise-induced muscle membrane damage by oestradiol. *Life Sci* 42: 2677-2680.

Belcastro AN, Shewchuk L and Raj DA (1998) Exercise-induced muscle injury: A calpain hypothesis. *Mol Cell Biochem* 179: 135-145.

Bemben DA and Langdon DB (2002) Relationship between estrogen use and musculoskeletal function in postmenopausal women. *Maturitas* 42: 119-127.

Chalmers RL and McDermott J (1996) Molecular basis of skeletal muscle regeneration. *Can J Appl Physiol* 21: 155-184.

Charge SBP and Rudnicki MA (2004) Cellular and molecular regulation of muscle regeneration *Physiol Rev* 84: 209-238.

Chung SC, Goldfarb AH, Jamurtas AZ, Hegde SS and Lee J (1999) Effect of exercise during the follicular and luteal phases on indices of oxidant stress in healthy women. *Med Sci Sports Exerc* 31: 409-413.

Clarkson PM and Hubal MJ (2001) Are women less susceptible to exercise-induced muscle damage? *Curr Op Clin Nutr Mebabol Care* 4: 527-531.

Clarkson PM and Sayers SP (1999) Etiology of exercise induced muscle damage. *Can J Appl Physiol* 24: 234-248.

D'eon, TM, Sharoff, C, Chipkin SR, Grow D, Ruby BC and Braun B (2002). Regulation of exercise carbohydrate metabolism by estrogen and progesterone in women. *Am J Physiol* 283: E1046-E1055.

Dernbach A, Sherman W, Simonsen J, Flowers K and Lamb D (1993) No evidence of oxidant stress during high-intensity rowing training. *J Appl Physiol* 74: 2140-2145.

Dubey, RK and Jackson EK (2001) Cardiovascular protective effects of 17b-estradiol metabolites. *J Appl Physiol* 91: 1868-1883.

Feng X, Li G and Wand S (2004) Effects of estrogen on gastrocnemius muscle strain injury and regeneration in female rats. *Acta Pharmacol Sin* 25: 1489-1494.

Grady D (2003) Postmenopausal hormones-therapy for symptoms only. *N Eng J Med* 348: 19-23

Greeves JP, Cable NT, Reilly T and Kingsland C. (1999) *Changes in muscle strength in women following the menopause: a longitudinal assessment of the efficacy of hormone replacement therapy.* 97: 79-84.

Grodstein F, Clarkson TB, Manson JE. Understanding the divergent data on postmenopausal hormone therapy. *N Eng J Med* 348: 645-650.

Harada H, Pavlick KP, Hines IN, Hoffman JM, Bharwani S, Gray L, Wolf RE and Grisham MB (2001) Effects of gender on reduced-size liver ischemia and reperfusion injury. *J Appl Physiol* 91: 2816-2822.

Hatae J. (2001) Effects of 17b-estradiol on tension responses and fatigue in the skeletal twitch muscle fibers of frog. *Japanese J Physiol* 51 : 753-759.

Hawke TJ and Garry DJ (2001) Myogenic satellite cells: physiology to molecular biology. *J Appl Physiol* 91: 534-551.

Hernandez I, Delgado JL, Diaz J, Quesada T, Teruel MJG, Llanos C and Carbonell LF (2000) 17b-Estradiol prevents oxidative stress and decreases blood pressure in ovariectomized rats. *Am J Physiol* 279: R1599-R1605.

Kadi F, Karlsson C, Larsson B, Eriksson J, Larval M, Billig H, and Jonsdottir I. (2002) The effects of physical activity and estrogen treatment on rat fast and slow skeletal muscles following ovariectomy. *J Muscle Res Cell Motil* 23: 335-339.

Kahlert S, Grohe C, Karas RH, Lobber K, Ludwig N and Vetter H (1997). Effects of estrogen on skeletal myoblast growth. *Biochem Biophys Res Comm* 232: 373-378.

Karas RH, Schulten H, Pare G, Aronovitz MJ, Ohlsson C, Gustafsson JA and Mendelsohn ME (2001) Effects of estrogen on the vascular injury response in estrogen receptor double knockout mice. *Circ Res* 89:534-539.

Koh TJ, and Tidball JG (2000) Nitric oxide inhibits calpain-mediated proteolysis of talin in skeletal muscle cells. *Am J Physiol* 279: C806-C812.

Komulainen J, Koskinen S, Kalliokoski R, Takala T and Vihko V (1999) Gender differences in skeletal muscle fibre damage after eccentrically biased downhill running in rats. *Acta Physiol Scand* 165: 57-63.

Kraemer RR, Johnson LG, Haltom R, Kraemer GR, Gaines H, Drapcho M, Gimple T and Castracane VD. (1998) Effects of horomone replacement on growth hormone and prolactin exercise responses in postmenopausal women. *J Appl Physiol* 84: 703-708.

Laughlin MH, Welshons WV, Sturek M, Rush JE, Turk JR, Taylor JA, Judy BM, Henderson KK and Ganjam VK (2003) Gender, exercise training and eNOS expresson in porcine skeletal muscle arteries. *J Appl Physiol* 95: 250-264.

Lemoine S, Granier P, Tiffoche C, Berthon PM, Thieulant ML, Carre F and Delmarche P (2002) Effect of endurance training on oestrogen receptor alpha expression in different rat skeletal muscle type. *Acta Physiol Scand* 175: 211-217.

Lemoine S, Granier P, Tiffoche C, Rannou-Bekono F, Thieulant ML and Delamarche P (2003) Estrogen receptor alpha mRNA in human skeletal muscles *Med Sci Sports Exerc* 35: 439-443.

MacIntyre DL, Reid WD, Lyster DM and McKenzie DC (2000) Different effects of strenuous eccentric exercise on the accumulation of neutrophils in muscle in women and men *Eur J Appl Physiol* 81: 47-53.

Malm C, Nyberg P and Endstrom M. (2000) Immunological changes in human skeletal muscle and blood after eccentric exercise and multiple biopsies. *J Physiol* 529: 243-262.

McCormick KM, Burns KL, Piccone CM, Gosselin LE and Braseau GA (2004) Effects of ovariectomy and estrogen on skeletal muscle function in growing rats. *J Muscle Res Cell Motil* 25: 21-27.

Meeuwsen IB, Samson MM and Verhaar HJ (2000) Evaluation of the applicability of HRT as a preservative of muscle strength in women. *Maturitas* 36: 49-61.

Moosmann B and Behl C (1999) The antioxidant neuroprotective effects of estrogens and phenolic compounds are independent from their estrogenic properties. *Proc Natl Acad Sci* 96: 8867-8872.

Nadal A, Diaz M and Valverde MA (2001) The estrogen trinity: membrane, cytosolic and nuclear effects. *News Physiol Sci* 16: 251-255.

Node K, Kitakaze M, Kosaka H, Minamino T, Funaya H, Masatsugu H (1997) Amelioration of ischemia- and reperfusion-induced myocardial injury by 17b-estradiol. *Circulation* 96:1953-1963.

Ogawa S, Chan J, Gustafsson J, Korach KS, Pfaff DW (2003) Estrogen increases locomotor activity in mice through estrogen receptor alpha: Specificity for the type of activity. *Endocrinol* 144: 230-239.

Pare G, Krust A, Karas RH, Dupont S, Aronovitz M, Chambon P, Mendelsohn ME (2002) Estrogen receptor-α mediates the protective effects of estrogen against vascular injury. *Circ Res* 90: 1087-1092.

Paroo Z, Dipchand ES and Noble EG (2002) Estrogen attenuates postexercise HSP70 expression in skeletal muscle. *Am J Physiol* 282: C245-C251.

Paroo Z, Tiidus PM and Noble EG (1999) Estrogen attenuates HSP72 expresson in acutely exercised male rodents *Eur J Appl Physiol* 80: 180-184.

Phillips SK, Rook KM, Siddle NC, Bruce SA and Woledge RC (1993) Muscle weakness in women occurs at an earlier age than in men, but strength is preserved by hormone replacement therapy. *Clin Sci* 84: 95-98.

Prorock AJ, Hafezi-Moghadam A, Laubach VE, Liao JK and Ley K. Vascular protection by estrogen in ischemia-reperfusion injury requires endothelial nitric oxide synthase. *Am J Physiol* 284: H133-H140.

Roth S, Martel G and Ivy F. (2000) High volume heavy-resistance strength training and muscle damage in young and older women. *J Appl Physiol* 88:1112-1118.

Salimena MC, Lagrota-Candido J, Quirico-Santos T (2004) Gender dimorphism influences extracellular matrix expression and regeneration of muscular tissue in mdx dystrophic mice. *Histochem Cell Biol* 122: 435-444.

Sarwar R, Beltran-Niclos B and Rutherford OM (1996) Changes in muscle strength, relaxation rate and fatiguability during the human menstrual cycle. *J Physiol* 493: 267-272.

Sayers SP and Clarkson PM (2001) Force recovery after eccentric exercise in males and females. *Eur J Appl Physiol* 84: 122-126.

Schlag MG, Harris K and Potter R. Role of leukocyte accumulation and oxygen radicals in ischemia-reperfusion-induced injury in skeletal muscle. *Am J Physiol* 280: H1716-H1721.

Seeley DG, Caouley JA, Grady D, Browner WS, Nevitt MC and Cummings SR (1995) *Arch Intern Med* 155: 293-299.

Shumate JB, Brooke M, Carroll J and Davis JE (1979) Increased serum creatine kinase after exercise: A sex-linked phenomenon. *Neurology* 29: 902-909.

Sipilä S and Poutamo J (2003) Muscle performance, sex hormones and training in peri-menopausal and post-menopausal women. *Scand J Med Sci Sports* 13: 19-25.

Sipilä S, Taafe DR, Cheng S, Puolakka J, Toivanen J and Suominen H (2001) Effects of hormone replacement therapy and high-impact physical exercise on skeletal muscle in post-menopausal women: a randomized controlled study. *Clin Sci* 101: 147-157.

Skelton DA, Phillips SK, Bruce SA, Naylor CH and Woledge RC (1999). Hormone replacement therapy increases muscle strength of adductor pollicis in post-menopausal women. *Clin Sci* 96: 357-364.

Sorensen MB, Rosenfalck AM, Hojgaard L and Ottesen B (2001) Obesity and sarcopenia after menopause are reversed by sex hormone replacement therapy. *Obes Res* 9: 622-626.

Sotiriadou S, Kyparos A, Mougios V, Trontzos C, Sidiras G and Matziari C (2003) Estrogen effect on some enzymes in female rats after downhill running. *Physiol Res* 52: 743-748

Squadrito F, Altavilla D, Squadrito G, Campo G, Arlotta M, Arcoraci V, Minutoli L, Serrano M, Saitta A and Caputi A (1997) 17b-oestradiol reduces cardiac leukocyte accumulation in myocardial ischaemia reperfusion injury in rat. *Eur J Pharmacol* 335: 185-192.

Sribnick EA, Swapan RK and Banik NL (2004) Estrogen as a multi-active neuroprotective agent in traumatic injuries. *Neurochem Res* 29: 2007-2014.

St. Pierre-Schneider, B, Correia L and Cannon J (1999) Sex differences in leukocyte invasion in injured murine skeletal muscle. *Res Nurs Health* 22: 243-250.

Stupka N, Lowther S, Chorneyko K, Bourgeois JM, Hogben C and Tarnopolsky MA (2000) Gender differences in muscle inflammation after eccentric exercise. *J Appl Physiol* 89: 2325-2332.

Stupka N, Tarnopolsky MA, Yardley NJ and Phillips SM (2001) Cellular adaptation to repeated eccentric exercise-induced muscle damage. *J Appl Physiol* 91: 1669-1678.

Stupka N, and Tiidus PM (2001) Effects of ovariectomy and estrogen on ischemia-reperfusion injury in hindlimbs of female rats. *J Appl Physiol* 91: 1828-1835.

Sugioka K, Shimosegawa Y and Nakano M (1987) Estrogens as natural antioxidants of membrane and phospholipid peroxidation. *FEBS Lett* 210: 37-39.

Teixeira PJ, Going SB, Houtkooper LB, Metcalfe LL, Blew RM, Flint-Wagner HG, Cussler EC, Sardinha LB, and Lohman TG. (2003) Resistance training in Postmenopausal women with and without hormone therapy. *Med Sci Sports Exerc* 35: 555-562.

Tiidus PM (1995) Can estrogens diminish exercise induced muscle damage? *Can J Appl Physiol* 20: 26-38.

Tiidus PM (1998) Radical species in inflammation and overtraining. *Can J Physiol Pharmacol* 76: 533-538.

Tiidus PM (2001) Oestrogen and sex influence on muscle damage and inflammation: evidence from animal models. *Cur Opin Clin Nutr Metabol Care* 4: 509-513.

Tiidus PM (2003) Influence of estrogen and gender on muscle damage, inflammation and repair. *Exerc Sport Sci Rev* 31: 40-44, 2003.

Tiidus PM and Bombardier E (1999) Oestrogen attenuates post-exercise myeloperoxidase activity in skeletal muscle of male rats. *Acta Physiol Scand* 166: 85-90.

Tiidus PM, Bombardier E, Hidiroglou N and Madere R (1998) Estrogen administration, post-exercise tissue oxidative stress and vitamin C status in male rats. *Can J Physiol Pharmacol* 76: 952-960.

Tiidus PM, Deller M and Liu XL (2005) Oestrogen influence on myogenic satellite cells following downhill running in male rats: a preliminary study. *Acta Physiol Scand* 184: 67-72.

Tiidus PM, Holden D, Bombardier E, Zachowski S, Enns D and Belcastro A (2001) Estrogen effect on post-exercise skeletal muscle neutrophil infiltration and calpain activity. *Can J Physiol Pharmacol* 79: 400-406.

Tiidus PM and Ianuzzo CD (1983) Effects of intensity and duration of muscular exercise on delayed soreness and serum enzyme activities. *Med Sci Sports Exerc* 15: 461-465.

Tiidus PM, Radke EA, Bombardier E, Gul M, Lewis G and SD Perry (2004) Strength training and hormone replacement positively influence gait and balance in older females: a pilot study. (Abs.) *Can J Appl Physiol* 29:S88.

Van der Meulen J, Kuipers H and Drukker J (1991) Relationship between xercise-induced muscle damage and enzyme release in rats. *J Appl Physiol* 71:999-1004.

Walden D, McCutchan J, Enquist e, Schwappach J, Shanley P, Reiss O, Terada L, Leff J and Repine JE (1990) Neutrophils accumulate and contribute to skeletal muscle dysfunction after ischemia-reperfusion. *Am J Physiol* 259: H1809-H1812.

Whiting KP, Restall CJ and Brain PF (2000) Steroid hormone-induced effects on membrane fluidity and their potential roles in non-genomic mechanisms. *Life Sci* 67: 743-757.

Wiik A, Glenmark B, Ekman M, Esjornsson-Liljedahl, Johansson O, Bodin K, Enmark E and Jansson E. (2003) Oestrogen receptor β is expressed in adult human skeletal muscle both at the mRNA and protein level. *Acta Physiol Scand* 179: 381-387.

Xing D, Miller A, Novak L, Rocha R, Chen YF and Oparil S. (2004) Estradiol and progestins differentially modulate leukocye infiltration after vascular injury. *Circulation* 109: 234-241.

Xu Y, Armstrong SJ, Arenas IA, Pehowich DJ, Davidge ST (2004) Cardioprotection by chronic estrogen or superoxide dismutase mimetic treatment in the aged female rat. *Am J Physiol* 287: H165-H175.

INDEX

concentration, vii, xi, 15, 31, 36, 37, 42, 49, 51, 55, 188, 195, 196, 197, 198, 199, 200, 201, 202, 203, 204, 205, 206, 207, 208, 209

conceptual model, 80

conditioning, xi, 157, 160, 162, 196, 209, 230

conduct, 126

confidence, 109, 112, 121, 184, 187, 189, 190

confidence interval, 184, 187, 189, 190

confidentiality, 128

conflict, 7, 176

confounders, viii, 60, 65, 66, 69, 135

connective tissue, 226

connectivity, 115

consciousness, 160

consensus, 6, 10, 63, 97, 100, 118, 134, 214

constipation, 11

construct validity, 172, 173

consumption, vii, 1, 2, 3, 4, 7, 9, 10, 12, 13, 15, 16, 22, 24, 30, 45, 46, 80, 86, 88, 90, 140

context, 26, 101, 118, 122, 124, 132, 148, 155, 157, 215

contingency, 162

control, vii, viii, 1, 2, 8, 10, 12, 13, 14, 17, 23, 26, 30, 31, 33, 34, 36, 37, 38, 46, 47, 49, 55, 74, 93, 96, 104, 107, 117, 119, 120, 125, 127, 128, 133, 135, 160, 162, 181, 189, 190, 193, 204, 211, 215, 218, 223, 224, 225, 226, 227

control group, 34, 119, 215, 223, 224, 226

controlled studies, 219

controlled trials, vii, xi, 49, 54, 55, 79, 213, 214, 215, 229

cooking, 5

coping, 128, 140, 142

coronary artery disease, 151

coronary heart disease, x, 3, 4, 19, 21, 22, 29, 79, 142, 147, 179, 191, 192

correlation, 19, 45, 46, 62, 78, 168, 169, 170, 199, 201, 207, 239

cortisol, 202, 203

cost saving, 58

costs, 50, 60, 103, 108, 110, 115, 147, 172

counseling, 112, 132, 137, 147

course work, 156, 160

coverage, 117

creatine, 233, 243, 246

credibility, 126

crime, 112, 116, 117

cross-sectional study, 75, 173, 180

CRP, 11, 13

crystals, 51

CT scan, 50

cues, 121

cultural differences, 171, 172

culture, x, 2, 107, 109, 120, 154, 155, 166, 172, 174

curriculum, 121, 122, 156

customers, 16

CVD, 179, 180, 181, 188, 191

cycles, 24

cycling, x, 114, 115, 119, 146, 147, 179, 180, 190, 206, 207, 208, 219

D

daily living, 180

damage, xii, 11, 211, 231, 232, 233, 234, 235, 236, 237, 238, 239, 240, 241, 242, 243, 244, 245, 246, 247

data analysis, 125, 126, 145

data collection, 124, 126, 159

database, 79, 215

dating, 4, 9

DBP, 186

death, 3, 18, 29, 101, 103, 112, 118, 145, 180, 189, 191

death rate, 3, 29, 103

decision making, 176

decisions, 109, 114, 126

defects, 225

defense, 6

deficit, 13, 14

definition, 65, 180

dehydration, 11

delivery, 11, 130, 177, 208, 223, 227

demand, 62, 83, 85, 87, 88, 90, 117, 131, 134, 189

democracy, 158

Denmark, 3, 98

density, viii, x, 11, 15, 59, 60, 61, 63, 66, 69, 70, 71, 72, 73, 74, 114, 115, 179, 180, 186, 188

Department of Health and Human Services, 150, 154, 155, 159, 177

dependent variable, 65, 82, 83, 84, 92, 165, 186, 187

depression, x, 11, 92, 112, 128, 154, 179, 214, 222, 227

depressive symptoms, 227

deprivation, 225

derivatives, 43

detection, viii, ix, 73, 77, 78, 82, 83, 84, 85, 88, 89, 90, 91, 93, 94, 96, 162, 237

developed countries, 29, 101, 102

diabetes, 8, 11, 14, 22, 23, 26, 29, 78, 79, 100, 103, 123, 145, 151, 180, 191, 192, 227

diabetic patients, 26

diastolic blood pressure, 185, 186, 187, 225

diastolic pressure, 221

diet, vii, 1, 2, 3, 4, 5, 6, 7, 8, 9, 10, 11, 12, 13, 14, 15, 16, 17, 18, 19, 20, 21, 22, 23, 24, 25, 26, 46, 50,

E

J

K

L

M

P

positive relationship, 67, 111
potassium, 240
poultry, 16
poverty, 116
power, 104, 124, 132, 160, 176
power sharing, 132
preadolescents, 156
precipitation, 159
prediction, 141, 173, 207
predictor variables, 168, 169
predictors, ix, 69, 73, 77, 82, 83, 85, 89, 92, 93, 94, 98, 145, 168, 169, 177, 193
preference, 148
pregnancy, xi, xii, 51, 213, 214, 215, 216, 217, 218, 219, 221, 222, 223, 224, 225, 226, 227, 228, 229, 230
premature death, 2, 103, 133
preparation, x, 16, 95, 154, 160, 168, 169, 172, 173, 210
preservative, 245
pressure, x, 4, 79, 97, 101, 108, 179, 188, 224, 225, 227, 229
preterm delivery, 226
prevention, viii, 3, 8, 19, 21, 22, 24, 45, 49, 50, 51, 52, 54, 55, 56, 57, 58, 73, 75, 78, 79, 94, 100, 101, 104, 117, 119, 139, 145, 149, 150, 151, 159, 191, 193
primacy, 9
principle, 218, 219
probability, 84, 85, 162
problem behavior, 81
problem behaviors, 81
problem-focused coping, 128
problem-solving, 119, 128
problem-solving strategies, 128
production, vii, viii, 2, 11, 31, 46, 49, 59, 62, 69, 72, 140, 225, 240, 241
productivity, 79, 96, 103
progesterone, xii, 231, 237, 238, 240, 241, 244
progestins, 247
program, 4, 8, 25, 50, 52, 57, 78, 79, 85, 93, 94, 95, 100, 101, 111, 112, 119, 120, 121, 123, 124, 125, 126, 127, 128, 129, 134, 136, 137, 141, 143, 145, 148, 161, 228, 229
prolactin, 244
proliferation, 237, 238
prophylactic, 51, 55, 57
prophylaxis, 55, 58
prostate, 4, 9, 78, 101, 136, 149
prostate cancer, 101, 136
protective factors, 149
protein folding, 234
protein synthesis, 234

proteins, xi, 195, 197, 198, 199, 200, 206, 207, 208, 209, 210, 212, 232, 239
proteolysis, 239, 244
proteolytic enzyme, 239
psychological stress, 83
psychological stressors, 83
psychological well-being, 101, 222
psychology, 107, 113, 127, 136, 155, 175
psychometric properties, 158, 161
public health, vii, 1, 2, 3, 11, 18, 50, 101, 104, 114, 115, 118, 120, 123, 134, 140, 142, 149, 155, 179, 180, 191
pulse, 104, 222, 225
purchasing power, 158

Q

quadriceps, 235, 236
qualitative research, 138, 150
quality control, 20
quality of life, 4, 101, 191
questioning, 18

R

race, 104, 109, 116, 117, 151, 159, 175, 212
range, vii, xii, 1, 12, 14, 44, 45, 51, 79, 83, 103, 116, 118, 182, 213, 223, 226, 232
ratings, 16, 116
reaction mechanism, 44
reactive oxygen, 212
reading, 127
recall, 110, 125, 135
receptors, 232, 239
recidivism, 13, 105
reciprocal relationships, 128
recognition, 120
reconcile, 161
reconstruction, 96
recovery, 50, 79, 101, 197, 198, 199, 200, 201, 202, 203, 206, 208, 212, 234, 235, 238, 240, 241, 246
recreation, 102, 113, 117, 123, 124, 129, 130, 134, 141, 142, 152, 160
recruiting, 126
recurrence, 3
redistribution, 225
reduction, vii, 3, 5, 7, 8, 12, 14, 25, 35, 36, 38, 39, 42, 44, 45, 49, 50, 52, 55, 56, 57, 78, 103, 110, 221, 225, 226, 234
refining, 161
reflection, 104
regeneration, 237, 238, 240, 243, 244, 245

S